FUNDAMENTALS OF ORNAMENTAL FISH HEALTH

FUNDAMENTALS OF ORNAMENTAL FISH HEALTH

Edited by

Helen E. Roberts, DVM

WILEY-BLACKWELL

A John Wiley & Sons, Ltd., Publication

Edition first published 2010
© 2010 Blackwell Publishing

Blackwell Publishing was acquired by John Wiley & Sons in February 2007. Blackwell's publishing program has been merged with Wiley's global Scientific, Technical, and Medical business to form Wiley-Blackwell.

Editorial Office
2121 State Avenue, Ames, Iowa 50014-8300, USA

For details of our global editorial offices, for customer services, and for information about how to apply for permission to reuse the copyright material in this book, please see our website at www.wiley.com/wiley-blackwell.

Library of Congress Cataloging-in-Publication Data

Fundamentals of ornamental fish health / edited by Helen E. Roberts.
    p. ; cm.
  Includes bibliographical references and index.
  ISBN-13: 978-0-8138-1401-8 (alk. paper)
  ISBN-10: 0-8138-1401-4 (alk. paper)
  1. Ornamental fishes–Diseases–Treatment.
2. Ornamental fishes–Health. I. Roberts, Helen E. (Helen Elizabeth), 1964–
  [DNLM: 1. Fish Diseases–diagnosis. 2. Fish Diseases–therapy. 3. Fishes–anatomy & histology. SF458.5 F981 2010]
  SF458.5.F86 2010
  639.3–dc22

                                    2009019201

A catalog record for this book is available from the U.S. Library of Congress.

Set in 9.5 on 12 pt Times Ten by
SNP Best-set Typesetter Ltd., Hong Kong
Printed in Malaysia.

1   2010

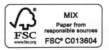

Dedication

This book is dedicated to the clients who have sought nonlethal diagnostics, a better understanding of pet fish disease, and requested more advanced treatment for their "wet pets"; pioneering colleagues who have laid the groundwork before me and those who will carry on the work ahead; my mother, who has always been my inspiration to try harder and leave the world a better place; and Kevin, who encouraged me all along the way.

Contents

Acknowledgments

While there are not many books available on clinical ornamental aquatic animal medicine, there are a number of great texts available on fish and invertebrate health. It is my hope that this text will complement those existing texts. Fish owners and hobbyists are increasing in numbers according to numerous industry studies. They are also searching for better ways to manage the health and well-being of their "wet pets." These owners are actively seeking medical care and advice for everything, from the goldfish they won at the county fair, to the show koi they paid several thousand dollars for, to the rare marine invertebrates they build a reef tank to support. It is an exciting time to be an aquatic health professional! The field of nonlethal aquatic diagnostics and medicine is still in its infancy but the knowledge base is rapidly expanding. I hope you, the reader, enjoy the practice of aquatic animal health as much as I do. And I do hope you learn something here you can use in your role in fish health.

Writing and editing a book is never a solitary process. The publication of this text would never have been possible without the involvement and assistance of many people. I would first like to thank all my colleagues who contributed chapters. No text would have existed without you. I hope you agree that this is a book we can all be proud of. I am grateful to Erica Judisch at Wiley-Blackwell for giving me the opportunity to develop, write, and edit this new text despite my relative lack of experience.

Researching new and innovative references is a time-consuming process and time management is not always easy for a private practitioner so I am extremely grateful to the wonderful group at VIN, especially Becky Lundgren, Mandy Grewe, Bonnie Simons, and Nicky Mastin in the document delivery system. You all made my life so much easier.

Chapter reviewers are able to look at documents that have been evaluated many times and still find those grammatical or technical errors that exist. Some reviewers even took the time to rewrite sections to achieve a better flow. Many thanks go to Mary Ellen Goldberg, Kami Rose Kernene, and Maureen Costello.

There are a few other people who deserve special recognition for the help they gave me in this endeavor. Jonathan Roberts, who answers my technical questions (despite the nontechnical way I ask them), who helped with the index, and who often serves as my photographer on house calls, many thanks! My business partner, Karen Fischer, thanks for always being supportive of the "different" activities I do, including this book. To my friends, thank you for all your support and the needed distractions! Willie Wildgoose has my sincerest gratitude for his encouragement and for offering realistic advice on what happens when you agree to a project of this magnitude. Thanks to Steve Smith for help with the editing—I owe you a sushi dinner! And Kevin, who understood the time commitments I had, tried very hard not to be jealous of the computer, and was 100% supportive of what I was trying to accomplish.

Finally, none of this would be possible without our clients giving us opportunities to treat their beloved pets. In helping them, we are able to learn more and continue to advance this field. I am especially grateful to those clients who offered their own pictures in the hopes that their pets can contribute to the knowledge base, even when the outcomes have not been favorable. Special mention goes to "Wendy," "Raven," "Gracie," "Lucky," "Mr. Cuddles," "Sadie Sky," "Bo-Bo," "Sushi," "Papa," "Ariel," and many more.

Contributor List

Jerry R. Heidel, DVM, PhD, DACVP
Veterinary Diagnostic Laboratory
College of Veterinary Medicine
Oregon State University
Corvallis, OR 97331

Timothy J. Miller-Morgan, DVM
Ornamental Fish Health Program
Oregon Sea Grant Extension
College of Veterinary Medicine
Hatfield Marine Science Center
Oregon State University
Corvallis, OR 97331

Brian Palmeiro, VMD, DACVD
Pet Fish Doctor
645 Pennsylvania Ave
Prospect Park, PA 19076
www.petfishdoctor.com

David J. Pasnik, DVM, MS
Aquatic Animal Health Research Laboratory
United States Department of Agriculture
Agricultural Research Service
118B Lynchburg Street
Chestertown, MD 21620

Drury Reavill, DVM, DACVP, DAVBP (Avian)
Zoo/Exotic Pathology Service
7647 Wachtel Way
Citrus Heights, CA 95610
www.zooexotic.com

Helen E. Roberts, DVM
Aquatic Veterinary Services of WNY
5 Corners Animal Hospital
2799 Southwestern Blvd Suite 100
Orchard Park, NY 14127

James L. (Jay) Shelton, Jr.
Associate Professor of Fisheries
D.B. Warnell School of Forestry and Natural
    Resources
University of Georgia
Athens, GA 30602

Stephen A. Smith, DVM, PhD
Professor of Aquatic Medicine/Fish Health
Department of Biomedical Sciences and
    Pathobiology
Virginia-Maryland Regional College of
    Veterinary Medicine
Phase II, Duck Pond Drive
Virginia Tech
Blacksburg, VA 24061-0442

Richard J. Strange, PhD
Professor of Fisheries
Department of Forestry, Wildlife and Fisheries
University of Tennessee
Knoxville, TN 37919

E. Scott Weber III, VMD, MSc with distinction
    (Aquatic Vet Sci/Pathobiology) Aquatic
    Animal Health
Professor of Clinical Studies
Companion Avian and Exotic Animal Service
VM: Medicine and Epidemiology
University of California, Davis
2108 Tupper Hall
Davis, CA 95616

William H. Wildgoose BVMS Cert FHP MRCVS
Midland Veterinary Surgery
655 High Road
London E10 6RA

FUNDAMENTALS OF ORNAMENTAL FISH HEALTH

Basics of
Fish Keeping

Chapter 1
Anatomy and Physiology

Richard J. Strange

Introduction

The study of fish anatomy and physiology is best approached as a comparison with the better-known mammalian model. The assumption is that fish share anatomical and physiological solutions to survival with mammals, but often, they do not; this chapter will highlight those differences. An organism has to live in its environment; the environment affects all aspects of form and function. The aquatic environment differs greatly from the terrestrial environment; that is the basis for differences in the anatomy and physiology of fishes. Since anatomy and physiology are shaped together as the organism adapts to the environment, the anatomical and physiological manifestations are discussed together.

Environment shapes form and function

As terrestrial organisms, we understand the constraints of the terrestrial environment but may have little appreciation of the aquatic environment. In the terrestrial environment, ambient temperature rapidly changes. Water has a high specific heat, which slows the rate it changes in temperature. Most bodies of water will change only a degree or two from day to night. The oceans might take weeks to change a degree. Similarly, the aquatic environment is buffered from seasonal fluctuations in temperature. The coldest that the aquatic environment can physically become is 0 °C (freezing), and because it is most dense at 4 °C, it freezes from the top down, so the aquatic habitat is preserved under a layer of ice in extreme cold.

While fish have less temperature change to cope with than terrestrial animals, they often suffer from a lack of oxygen availability. The concentration of oxygen (O_2) in air is always 260 mg/l. The concentration of available (dissolved) oxygen (DO) in water is usually about 8–14 mg/l (air saturation) and may be much less, even 0, and rarely, even more, depending on a variety of circumstances, including temperature and biological activity. As a consequence, fish must be able to function with less oxygen than terrestrial animals. While the concentration of oxygen in the water is a fraction of that in the air, the pressure of the gas is usually equal, often less, and rarely more; this has important physiological consequences and will be discussed in a following section. Gravity is the same in terrestrial and aquatic environments, but the effect of gravity on fish is much less because of buoyancy. There are large differences between air and water in light transmission and density (which affects viscosity and pressure waves) that have a profound effect on sensory function and locomotion. Finally, the air is chemically uniform, while water varies in pH, salinity, and other dissolved substances, which make the maintenance of homeostasis more difficult.

Mammals and fish have similar needs for homeostasis, but their external environments (terrestrial vs. aquatic) differ greatly, and this demands differences in their anatomy and physiology.

Respiration and gill structure

Respiratory pump in fish

In mammals, birds, and other terrestrial animals, the respiratory pump is bidirectional. Air moves

Phase I - Expanding

Midpoint

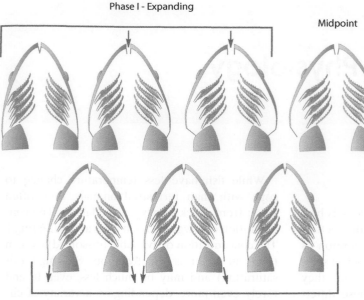

Phase II - Contracting

Fig. 1.1 Sequence of the dual phase buccal/opercular respiratory pump in fish. Arrows indicate the direction of water flow.

in and out of the same opening into and out of the lungs. This is not the most efficient system because there is some mixing of fresh and respired air and there are pockets in the lungs that may never, or hardly ever, get fresh air. Such an inefficient system is not a problem for terrestrial animals because of the rich concentration of oxygen in the air and the consistently high partial pressure of oxygen (PO_2).

Fish need a more efficient method due to lower amount of oxygen in water and variable PO_2. In most fish, the system is unidirectional; water always moves through the mouth and one way across the gills, then out through the operculum. There is no mixing of fresh and respired water, maintaining as high a PO_2 at the gill surface as possible. When the fish is moving rapidly or in a strong current, it may ram ventilate by holding its mouth open and letting the water flow over the gills without any respiratory pumping. This is an effective and energy-efficient system of ventilation. However, if the fish is not moving rapidly and in still water, it must use respiratory pumping.

The sequence of events in respiratory pumping is as follows. Water is drawn through the mouth into the buccal cavity by expansion of the buccal and opercular cavities while the opercula are closed. Then, the mouth and oral valve close, the opercular valve opens, and the buccal and opercular cavities contract, forcing the water across the gills and out the opercula (Fig. 1.1).

The respiratory pump is sometimes called the dual pump because the pumping takes place in two phases:

- Phase I: mouth open, opercula closed, buccal cavity expanding, opercula cavity expanding. (Buccal and opercular expansion are almost simultaneous, but buccal expansion may occur slightly ahead of opercular expansion.)
- Phase II: mouth closed, opercula open, buccal cavity contracting, opercula cavity contracting. (Again, the contractions are almost simultaneous, with the buccal cavity contracting slightly ahead of the opercular contraction.)

Gill structure

All modern fishes have four respiratory gill arches and a fifth nonrespiratory arch on each side of the buccal cavity (Fig. 1.2). Each respiratory arch is composed of a cartilaginous supporting structure that bears gill rakers in the front and respiratory tissue in the rear. The gill rakers act like a strainer

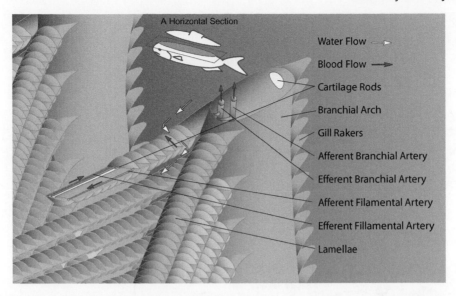

A Horizontal Section

Water Flow →
Blood Flow →
Cartilage Rods
Branchial Arch
Gill Rakers
Afferent Branchial Artery
Efferent Branchial Artery
Afferent Filamental Artery
Efferent Fillamental Artery
Lamellae

Fig. 1.2 Illustration of a section of the respiratory arch showing structure and flow of water and blood (magnified).

to keep food items from passing through the gills. Piscivorous fish have short, stubby rakers, while planktivorous fish have gill rakers that are fine and feathery. The respiratory tissue is comprised of a paired series of filaments, similar to a feather. There are two series of filaments on each arch. One series of filaments is termed a hemibranch, while both together are termed a holobranch.

There are numerous platelike lamellae on each filament. The lamellae are the site of blood/water exchange. In a healthy gill, the blood is separated from the water by two layers of epithelial cells. Gill irritation causes epithelial hyperplasia reducing exchange efficiency. Fishes have a countercurrent system where blood and water flow on opposite directions at the lamellae. This greatly increases exchange efficiency.

Lamellar structure

Blood flows from the heart toward the head in the ventral aorta. From the ventral aorta, afferent branchial arteries branch off to each gill arch and run up the center of the cartilaginous arch, where another branch comes off at each filament and is called the afferent filamental artery. Blood then flows through the lamellar lacunae where the exchange of respiratory gases takes place. Pillar

cells connect the sides of the lamellae, preventing it from ballooning due to blood pressure. Pillar cells also direct most of the blood flow into the marginal channel, where the water flow is greatest and, therefore, gas exchange most efficient. Microscopic anatomy indicates that some blood may flow between the pillar cells and also into a central compartment (central venous sinus). This central sinus probably serves a nutritive function for the gill. From the lamellar lacunae, the oxygenated blood flows into the efferent filamental artery and into the efferent branchial artery and then to the dorsal aorta out to the body (Fig. 1.3).

Lamellar anatomy is quite variable between species. For example, in tuna, the arrangement of the pillar cells forms not one, but several channels. Moreover, the lamellae of one filament are connected to the lamellae of the other filament so the filaments cannot separate, thus the hemibranch is like a sieve. This allows the tuna to ram ventilate at high swimming speeds without blowing the filaments apart.

Much speculation and research has centered on whether a nonrespiratory shunt exists in the gills of fish. Such an alternative pathway for blood flow would be beneficial since during times of low respiratory need, the fish could direct blood away from the water, minimizing osmoregulatory loss

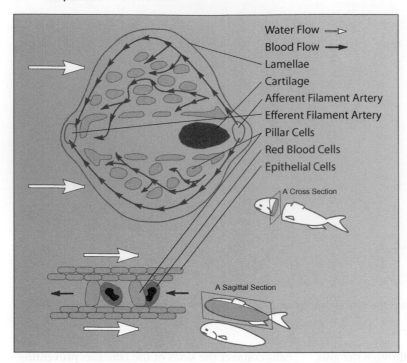

Fig. 1.3 Sections of the respiratory lamellae showing structure and flow of water and blood (highly magnified).

or gain (see "Osmoregulation" section in this chapter). Evidence favors the existence of a non-respiratory pathway, at least in some species. One mechanism may involve contraction of the pillar cells to redirect blood to and away from maximum exposure to the water as it circulates through the lamellae.

Countercurrent versus parallel flow

The countercurrent system maximizes the extraction of oxygen from the water and excretion of wastes. Organisms use countercurrent systems in different ways. For example, fishes also use a countercurrent system to inflate their swim bladders, but in the gill, it is used to increase blood/water exchange.

Oxygen in water flowing over the gill will diffuse from an area of high pressure into the blood, an area of low pressure, until the oxygen content of both water and blood is equal. A countercurrent system places the water with the highest oxygen content in contact with the blood with the highest oxygen content and as blood and water flow through lamellae, exchange occurs over the entire respiratory surface. This maintains the greatest pressure gradient possible over the entire blood/water interface, maximizing the flow of oxygen into the blood.

A parallel (noncountercurrent system) puts the water with the highest oxygen pressure immediately into contact with the blood with the lowest oxygen pressure and does not maintain a continual gradient. A parallel system has a maximum transfer efficiency of 50%. If contact time is long enough, half the pressure difference between the incoming water and blood can be transferred, that is, the oxygen diffuses until the pressures meet in the middle. On the other hand, a countercurrent system can have a transfer efficiency of 80% or more, depending on contact time.

Some unique adaptations

Skates and rays have gill openings on the underside of the body and have two spiracles on top of the head that bring water into the buccal cavity when the mouth is buried in the sand. In halibut and flounder, water is taken in on the side of the mouth and channeled through the dorsal operculum.

Blood gases and gas bladder function

Oxygen (O_2) in blood

Hemoglobin (Hb)

Hb is a complex protein molecule. It consists of four separate polypeptide chains called protein subunits. Each Hb molecule can attach to four O_2 molecules. The importance of Hb is that when O_2 is bound to Hb, the O_2 is no longer in solution and does not affect partial pressure. Hb increases the carrying capacity of the blood for oxygen by 15 to 25 times. Carbon monoxide (CO) also binds with Hb. Blood fully saturated with CO can carry only 1/20th of the normal amount of O_2. This is why CO can be quickly lethal for most animals. Fish at very cold temperatures ($<5\,°C$) can survive CO poisoning; in fact, Antarctic icefish have no erythrocytes or Hb in their blood (they have white gills) and live quite well moving oxygen in simple solution in their blood plasma.

Dissociation curves

An oxygen dissociation curve for Hb describes the relationship between partial pressure and the amount of oxygen bound on the Hb. At higher partial pressure more oxygen is forced into binding with Hb, and at lower partial pressure less oxygen is bound. Dissociation curves are not linear but sigmoid. The defining attribute of a given dissociation curve is its P50. The P50 of Hb differs among species.

There is adaptive significance to each species' P50. There are advantages to a high P50 and advantages to a low P50—it all depends on the animal's environment and way of life. Consider the difference between the P50 of a trout and a carp (Fig. 1.4).

A trout in water with low oxygen (5–20 mm Hg partial pressure) cannot load its Hb; therefore, its tissues will suffocate and it will die. But carp Hb has a higher affinity for O_2. Therefore, a carp can load oxygen at a lower PO_2 and live in a lower-O_2 environment; however, both the trout and the carp Hb will hold the same amount of oxygen. The dissociation curve of carp indicates that their Hb can fully load at a PO_2 of about

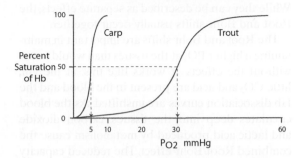

Fig. 1.4 Hemoglobin dissociation curves for carp and trout showing P50's. PO_2, partial pressure of oxygen.

20 mm Hg (about 1 mg/l of DO), while it requires about 50 mm Hg (3 mg/l) to fully load a trout's Hb. Why does a trout's Hb have a low affinity if that limits the amount of oxygen necessary for it to live? The advantage is that a higher P50 results in the Hb unloading the oxygen at the tissue level at a higher pressure. Therefore, a trout has a higher PO_2 in its tissue than does a carp. Higher PO_2 in the trout's tissue means that oxygen flows more quickly into the mitochondria and so a higher rate of metabolism is possible, thus the trout can maintain a higher level activity than a carp. It is a trade-off, and the advantage of each approach depends on the fish's environment and the way it lives.

Dissociation curves are determined *in vitro* and *in vivo*. PO_2's in the water need to be higher than the P50 of the Hb to support fish life because a certain amount of pressure differential is required to move O_2 from the water across the gill epithelial cells into the plasma, then into the red blood cells (RBCs), and finally into the Hb. In life, trout tend to suffer from hypoxia in water containing less than 4–5 mg/l DO.

Root and Bohr effects

An increase in the partial pressure of carbon dioxide (PCO_2) in the blood decreases the Hb's capacity for oxygen. This is termed the Root effect or shift. At high PCO_2, the Hb's capacity to bind oxygen can be decreased as much as 50%.

A decrease in pH has a different effect on Hb; it causes a decreased affinity for oxygen. This is termed the Bohr effect or shift. At low pH, the

Hb's affinity for O_2 can decrease two to three times. While they can be described as separate effects, the Root and Bohr shifts usually occur together.

The Root and Bohr shifts are important in maintaining a higher PO_2 at the tissues than would occur without the effects. It works like this: at the gill, little CO_2 and acid are present in the blood and the Hb dissociation curves are unshifted. As the blood circulates deep into the tissues, carbon dioxide and lactic acid produced by metabolism cause the combined Root/Bohr effect. The reduced capacity and decreased affinity causes the Hb to "dump" oxygen, increasing the PO_2. As the blood circulates between the gill and tissues and back, the combined shifts occur back and forth again and again. The result is a higher PO_2 at the tissues than would occur in the absence of the effects.

This works well for the fish in habitats with high oxygen content and low carbon dioxide. In habitats with low oxygen and high carbon dioxide (e.g., swamps), it can be counterproductive because carbon dioxide prevents a shift back at the gill (CO_2 causes the Bohr as well as the Root effect because it reacts with water to form a weak acid). Fishes such as bullheads, carp, bowfin, and lungfishes, which are adapted to swamp life and slow water habitats where low oxygen and high carbon dioxide content are normal, have blood with weak Root/Bohr effects. Fish that normally engage in vigorous burst swimming have some Hb that lacks the Root/Bohr effects because during periods of strenuous exercise blood acidosis may occur, preventing the shift back at the gill. By having Hb's with and without the effects, they "hedge their bets" physiologically.

Temperature effect

With each degree centigrade increase in blood temperature, there is a decrease in affinity equal to an increase in the P50 of 1 mm Hg. While this effect is slight compared with the Root and Bohr effects, it is adaptive since active muscles tend to be warmer than the water at the gill.

Carbon dioxide

Carbon dioxide is more soluble in water than oxygen and is reactive with water, forming carbonic acid (H_2CO_3). Carbonic acid quickly dissociates to form H^+ (hydronium ion) and HCO_3^- (bicarbonate ion). Carbon dioxide that reacts with water to form carbonic acid no longer contributes to the partial pressure (PCO_2). For both of these reasons, there is more inorganic carbon (CO_2 and H_2CO_3) in water at a given partial pressure than oxygen. Also, there is much less CO_2 in the atmosphere than O_2 (0.035% vs. 21%), so there is usually a tiny fraction of the pressure (0.25 mm Hg at air saturation) of CO_2 in water compared with O_2 (150 mm Hg).

Aerobic metabolism produces a molecule of CO_2 for each molecule of O_2. So the same amount of CO_2 as O_2 must be carried by the blood and diffuse across the gill. Since CO_2 is very soluble and, more importantly, reactive, the blood easily carries all that is produced by metabolism at low partial pressure (about 2 mm Hg) without the necessity of a specific carrier molecule (Hb) that oxygen requires. That is not to say that RBCs and Hb do not play a role in CO_2 transport. RBCs and gill epithelial cells contain an enzyme, carbonic anhydrase (CA), that catalyzes the reaction (both ways) between water and CO_2. The CA in the RBCs of venous blood converts the vast majority (95%) of the CO_2 into bicarbonate. Of the remaining CO_2, a small amount is in solution and some is bound to the Hb. When the blood reaches the gill, the Haldane effect causes much of the bicarbonate to shift rapidly back to CO_2, increasing the partial pressure. However, the partial pressure gradient between blood and air at the gill for CO_2 is still relatively small compared with that for oxygen. In addition to CA and the Haldane effect, there is an enzyme system that is powered by ATP that actively pumps the bicarbonate ion out of the cell. This is independent of both partial pressure and osmotic gradients. The export of bicarbonate (HCO_3^-) is coupled with an import of chloride (Cl^-). Once the bicarbonate ion is pumped out into the water, much of it will split back to CO_2 and H_2O, thus potentially lowering the already small pressure gradient for carbon dioxide between the water and the blood. However, since there is no CA in the water, the reaction back to CO_2 is relatively slow, and by the time much of the carbon dioxide has formed, the water has passed out of the gills. So, practically, the bicarbonate pump has little effect on the carbon dioxide gradient.

In summary, a fish must move as much CO_2 out of the blood at the gill as it moves O_2 into the blood. The problem is that the high solubility and reactivity of CO_2 makes for a much low partial pressure gradient than that exists for O_2; diffusion alone will not move the CO_2 as rapidly as O_2. This is addressed by the enzyme CA and the Haldane effect that temporarily boost the PCO_2 as the blood enters the gill and the bicarbonate pump that acts independently of partial pressure.

Swim bladder (gas bladder, air bladder) anatomy and function

Buoyancy

In most fish, the swim bladder is a hydrostatic organ. It evolved from a primitive lung and still has respiratory function in lungfish, gars, and bowfins. Fish have a specific gravity of about 1.06–1.09. The specific gravity of freshwater (FW) is 1.00, and as saltwater (SW) is slightly denser because of dissolved salts, it is about 1.03. Most fish would sink if they did not have some kind of hydrostatic compensation. It is advantageous to be neutrally buoyant, that is, have a specific gravity of 1.00, so that it is not necessary for the fish to expend energy to keep itself up in the water column. The swim bladder lies just below the spinal column at the top of the body cavity in most fish. This puts it a little bit above the midline, so the fish has more of its weight below the air bladder and tends to float right side up. There is a South American catfish that normally swims upside down. The gas bladder in this fish is located more ventrally.

Physostomous swim bladder

Since it evolved from a lung, the most primitive condition is where a direct connection, the pneumatic duct, exists between the swim bladder and the esophagus, and is termed physostomous. In the phylogenetic hierarchy of the bony fishes, all groups up through the salmonids are physostomous. This includes the eels and herrings.

It is unclear how much the duct is routinely used to move gas in and out of the swim bladder.

Physostomes such as gars and bowfins that use the swim bladder for respiration obviously use the duct to move air in and out. It appears that when physostomous fish fry, such as trout, "swim up," or become free living after absorbing their yolk sac, they gulp air to fill the swim bladder. It also seems likely that when a physostome swims rapidly upward in the water column, the duct is used to vent the expanding gas. If a physostome were to stay neutrally buoyant below 3 or 4 m, however, it would need to fill the swim bladder to above 1 atm (see Fig. 1.5), which could not be accomplished through the duct, but only with a gas gland and rete mirabile. The degree of gas gland and rete development in physostomes is variable, with some advanced types (e.g., eel) having them well developed, while others show less anatomical evidence of gas gland function. The physostomes with a well-developed gas gland and rete also have a resorptive area for the removal of gas. The ability to fill and empty the swim bladder through the blood calls into question the routine use of the pneumatic duct by these advanced physostomous fish.

Physoclistous swim bladder

There is no duct between the bladder and the esophagus in physoclistous fishes (all teleosts above salmonids), so there must be a well-developed gas gland/rete and resorptive area in order to fill and empty the swim bladder. Resorption of gas is more straightforward because the pressure in the swim bladder will never be lower than 1 atm, and therefore, will always be higher than the blood. In order to reduce pressure in the swim bladder, the fish needs only to allow the gas to flow into the blood and then out into the water at the gill. At low pressures, this is easily accomplished by simply increasing the blood flow to the capillary bed in the resorptive area to decrease pressure or decreasing blood flow to allow the gas gland to increase pressure. However, when pressure in the gas bladder rises, and it may rise to 10 atm or more in moderately deep-dwelling ocean fishes, a more effective barrier must be created to prevent outgassing. Physoclists that maintain high gas pressure in the air bladder have an out-pocketing of the bladder, called the oval,

Physostomous Gas Bladder

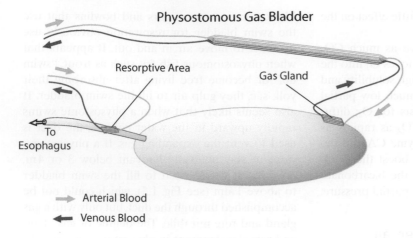

Physoclistous Gas Bladder

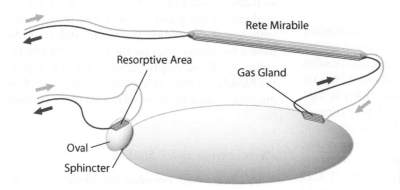

Fig. 1.5 Two types of gas bladders showing structure and blood flow.

with a muscular sphincter at its neck that physically prevents the gas from entering the bloodstream when it is contracted. When gas is to be resorbed, the sphincter is relaxed and gas enters the pocket to be taken up by blood circulating through the capillaries of the resorptive area.

Gas gland and rete

The gas gland is a highly vascular area on the inside of the air bladder, where capillaries allow for exchange between the blood and lumen of the swim bladder. The rete mirabile feeds the gas gland, and the countercurrent system in the rete maintains a pressure differential between the blood and gas bladder. The rete has a barrier effect that keeps high pressure in the bladder and prevents the bladder from losing gas into the blood, and then into the water at the gill. The

barrier is maintained by long parallel capillaries, which are arranged so that gas can diffuse from higher pressure in the efferent capillary to lower pressure in the afferent capillary. Over a long-enough distance, this will result in blood exiting the rete with the same low gas pressure as the blood entering.

Pressure is increased in the swim bladder by aerobic and anaerobic metabolism in the gas gland cells that result in the excretion of carbon dioxide and lactic acid. The CO_2 induces the Root effect, and the lactic acid induces the Bohr effect. These shifts cause the Hb to release bound O_2, which increases the partial pressure of the blood. Moreover, the presence of lactic acid in the blood causes a "salting out" effect that reduces the solubility of the plasma water for all gases, thus increasing the partial pressure of both O_2 and N_2. All of these increases in pressure are small, but they may occur in blood that already has very high gas pressure due to the high pressure in the bladder. These incremental elevations in gas pressure are preserved by the rete and, slowly, the fish is able to pump up pressures in the gas bladder to remarkable levels. This is termed the multiplier effect. Because the Hb shifts are more important in the multiplier effect than salting out, the predominant gas in the swim bladder of fish with high bladder pressure is O_2.

Swim bladder performance

Inflation and deflation

Performance of the swim bladder is an area that seems counterintuitive for many people. There are two things to remember. First, for a fish to remain neutrally buoyant, the swim bladder must always remain the same size. It would only change

size as the fish grows or changes mass in some other way, like eating a large meal. Second, as the fish swims up and down in the water column, the hydrostatic pressure changes greatly (1 atm for every 10 m of depth). Since the bladder comprised relatively soft, pliable tissue, the swim bladder pressure pushing out will always equal the hydrostatic pressure pushing in. Unless the amount of gas in the bladder is increased or decreased, it will change size as the hydrostatic pressure changes. The only way for it to remain the same size as the external hydrostatic pressure on the fish increases or decreases is for the fish to increase or decrease the amount of gas in the bladder. The reason that this is counterintuitive is that most people would guess that a fish would deflate and release gas from the bladder to go deeper, and inflate and add gas to the bladder to come up, but in fact, it is the opposite (Fig. 1.6).

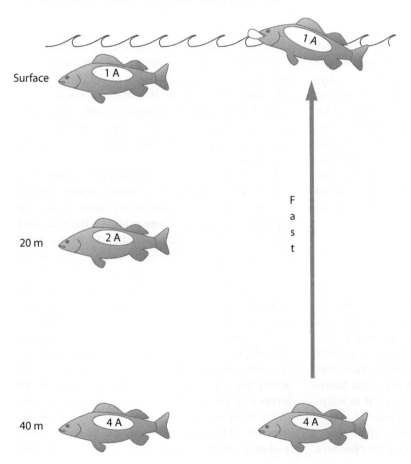

Fig. 1.6 Function of swim bladder showing gas pressure at depth.

When a fish swims down, there will be more pressure pushing in on the fish and squeezing the gas bladder smaller. At 10 m, there will always be 2 atm pressure in the bladder; the pressure in the elastic bladder pushing out must equal the pressure pushing in. If the fish does not put more gas into the bladder as it swims down, the bladder will shrink, the gas compressing until it reaches 2 atm, and the fish will be less buoyant. It will then begin to sink, which will further compress the bladder and accelerate the sinking until the fish is resting on the bottom, denser than the water. The reverse would occur when the fish swims up. If it did not decrease the amount of gas in the bladder, the decreasing hydrostatic pressure would allow the elastic bladder to balloon, making the fish more buoyant, and it would pop up to the surface over-inflated and unable to swim down. So, fish inflate (put more gas into the bladder) as they swim down and deflate (resorb gas from the bladder) when they swim up.

An actual example of this phenomenon occurs in deepwater fishing. A fish hooked and brought up rapidly is unable to deflate the gas bladder quickly enough and the fish is bloated with a greatly expanded bladder, sometimes protruding out of the mouth. If the fish is released without the angler deflating the gas bladder it will flounder on the surface, unable to swim down. The need to add and subtract gas from the bladder as the fish moves up and down in the water column limits the speed with which a fish can move up and down. There must be enough time for the fish to adjust bladder pressure through the rete and gas gland or resorptive area.

Fish without swim bladders

Agnathans and elasmobranchs do not have swim bladders; neither do some bottom-dwelling teleosts such as the darters (small percids). Darters live on the bottom, often in swift water. The absence of a bladder makes them negatively buoyant (heavier than water) and helps them stay in place. It should be noted, however, that this is the exception, and that in most cases, it is adaptive even for bottom dwelling fish such as catfish (ictalurids and silurids) and suckers (catostomids) to be neutrally buoyant. Sharks lack air bladders, but because of a cartilaginous skeleton and a large, fatty liver, they are only slightly heavier than seawater. Still, they must swim continually or slowly sink. Angled pectoral fins and a heterocercal tail help push them up as they swim forward.

Circulatory system

Heart

Teleosts

The teleost heart has four chambers. The generalization often learned in freshman biology, that fish have a two-chambered heart, means that they have only two pumping chambers, the atrium and the ventricle, but they also have a sinus venosus and a bulbous arteriosus (Fig. 1.7). Blood returning from the fish's body enters the sinus venosus, a thin-walled sac where the major veins coalesce. Expansion of the weakly muscular atrium pulls blood from the sinus venosus. Blood then flows from the atrium to the ventricle; strong contractions of the ventricle's thick muscular wall send the blood under pressure into the elastic bulbous arteriosus. From there, the blood flows into the ventral aorta and on through the gills. There are three valves in the heart to prevent backflow during the expansion (diastole) of the pumping chambers.

Fish have a very low-pressure circulatory system. There is very little blood pressure in the venous system and return to the heart is aided in all species by skeletal muscular contraction, and in some species by accessory hearts. By the time the blood reaches the sinus venosus, pressure is essentially zero. Contractions of the atrium draw the blood from the sinus venosus and help fill the ventricle. Ventricular contractions generate the pressure to move the blood through the body.

The bulbous arteriosus is neither contractile nor valved, but elastic. It expands with each ventricular contraction as it fills with blood and maintains aortal pressure during ventricular diastole. In terms of pressure, the gills are somewhat restrictive, with blood cells meeting resistance within the lamellae. When the ventricle contracts, it sends a charge of blood into the bulbous; when the

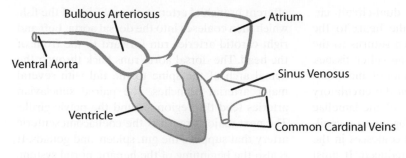

Bulbous Arteriosus — Atrium

Ventral Aorta

Sinus Venosus

Ventricle

Common Cardinal Veins

Ventricular Diastole

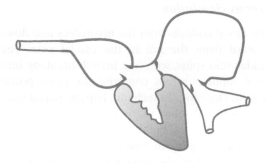

Ventricular Systole

Fig. 1.7 Teleost heart showing chamber enlargement and valve function at ventricular diastole and systole.

ventricle expands, the valve between the bulbous and the ventricle keeps the blood from going back into the ventricle. Coupled with the resistance of the gills, this causes the elastic bulbous to expand. As the blood continues to flow through the gills, the bulbous begins to "deflate," then comes another charge of blood from the ventricle. The bulbous functions to average out the pressure extremes and keep a steadier flow of blood going through the gills.

If teleosts did not have a bulbous, then the blood would strongly pulse over the gills. It appears to be adaptive for the fish to move the blood across the gills at a more constant rate. However, there is some pulsing even with the bulbous, and fish actually synchronize their heartbeat with their opercular movements in order to match peak blood flow with the water pulses associated with the buccal pump. This is especially evident when fish are subjected to hypoxia.

Other fishes

In elasmobranchs, agnathans, and holosteans, the fourth chamber, termed conus arteriosus, is not elastic, but fairly rigid, and its wall contains a series of valves to prevent backflow of blood. Since the conus is a more primitive condition, we can think of teleosts having the conus reduced to one valve (between bulbous arteriosus and ventricle), with the bulbous arteriosus evolved from the ventral aorta. In lungfish and amphibians, there is a septum dividing the atrium into two chambers, but not the ventricle.

Vascular system

Single-circuit circulation

Fish have single-circuit circulation. That is, blood leaves the heart, travels through the gills and the body, and then returns to the heart. Mammals (and reptiles and birds) have dual-circuit circulation: blood is pumped by the heart to the lungs and is oxygenated and then returns to the heart to be pumped again to the other tissues. The two-circuit (mammalian) model maintains higher blood pressure throughout the circulatory system. In fish, the lacunar space of the lamellae is a high-resistance system, analogous to a capillary bed. By the time the blood coalesces in the dorsal aorta, blood pressure is reduced. It must then flow through the capillary beds of the tissues. Fish blood always has to go through two high-resistance areas, that is, it always goes through the gills and the systemic circulation. Moreover, fish have two portal systems: a renal portal and a hepatic portal. The fish kidney, unlike the mammalian kidney, which is entirely supplied by the arterial system, is largely fed from the venous system. So, fish blood must always pass through two, and sometimes more, high-resistance areas during circulation. The consequence is relatively low blood pressure compared with mammals.

Mammals are subject to gravity, while the effect of gravity on fish is essentially zero. Gravity requires that mammals expend more energy when stationary or during slow movement than fish, and the blood itself must be pumped upward against gravity as well. The regulation of body temperature in mammals also requires a higher metabolic rate compared with that in ectothermic fish. These two differences mean that a high-pressure, rapid circulation is necessary in homeotherms to replenish the cells with oxygen and nutrients. Homeotherms have lower-affinity oxygen dissociation curves than fish for the same reason. On the other hand, fish have lower metabolic rates than homeotherms, and in some cases they must, because the PO_2 in the aquatic environment is often less than air, and with less oxygen pressure, fish cannot maintain as high a metabolic rate.

Arterial circulation

Circulation patterns vary widely in the fishes, but in general, unoxygenated blood flows from the bulbous arteriosus to the ventral aorta and branches off into the four afferent branchial arteries on each side of the fish's head. Blood becomes oxygenated at the gill and collects in the four efferent branchial arteries on each side of the fish, which then coalesce into the dorsal aorta. Left and right carotid arteries run forward to the front of the head. The dorsal aorta runs back through the hemal arch of the spine to the tail with several major arterial branches. The paired subclavian arteries feed the region around the pelvic girdle. The next major branch is the coeliacomesenteric artery that supplies the gut, spleen, and gonads. It is also the beginning of the hepatic portal system. The renal artery supplies the kidney with arterial blood. The dorsal aorta runs on to the tail, with branches at each myotome (Fig. 1.8).

Venous circulation

The blood collects from the myotomes and flows forward from the tail in the caudal vein. The caudal vein splits, with one branch breaking into renal capillaries that comprise the renal portal system. The other branch, the hepatic portal vein, collects blood from the gut, spleen, and gonad capillaries before breaking into liver sinusoids and coalescing again into the hepatic vein that returns blood to the sinus venosus of the heart. The dorsal and anterior part of the fish is drained by a system of paired veins, the cardinals. The left and right postcardinal veins drain the kidney and flow forward, joining the precardinal veins to form the common cardinals that feed into the sinus venosus. The precardinals along with jugular veins drain the head and the subclavian veins drain the pectoral area. Venous return in fish, like in mammals, is aided by muscular contraction, especially so in fish since they have such a low-pressure system. The veins in fish also have valves, like in mammals, to prevent backflow of blood. Some fish have accessory hearts (valved sacs) in the caudal region that are weakly contractile to aid venous return.

Vascularization of muscle

Muscle in fish is segregated into poorly vascularized white muscle and richly vascularized red muscle. A skinned fish shows a large bulk of the muscle to be white, while a stripe of red muscle runs along each side. Red muscle is highly vascularized because it is the muscle that is used for

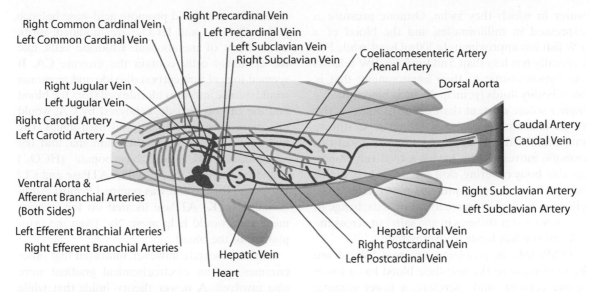

Fig. 1.8 Schematic of a typical teleost circulatory system.

continuous swimming; the white muscle is used only in bursts of activity. Red muscle relies on the efficient, aerobic respiration of oils to generate ATP, while white muscle uses much less efficient anaerobic fermentation of glycogen to create ATP. Glycogen has about half the calories per gram of oils, and anaerobic glycolysis harvests only a tiny fraction of that energy. The rest is tied up in lactic acid (lactate), which can only be further metabolized aerobically. Since white muscle is poorly vascularized, the lactate is oxidized very slowly. While white muscle is an inefficient producer of mechanical energy from food, it does provide a mechanism for fish to be highly active for brief periods despite a low-pressure circulatory system.

There is a strong correlation between routine swimming activity and the amount of red muscle in fish species. Sedentary fishes have very little red muscle, while fish that swim continually have much more, although all fish have more white than red. Constant fast swimmers such as tuna have a large mass of red muscle; moreover, a counter-current system of blood vessels feeding the red muscle conserves the heat generated by muscle contractions and allows the muscle to reach a temperature much higher than the surrounding ocean water, allowing for a faster rate of metabolism. Since red muscle is oily and oils retain a "fishy"

flavor, red muscle is routinely discarded when fish is prepared for food. For example, tuna red muscle is used in canned cat food and the white in canned tuna for human consumption.

Blood cells

Like other vertebrates, fish have red (erythrocytes) and white (leukocytes) blood cells. Fish erythrocytes retain their nucleus. While the density of erythrocytes in fish blood varies greatly among species, a typical hematocrit in fish is about 30%, much less than the 50% usually found in mammals. Fewer RBCs are needed in fish because they have lower metabolism and thus need to move less oxygen. In very active fish such as tuna, the hematocrit approaches 50%. Like other vertebrates, the leukocytes in fish have a variety of types that function in different ways from immune reaction to clotting.

Osmoregulation

Gill function

Basic problem

The process of osmosis makes the blood of FW fishes have a higher osmotic pressure than the water in which they swim. Osmotic pressure is expressed in milliosmoles, and the blood of a FW fish has approximately 300 mOsm/l, while FW generally has less than 5 mOsm/l. So, FW teleosts are hyperosmotic to their environment; that is, their bodily fluids (principally their blood) have a higher solute content than the environment. The result is a strong tendency for water to diffuse into the FW fish and salt out. Fish can resist this osmotic movement by having a relatively impermeable body covering, skin and scales help in this regard; however, the epithelial membrane of the gill must be highly permeable for gas exchange to occur. So, water diffuses in and salts out across the gill and the fish tends to overhydrate.

In SW fish, the problem is reversed. SW fish are hypo-osmotic to the sea; their blood has a lower solute content, and therefore, a lower osmotic pressure (about 400 mOsm) than seawater (about 1000 mOsm). SW fish suffer a passive loss of water at the gills and a passive gain of salts. SW fish tend to dehydrate.

The gill's role in osmoregulation in FW fish

In order to maintain 300 mOsm/l in its blood despite the osmotic tendency to gain water and lose ions, a FW fish must actively scavenge ions from the environment and excrete water from its body. It accomplishes this by (a) stopping the salt outflow at the gills and (b) producing copious, dilute urine. FW fish never drink as they gain all (and more) of the water they need passively over the gill.

The accepted theory of how FW fish reverse the flow of salt at the gills has evolved over time. Early research indicated enzymes (ATPases) in gill tissue split ATP and moved salts against the osmotic gradient with the energy that was released. It was presumed that most of this activity occurred in specialized cells in the gill epithelium termed beta chloride cells (to differentiate them from the anatomically different alpha chloride cells found in SW fish). Chloride cells have many mitochondria, capable of producing a lot of potential energy in the form of ATP that can be used by ATPases. This theory was intuitively appealing because the ATPases could exchange Na^+ for NH_4^+ and Cl^- for HCO_3^-. The exchange

of like charges would promote acid–base balance and both NH_4^+ and HCO_3^- are modified, waste by-products of metabolism. Chloride cells, like the epithelial cells, contain the enzyme CA. It seemed logical that carbon dioxide and ammonia would diffuse into the chloride cell from the blood and the carbon dioxide, catalyzed by CA, would dissociate into bicarbonate and hydronium. The hydronium would ionize the ammonia, and the ammonium (NH_4^+) and bicarbonate (HCO_3^-) would be excreted by Na^+/NH_4^+ ATPase and Cl^-/HCO_3^- ATPase as salt was pumped inward. Additionally, Na^+/K^+ ATPase located on the interior membrane would help move Na^+ from the cytoplasm into the blood.

Further research, however, indicated that other enzymes and an electrochemical gradient were also involved. A newer theory holds that while all of the above described movements no doubt occur, Na^+ also follows an electrical gradient (the cell being more negatively charged than the water) into the cell. The combined effect of the electrical gradient and the opposite osmotic gradient is termed the electrochemical gradient, and it is close to 0 for FW fish, stopping the outflow of salt at the gill. This electrical potential is maintained by a different ATPase that pumps H^+ out of the cell into the water and Na^+/K^+ ATPase that exchanges three Na^+ for two K^+ at the interior membrane. It is unclear which of these movements may occur in the chloride cell and which may be located in epithelial cells.

Most of the carbon dioxide is already in the form of bicarbonate by the time it reaches the gill because at the pH of blood, HCO_3^- is the predominate ion and the reaction from CO_2 to HCO_3^- is catalyzed by the enzyme CA in the RBCs. The chloride cell also contains CA to catalyze any remaining CO_2 to HCO_3^-. Obviously, the HCO_3^- already in the blood simply diffuses directly to the ion pump and is exchanged for Cl^-. Since there is no CA in the water, the slow conversion back to CO_2 does not occur until the water has exited the gill.

The gill's role in osmoregulation in SW fish

In order to maintain 400 mOsm despite a passive gain of salts and loss of water, SW fish must (a) stop the inflow of salt and actively secrete it at the gill and (b) drink seawater and hydrate themselves with it. SW fish excrete very little urine; in fact, some SW fish do not even have glomeruli in their kidneys.

While FW and SW fish face similar osmotic gradients (300–400 mOsm) between their blood and environment, the ATPase activity in the SW fish's gill is relatively higher. The reason for this is that salt must be actively pumped into the fish at the gut (discussed in detail later in this section) for hydration to occur. So, at the gill, SW fish must rid their body of both actively and passively gained salt. Additionally, it may be necessary for SW fish to employ ATPase pumping of Na^+ in exchange for NH_4^+ to rid themselves of nitrogenous waste, at times. Obviously, Na^+/NH_4^+ ATPase and Cl^-/HCO_3^- ATPase are not going to aid in osmoregulation in SW fish as they are presumed to do in FW fish.

It is believed that electrical gradients in a SW fish's gill move the necessary ions. In this gradient, the SW is negatively charged, the alpha chloride cell is more highly negative, and the blood is positively charged. The electrical gradient is maintained by Na^+/K^+ ATPase located in an extensive microtubule system schematically represented in the illustration as a single large indentation. The active pumping of Na^+ out of the chloride cell results in an Na^+ gradient (higher in the blood than in the chloride cell) that drives a Na^+/Cl^--linked carrier system increasing the Cl^- content of the cell, and thus the electronegativity of the chloride cell. The highly negative chloride cell causes Cl^- to move to less negatively charged seawater along the electrical gradient. The positively charged Na^+ will follow the gradient from positively charged blood to negatively charged seawater outside the chloride cell. Since this ion-moving mechanism is powered entirely by Na^+/K^+ ATPase, it is not surprising that this enzyme increases dramatically as euryhaline fish move from FW to SW.

Drinking in SW fish

Ingesting SW will not hydrate an animal unless that animal has a mechanism to move the water molecules from the gut into the blood against an osmotic gradient. Organisms cannot pump water

directly. The only way they can move water is to move salts, thus creating an osmotic gradient that water will follow. The cells of the gut lining in SW fish use Na^+/K^+ ATPase to create an electrochemical gradient similar to the chloride cells of the gill (but in the opposite direction) that move NaCl into the tissue surrounding the gut, creating a localized area of where the osmolality is greater than seawater, which causes water to flow into the blood of the fish. The final step in this hydration is the excretion of the salt by the chloride cell of the gill.

Kidney function

General

In mammals, the kidney is important in both osmoregulation and excretion of nitrogenous waste in the form of urea. In fish (teleosts), however, the kidney only serves an osmoregulatory function; the excretion of nitrogenous waste occurs at the gill, where ammonia is excreted as quickly as it is produced. The functional unit of the kidney is the nephron, which is composed of the glomerulus and renal tubule. The glomerulus is a tuft of capillaries through which the glomerular filtrate is passed. In fish, the tubule is divided into a Bowman's capsule that surrounds the glomerulus, followed by a series of segments (proximal I, proximal II, distal, and collecting duct) that perform different functions.

Teleosts

In FW teleosts, the kidney is of major importance. It removes water that passively entered at the gill through generation of dilute urine. In SW teleosts, the kidney is only of minor importance. It helps rid the fish of divalent cations (Ca^{++} and Mg^{++}), excess hydronium ions, and a few other minor waste products, but plays no role in water balance. Since SW fish need to retain water and the piscine kidney cannot produce urine more concentrated than body fluids, urine flow is kept to a minimum.

The first step in urine formation is the production of glomerular filtrate. This occurs when the permeable capillaries of the glomerulus "leak" water, salts, glucose, amino acids, and small

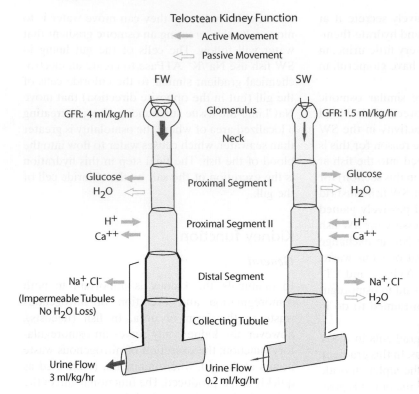

Fig. 1.9 Schematic of the euryhaline teleost kidney tubule (nephron) showing changes between freshwater (FW) and saltwater (SW) adaptations. GFR, glomerular filtration rate.

protein molecules. Some marine teleosts lack glomeruli, and therefore produce almost no filtrate and no urine. The filtrate is collected in the Bowman's capsule and proceeds down the tubule. The function of the tubule is to selectively add and remove solutes, and therefore water, to turn a general blood filtrate into urine waste.

After passing through the neck, which may be ciliated to help move the filtrate, the filtrate enters proximal segment I (PSI) (Fig. 1.9). In PSI, glucose and other desirable larger molecules are scavenged out of the filtrate, and to a lesser extent, anionic organic waste products are pumped in. The larger molecules are retrieved by pinocytosis, while the ions are moved by ATPases. This occurs in both FW and SW fish. In PSI (and PSII), the tubule is permeable to water, water follows the solutes out of the filtrate, and as a result, there is no change in the osmotic pressure of the filtrate. PSII is responsible for handling divalent cations. In salt-starved FW teleosts, the divalent cations in the filtrate are recovered, and in ion-rich SW teleosts, additional cations are excreted into the waste

stream. In at least some FW fish (e.g., eels), Na^+ and Cl^- are secreted into the filtrate in the proximal segments so water will follow and increase urine flow (the ions will be recovered later).

The distal segment (DS) and collecting tubule (CT) are where Na^+ and Cl^- are pumped back out of the filtrate. FW teleosts do this to recover the ions, while SW teleosts do not need the ions, but pump the salt to move the valuable water back out of the filtrate. FW and SW teleosts differ in the permeability of the DS and CT. In FW teleosts, the walls are impermeable to water, so ions can be recovered without water following, while in SW teleosts the walls are permeable so water will follow the salts. This impermeable section allows FW teleosts to excrete urine that is much more dilute than the blood. In SW teleosts, the tubules are permeable throughout the nephron so the urine, while having a different ion makeup than the filtrate, will differ little in osmotic pressure.

In summary, FW and SW fish differ in their kidney function in that (a) glomerular filtration rate (GFR) is higher in FW teleosts, (b) in PSII,

FW fish pump divalent cations out of the filtrate, while SW teleosts pump them in, and (c) the DS and CT are impermeable in FW fish and permeable in SW fish. It should be noted, that it is necessary for euryhaline fish to change kidney function in these three ways as they move from FW to SW and back. GFR and the divalent ion pump can be changed fairly rapidly, requiring only a day or so to adapt to the new environment. Changing the permeability of the DS and CT involves cell mitosis and takes several days.

Contrasts with mammals

There are interesting contrasts in kidney function between fish and mammals. First, GFR is much higher in mammals (about 650 ml/kg/hr); the average human produces 50 gallons of filtrate a day. GFR in mammals is higher because their glomerulus is fed by high-pressure arterial flow, while fish (with lower blood pressure to begin with) have their glomerulus supplied with venous blood from the renal portal system. Another difference is in urine flow. Urine flow in mammals is quite variable, of course, and depends on the amount of liquid the animal has imbibed. Mammals are capable of varying the osmolality of their urine as their state of hydration requires. FW fish, on the other hand, have a steady state of hydration because the water flow in through the gills remains fairly constant, which results in less fluctuation in urine flow. Finally, fish are unable to produce urine with a higher osmotic pressure than their blood, while dehydrated humans can concentrate urine to 1200 mOsm and desert rodents can produce urine with over 2000 mOsm, five to six times saltier than their blood. Mammals can do this because of the special structure of their kidneys. Mammalian kidney tubules form a loop in the medullary region of the kidney termed the loop of Henle. In the ascending part of the loop, salt is pumped out, but water cannot follow because the tubule is impermeable to water. This maintains a high osmotic gradient in the medullary region. When the CT, which is permeable to water, passes back through this salty region, the water is drawn out of the urine. Mammals can control the osmolality of the urine by regulating the permeability of the CT with hormones.

Senses

Usual senses

Overview

Fish have the usual senses (vision, hearing, tactile, taste, and smell) that terrestrial animals do, but they may be modified by adaptations to the aquatic environment. Additionally, the aquatic environment makes possible some unusual senses unknown in terrestrial animals. All sensory perceptions require a "sending unit" that translates physical stimuli such as light and sound into nerve impulses that are sent to the brain, where the impulses are interpreted as sight or sound.

Vision

Most fishes can see to some extent and some have good vision like most terrestrial animals. However, the aquatic environment tends to be dimmer and murkier than air, and the longer wavelengths of light (red-orange) are rapidly absorbed by water, leaving only bluish light at depth. As a consequence, sight is often of limited value underwater and many fishes rely heavily on nonvisual senses. A few fish have lost functional eyes through adaptation to permanently dark cave habitat

Some fishes need to be able to see up into the air through the surface of the water in order to detect predators and prey. Light rays bend as they pass from air into water because of the difference in refractive index, so a fish's view upward into the air is distorted. While everything is visible from horizon to horizon, only objects directly overhead appear accurately. Other objects appear to be higher off the horizon then they actually are. This type of view is seen in a photo taken with a "fish-eye" lens, hence the name. Note that fish only have a "fish-eye" view when looking through the surface, not when seeing underwater. A few fish have special adaptations to minimize this distortion. For example, *Anableps* is termed the four-eyed fish because each eye is divided into an upper and lower part, with a divided iris. The corneas and lenses of the upper and lower parts are modified to compensate for the different refractive indices of air and water. *Anableps* swims with the water's surface at the division.

Fish have both rods and cones in the retina, although rods predominate in fish from dim, deepwater environments. The presence of cones, and pigments that absorb different wavelengths, suggests that fish can see color. Behavioral experiments with a limited number of species confirm this. Sharks accommodate for changing light intensity by dilation and contraction of the iris. Teleosts, however, rely on retinomotor light adaptation, that is, moving the pigment layer and light-sensitive rods as light intensity changes.

Hearing

Sound travels well underwater, and because water is so dense, fish tend to hear well. They have no external ear canals, eardrums, or middle ear bones; therefore, sound waves must reach the inner ear by traveling through the body. The innervated cilia that pick up the physical vibrations and transmit a nerve signal to the brain are located in inner ear sacs and have otoliths resting on them. The sound vibrations move the otoliths and the surrounding fish tissue differently. The cilia sense the relative motion and the brain interprets this as sound. Fish do not have a spiral cochlea and so they presumably cannot distinguish frequencies as well as humans can. The ostariophysan fishes (minnows and catfish) have a mechanical connection of connective tissue, muscle and bone between the swim bladder and the inner ear. This Weberian apparatus serves to amplify sound because the relative motion between the gas in the air bladder and the fish caused by sound waves is greater than between the fish and the otolith. The Weberian apparatus transmits this stronger vibration to the inner ear.

It is sometimes suggested that ice on a koi pond should be slowly melted rather than broken because the loud noise can kill the fish under the ice. There is no scientific information to support this concern. While loud noises can be stressful to fish, for fish to actually die of stress, the stressor must persist for at least 12 hours; moreover, fish at frigid temperatures found under ice have a much attenuated stress response. This concern may have originated when fish dead or dying of winter kill (hypoxia) were discovered under broken ice.

Chemoreception

In terrestrial animals, chemoreception is usually divided into taste and smell. The difference being that taste is waterborne and smell is airborne. In fish, all chemical stimuli are carried in the water, so the distinction is blurred. There remains in fish the division of receptors into those in the nasal cavity (smell) and all others (taste) that may occur in the mouth, on barbels, or elsewhere on the body. Fish use chemoreception for finding food, of course, and the ability of sharks and catfish to detect a meal they cannot see is well known. Less appreciated is the role of chemoreception in behavior and orientation. Detection of pheromones is important in breeding and schooling. Some fishes (e.g., minnows) release an alarm substance (termed "Schreckstoff" in German) when they are injured that alerts others nearby of danger.

The acuity of chemoreception in homing salmon rivals bloodhounds. It has been shown experimentally that salmon find their way from the main stem of a river to their natal stream by chemoreception. When salmon are small (smolts) in their home stream, they imprint on the subtle unique odors that the watershed gives that particular stream. After migrating downstream and living for years in the ocean, they are able to "sniff" their way home. If the natural stream odors are overwhelmed by a smelly substance, the salmon will imprint on that and later home to wherever the researchers dispense the odoriferous substance. Another experiment showed that blinded salmon could find their way home, but salmon with their nares plugged could not.

Unusual senses

Lateral line

Because water is so dense, it propagates pressure waves very well. Fish have evolved a lateral line sense that detects and interprets pressure waves. This sense allows fish to detect very low-frequency vibrations such as those generated by a tail beat or nearby relative movement. To understand the detection of relative movement by pressure wave perception, move your hand slowly toward the top of your desk without quite touching it. If the air was dense enough, and your hand was sensi-

Lateral Line System

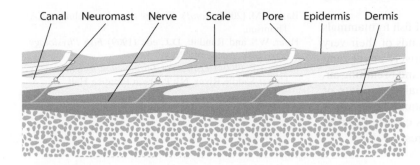

Canal   Neuromast   Nerve   Scale   Pore   Epidermis   Dermis

Fig. 1.10 Anatomy of the lateral line canal.

tive enough, you could feel the higher pressure above the desk relative to the lower pressure at the edge where the air could flow away. This is how the lateral line works in fish and why it has been termed "distant touch." For the lateral line sense to work, either the fish, the object it is detecting, or both must be moving. Experimental evidence suggests that the lateral line sense can be quite precise in detecting relatively small objects, but primarily at close range. Under poor visibility conditions, which are quite common underwater, the lateral line sense is quite valuable in feeding (Fig. 1.10).

The receptor for the lateral line system is the neuromast. This small structure consists of a flexible, jellylike cupula resting on a mass of sensory cells. The sensory cells have hairs embedded in the cupula. A pressure wave causes the cupula to move and the hairs transmit the direction and extent of movement to the sensory cells, which then generate nerve impulses, carrying this information to the brain, where it is interpreted. Neuromasts may be located on the skin, in pits, or in canals that run in the superficial bone of the head and through the scales along the side of the fish (hence lateral line sense).

Weak electrical senses

Water is an excellent conductor of electricity. It is not surprising then that many fish have the ability to sense low levels of electrical current such as those generated by muscle contractions and movement through the earth's magnetic field. Electrical reception in many fish is accomplished by pit organs in the skin. Sharks have a highly developed electrical detection system consisting of canals of electrical conducting gel joining many sensory pits, termed ampullae of Lorenzini. Interestingly, electrical reception is more widespread in primitive fishes such as lampreys and sharks than in teleosts.

A few teleosts have taken weak electrical sense a step further. Members of the family Gymnotidae (knife fish) and Morymidae (elephant fish) not only receive electrical signals but transmit them as well. Elephant fish typically live in turbid environments, where sight is of limited value, and feed on small worms buried in the substrate. Elephant fish generate a weak electrical field from electric organs located in the caudal region. This field has a potential of only about 10V, far less than the hundreds of volts that strongly electric fishes (eels and catfish) use to stun their prey. The elephant fish transmits and receives its own signal and is able to tell when a hidden body, with a different conductivity than water or mud, changes the shape of the field. In this way, it uses the electrical field as a probe for food. It apparently takes a lot of neural processing to execute this type of detection because morymids have the largest relative brain weight of any fish, even exceeding humans. The bulk of this brain mass is in the cerebellum.

Form and function follow habitat

As we have seen in the preceding pages, many attributes of the anatomy and physiology are similar to mammals, but differences abound.

Some of the differences are related to gill breathing, some to locomotion by swimming, and many to their ectothermy.

Ultimately, all the contrasts of fish to mammals can be traced back to the demands of their very different habitat. Humans intuitively understand the constraints of living on land and breathing air. Only by appreciating the special constraints of the aquatic habitat and understanding the fish's adaptations to these constraints can we begin to keep fish healthy and free of stress.

Further reading

Barton, M. (2007) *Bond's Biology of Fishes*. Belmont, CA: Thomson.

Hoar, W.S. and Randall, D.J., eds. (1969) *Fish Physiology*. New York: Academic Press.

Moyle, P.B. (2004) *Fishes: An Introduction to Ichthyology*. Upper Saddle River, NJ: Pearson Prentice Hall.

Chapter 2

A Brief Overview of the Ornamental Fish Industry and Hobby

Tim Miller-Morgan

Introduction

Ornamental or pet fish keeping is an activity that has existed for thousands of years, with evidence suggesting it dates back as early as 500 BCE. The ancient Romans in the 2nd century maintained elaborate ornamental marine fish ponds, and many of them became quite attached to their pet fish (see Fig. 2.1) (Higginbotham, 1997; Brunner, 2003). The Chinese developed the practice of breeding and keeping goldfish perhaps as early as the T'ang dynasty (AD 619–907), and by the year AD 960, there are writings that indicate that goldfish were kept as household pets in ponds (Hervey and Hems, 1948). Beginning about 1276, goldfish were being maintained indoors in fancy bowls, and by 1548, fancy goldfish keeping was a popular hobby throughout China (Balon, 2004).

Goldfish keeping in Europe began in the early 1600s, probably in Portugal, and had spread to Great Britain by 1691. By the 1700s, goldfish keeping was a popular hobby throughout Europe and Britain (Brunner, 2003). Goldfish keeping did not reach the United States until the mid-1850s and may have been popularized by Phineas T. Barnum, who is said to have brought back some specimens from his travels in Europe. In 1865, goldfish were being sold in a New York City pet shop. Hugo Mullert, who many consider the father of the aquarium hobby in America, started the first commercial goldfish hatchery in 1883 in Cincinnati, Ohio (Brunner, 2003; Klee, 2003).

Modern aquarium keeping, maintaining fish in "balanced" glass aquaria, has its origins in Victorian England in the mid-1800s. This pastime was initially popularized by the publication of two popular books in Britain: *The Aquarium: Unveiling the Wonders of the Deep Sea*, by Phillip Henry Gosse, in 1854, and the publication of *Rustic Adornments for Homes of Taste*, by Shirley Hibbert, in 1856. These books and many later works popularized the keeping of fish in aquariums in Britain, Europe, and the United States (Klee, 2003). The world's first aquarium magazine, the *New York Aquarium Journal*, was published in 1876. With the turn of the century, there began a large expansion of the hobby and the industry throughout Europe and the United States. The development and popularization of aquarium societies, ornamental fish exhibitions, competitions, and many more aquarium and pet fish keeping magazines served to rapidly increase the awareness and interest in aquarium fish keeping (Brunner, 2003; Klee, 2003).

The hobby and industry continued to expand throughout the 20th century with increasing imports of wild exotic fishes, tank breeding and farm production of many species, and improved techniques for shipping fish over long distances (Brunner, 2003; Klee, 2003).

Exports of Amazonian fish began in the 1930s and expanded greatly in the 1950s. Exports of freshwater fish from South Asia were recorded in the 1920s and 1930s. Small numbers of marine fish began to be exported out of Sri Lanka in the 1930s (Wijesekara and Yakupitiyage, 2000; UNEP-WCMC, 2007). This early trade was primarily based upon wild-caught specimens; however, captive-bred specimens from ornamental fish farms began to play an increasing role in the freshwater aspects of this industry.

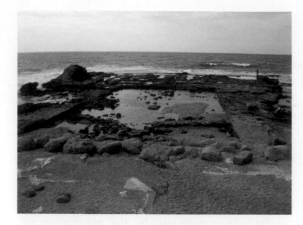

Fig. 2.1 Example of a Roman fish pond in Caesarea, Israel (1st century AD).

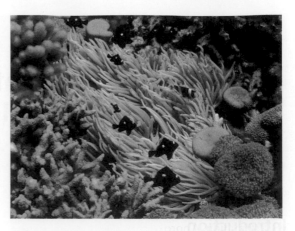

Fig. 2.2 Wild marine fish photographed on a reef in Indonesia. These are examples of some fish species commonly collected for the marine ornamental sector of the industry.

Today, the majority of the ornamental freshwater fish are captive bred, primarily in Asia and Florida, while the majority of marine species are still wild caught (Andrews, 1990; Oliver, 2001; Wood, 2001; Wabnitz et al., 2003; UNEP-WCMC, 2007).

The increased availability of cheaper international air transport, the development of the plastic shipping bag, and the improvement in aquarium equipment in the years following World War II are some of the important factors that led to the rapid expansion of the industry and hobby in the late 20th century (Axelrod, 2001; Vitko, 2004; UNEP-WCMC, 2007).

An expanding area of the industry and hobby today is the interest in keeping tropical reef aquariums. Reef tanks are saltwater aquariums principally focused on coral reef invertebrates, with a minimal number of fish (see Fig. 2.2). Typical reef tanks will contain live rock, hard and soft corals, and various other invertebrate species such as mollusks, crustaceans, echinoderms, and a few reef fish (Livengood and Chapman, 2007).

The increased interest in the keeping of reef aquariums has resulted in a significant rise in the number of countries exporting and culturing ornamental fish and invertebrates over the past two decades (Wabnitz et al., 2003; Livengood and Chapman, 2007).

Today, ornamental fish are the world's most popular pets, and ornamental fish keeping is second only to photography as the most popular hobby.

Ornamental fish keeping is primarily practiced in the industrialized countries because it is still a relatively costly hobby (Oliver, 2001). It can be divided today into three main sectors: tropical freshwater fish, tropical marine fish and invertebrates, and ornamental pond fish (primarily goldfish and koi), although it is not uncommon for hobbyists to maintain fish from multiple sectors (APPMA, 2007).

Current status and scope of the ornamental fish industry

Today, ornamental fish comprise a very large and diverse global industry, with trading in over 4500 species of freshwater fish, 1450 species of marine fish, and over 650 species of corals and other marine invertebrates.

More that 50% of the ornamental fish supply originates in Asia. Eighty percent of these are farm-raised freshwater fish, and 15% and 5% are wild-caught marine and freshwater species, respectively. Singapore specializes in farming freshwater species but also serves as a major reexporter of fish from other Asian countries. A number of other Asian countries also specialize in farming freshwater ornamental fish. These include Thailand, Japan, China, Malaysia, and Sri Lanka (Oliver, 2003).

The United States—Florida, in particular—farms primarily freshwater species, but some marine species are also captured in the wild. The United States also imports most of the ornamental fish exported from South America. The majority of these species are wild caught, and then reexported to Canada, Europe, and Japan. Israel is a significant exporter of farm-raised fish, as is the Czech Republic, which specializes in farming freshwater species (Oliver, 2003).

Since 1985, the value of the industry has grown by an average of 14% per year, and recent estimates place the value of live ornamental fish at US$900 million. Approximately 90% of this value can be attributed to freshwater species, and the remaining 10% to marine species. The value of global industry, including retail sales, associated materials, wages, and nonexported products, is estimated to be worth US$15 billion (Oliver, 2001, 2003; Wabnitz et al., 2003; Bartley, 2005; UNEP-WCMC, 2007; Whittington and Chong, 2007).

Table 2.1 shows the major ornamental fish exporting and importing countries. Approximately one billion ornamental fish and invertebrates captive bred and wild caught are exported annually from over 100 countries.

While most of the freshwater species are farm raised, significant numbers are wild caught. The major centers for wild-caught freshwater fish include the Amazon River basin, the Congo River basin, and major rivers in Southeast Asia. Since there is a dramatic disparity between the numbers of freshwater fish exported compared with marine fish, it is possible that the actual numbers of wild-caught freshwater species may exceed the number of wild-caught marine fish species.

Approximately 98% of marine species are wild caught, with the remaining 2% farm raised. The primary import markets for ornamental fish are the United States, Western Europe, and Asia. In the last few years, there have also been increased imports to Australia, Brazil, Israel, and South Africa, indicating the growing presence of ornamental fish keepers in these countries (Andrews, 1990; Oliver, 2003; Gerstner et al., 2006; UNEP-WCMC, 2007).

Components of the ornamental fish industry

The distribution network that has developed for the modern ornamental fish industry is a complex, diverse, highly interrelated mix of industry, regulatory (governmental and nongovernmental), and support businesses (Fig. 2.3). Components of this network can be found on every continent except Antarctica.

Fishermen or collectors

The collectors are generally small-scale fishermen in tropical countries who tend to work alone or in small groups (Fig. 2.4). They typically work with basic equipment and often collect fish by hand.

Table 2.1 Major ornamental fish exporting and importing countries.

Exporting country	Importing country
Singapore	United States
United States	Japan
Malaysia	Germany
Czech Republic	France
Sri Lanka	Belgium
Japan	Italy
Philippines	Singapore
Israel	The Netherlands
	China, Hong Kong
	Canada

Source: Oliver (2001).

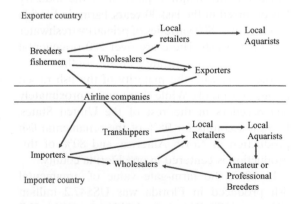

Fig. 2.3 This diagram illustrates the international ornamental fish distribution network.

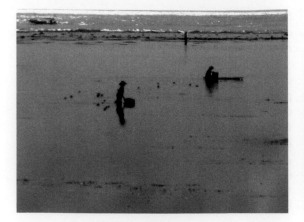

Fig. 2.4 Ornamental fish collectors harvesting fish from a shallow reef in Indonesia.

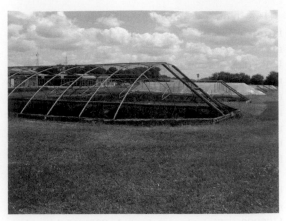

Fig. 2.5 A typical ornamental fish farm in Florida (photo courtesy of Dr. Roy P. Yanong).

They are the first link in the "chain of custody" for ornamental fish. Most work for exporters of wholesalers and are paid for the number of fish they collect (Oliver, 2003).

Breeders or farmers

The majority of ornamental fish breeders are located in Asia, but there are a significant number in North America—primarily in Florida—South America, the Czech Republic, and Israel. Most of these fish are reared in outdoor ponds or tanks (Oliver, 2003).

Florida is an excellent example of the success that can be associated with ornamental fish farming (Fig. 2.5). The industry dates to the early 1930s, but the major expansion in the industry has occurred in the last 30 years. Farms in Florida produce over 800 varieties of primarily freshwater ornamental fish. There are over 200 ornamental fish breeders concentrated in the southern part of the state, with the majority of the fish raised in outdoor ponds. While there are approximately 500 breeders in the rest of the United States, Florida accounts for 95% of the ornamental fish production in North America, and 80% of this production is centered in one Florida county.

In 2003, the farm-gate value of ornamental fish produced in Florida was US$47.2 million (Watson, 1999; Watson and Shireman, 1996; Hill et al., 2002; Oliver, 2003).

Wholesalers

Wholesalers in exporting countries buy from the collectors, breeders, and importers, and sell to the exporters. In importing countries, the wholesalers buy directly from the importers and sell to the retailers. Many wholesalers are disappearing due to the introduction of transshipping and the development of Internet-based sales (Oliver, 2003).

Exporters

Exporters buy directly from multiple wholesalers or fish collectors. Some exporters may also employ their own collectors. An exporter typically will assess the quality and health of the fish prior to purchase. They may quarantine their fish before shipment. Utilization of quarantine will depend upon their sales volume, facility capabilities, the value of various fish species, and pertinent regulations. The quarantine period may last from a few days to months, depending on the previous factors. Many export facilities will have substantial infrastructure, which may include single to multiple warehouses, with hundreds of holding tanks, single or multiple water treatment systems, a fish health laboratory, food storage, packing areas, and sales offices (Fig. 2.6).

The fish will typically be packed in plastic shipping bags partially filled with water, with oxygen filling the remaining space. These bags will be packed in insulated Styrofoam shipping

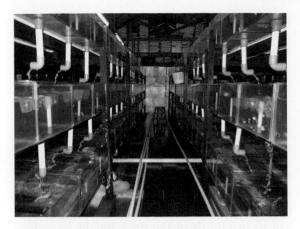

Fig. 2.6 An export facility in Indonesia.

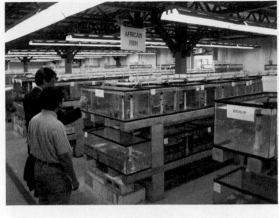

Fig. 2.7 A typical ornamental fish import facility in North America.

containers and packed in cardboard shipping boxes. Heat or cold packs may also be added to the boxes, depending on the time of year and destination. The packing density in each bag varies with the species, size, and duration of the shipment. Freshwater fish are generally packed at high densities, while marine species are packed at very low densities (Cole et al., 1999; Lim et al., 2003; Wabnitz et al., 2003).

Exporters must also obtain licenses for each shipment, as well as customs declarations and, in some cases, health certifications before the shipment may leave its country of origin. Each importing country may also have additional customs and health certification requirements (Oliver, 2003).

Importers

Importers generally purchase their stock from multiple exporters or transshippers. Shipments are typically received with the appropriate health, customs, and Convention on the International Trade in Endangered Species (CITES) certificates. Once these are reconciled, the fish will be unpacked, acclimated to the new environment, and assessed for overall health. These animals may also be quarantined, depending on the same factors mentioned above for the exporters. Once the health status and feeding of these animals is assured, importers will sell their animals to wholesalers or directly to retailers (Fig. 2.7). The shipping and packing practices are similar to those

used for exporters above, although in many cases there is a shorter shipping duration. In some cases, they will reexport these animals to other countries. For example, Singapore imports much of the Asian production but then reexports worldwide (Oliver, 2001; Wabnitz et al., 2003).

Transshipping

Transshipping began in the mid-1970s to reduce the overall import cost of the fish and has significantly changed the global ornamental fish sales network. Transshippers will group a number of orders from several retailers or importers together, collect the fish at the airport, and redistribute them to their customers. If the boxes are opened upon arrival, the transshipper may do a water change and reoxygenate the shipping bags. Transshippers do not generally acclimate the fish or check their health status. The customer takes all responsibility for the animals in the shipment, including animals that may have died during the transport. While the quality of transshipped fish is often lower than that of fish moved through an import or wholesale facility, the price may be half the cost of fish from those facilities (Oliver, 2001, 2003).

Retailers

Retailers generally buy their fish directly from a wholesaler, importer, or transshipper. They may

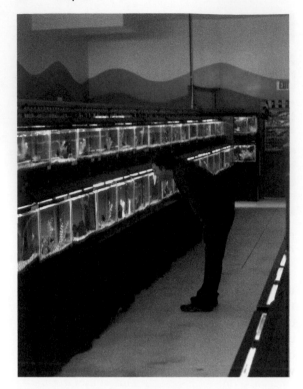

Fig. 2.8 An ornamental fish retail facility in Portland, Oregon.

also set up their own transshipments. If they order through a transshipper, they will need to acclimate the fish themselves, but if they buy from a wholesaler or importer, the fish are often acclimated and will generally be ready for sale (Fig. 2.8).

Increasingly, there has been a tendency for retailers to bypass the exporters, wholesalers, and importers and buy their fish directly from the breeders and collectors. However, there are a number of emerging diseases that often could be identified during quarantine at the export, wholesale, and import facilities. Bypassing these facilities may expose the retailer to more disease risk, and it may be advantageous for the retailer to establish their own quarantine and health assessment protocols (Oliver, 2001; Miller-Morgan and Hartman, 2007).

Airlines

International airlines currently transport all of the fish from exporting to importing counties, becoming key players in an industry in which the quality of the air transport reflects in the final quality and health of the fish.

Airline transport associations, such as the International Air Transport Association, have developed guidelines for the packaging and transport of these animals, and the packing techniques mentioned previously were developed in consultation with these associations.

The transport of ornamental fish has become a highly profitable area for the airlines. Due to the weight of the shipping water, the freight charge for these shipments may represent more than one-half to two-thirds of the price for the importer. The fish may only represent 1% of the total shipment weight (Oliver, 2001; Wabnitz et al., 2003).

Governments and international bodies

Many governments of ornamental fish exporting countries are directly involved in the industry. They may provide financial assistance to the local industry, assist with the development of improved management schemes, sponsor international trade shows or conferences, fund applied research, or enact improved trade regulations to foster the local industry. In some cases, the government will set fishing quotas, limited collection areas, or prevent certain fishing practices such as dynamite or cyanide fishing (Oliver, 2001).

A number of species are protected under the CITES. Some species are completely prohibited from export to prevent further exploitation, while others may be exported in limited numbers, primarily corals, as long as proper permits have been obtained. Import of such species without the proper documentation will generally result in confiscation by customs officials at the port of entry (Oliver, 2003; Wabnitz et al., 2003).

The Marine Aquarium Council (MAC) is a nongovernmental organization that has developed a certification scheme to track marine ornamental fish and invertebrates from the collector to the hobbyist. The program, created in 1996, has developed standards to ensure animal quality and health, sustainable wild harvesting practices, and sustainable, healthy, and humane culture practices. There is a system of independent evaluators to certify compliance with these standards. The goal is to create a demand within the marine ornamental hobby for certified products. The MAC has developed a network of stakeholders in over 60 countries (Wabnitz et al., 2003; MAC, 2007).

Ongoing issues within the ornamental fish industry

There are a number of issues that continue to challenge the ornamental fish industry. While multiple efforts are ongoing to improve many of these problems, until they are adequately addressed they will continue to impact the overall quality and health of animals within the industry.

One of the more pressing issues is the lack of qualified staff within the distribution chain and at the retail level. This leads to poor quality, poor health, and increased mortality of the animals throughout the chain of custody.

At the retail level, this lack of professionalism and training often leads to poor advice and information given to the customer. As a result, the animals may do poorly in captivity, and the consumer often starts to view these animals as disposable commodities. For example, koi and goldfish bought in garden centers often are not quarantined and are carrying diseases that have not been identified or treated. These fish may then infect the fish in the hobbyist's pond.

There is a recurrent problem of insufficient veterinary oversight, care, and availability for these species. This is primarily due to a lack of specific training in fish and invertebrate medicine within the veterinary curriculum and a poor understanding of the value of veterinary involvement within the ornamental fish industry (Oliver, 2003; Miller-Morgan, 2006).

There are significant concerns about the sustainability of wild harvesting within both the freshwater and marine sectors. While there are a number of organizations addressing this issue— most notably Project Piaba in the Amazon basin and the MAC—this will remain a significant concern until these issues are resolved (Chao et al., 2001; Wood, 2001; Corbin et al., 2003; Oliver, 2003; Wabnitz et al.,2003).

Many of the problems are exacerbated by the traditionally poor organization and communication within and among all sectors of the industry. Improved communication and increased transparency will be required to improve the general awareness of these problems and to develop incentives to address these issues (Oliver, 2003).

In spite of these problems, ornamental fish keeping as a hobby continues to improve and develop. Furthermore, the industry has begun to develop trade associations in many countries to take a proactive approach to many of these issues. Tropical freshwater fish continue to be the mainstay of the industry and hobby. In the past few decades, there has been an increased emphasis within the ornamental marine and pond fish sector. Ornamental fish keeping will continue to develop and gain a higher profile worldwide, and this continued and growing interest should drive expansion and improvement within the industry (Oliver, 2003; Wabnitz et al., 2003).

References and further reading

Andrews, C. (1990) The ornamental fish trade and fish conservation. *Journal of Fish Biology* **37** (Suppl. A): 53–59.

APPMA. (2007) APPMA National Pet Owners Survey. Greenwich, CT: National Pet Owners Manufacturers Association.

Axelrod, H.R. (2001) Discovery of the cardinal tetra and beyond. In *Conservation and Management of Ornamental Fish of the Rio Negro Basin, Amazonia, Brazil—Project Piaba* (Chao, N.L., Petry, P., Prang, G., Sonneschein, L., Tlusty, M., eds.), pp. 17–26. Manaus, Brazil: Editora Da Universidade, Do Amazonas.

Balon, E.K. (2004) About the oldest domesticates among fishes. *Journal of Fish Biology* **65** (Suppl. A): 1–27.

Bartley, D. (2005) Topics Fact Sheets. Ornamental fish. In *FAO Fisheries and Aquaculture Department*. www.fao.org/fishery/topic/13611/en.

Brunner, B. (2003) *The Ocean at Home: An Illustrated History of the Aquarium*. New York: Princeton Architectural Press.

Chao, N.L., Prang, G., and Petry, P. (2001) Project Piaba—maintenance and sustainable development of ornamental fisheries in *the Rio Negro Basin, Amazonas, Brazil. In Conservation and Management of Ornamental Fish of the Rio Negro Basin, Amazonia, Brazil—Project Piaba* (Chao, N.L., Petry, P., Prang, G., Sonneschein, L., Tlusty, M., eds.), pp. 3–14. Manaus, Brazil: Editora Da Universidade, Do Amazonas.

Cole, B., Tamaru, C.S., Bailey, R., et al. (1999) *CTSA Publication 131, Shipping Practices in the Ornamental Fish*

Industry. Honolulu, HI: Center for Tropical and Sub-tropical Aquaculture.

Corbin, J.S., Cato, J.C., and Brown, C.L. (2003) Marine Ornamentals Industry 2001: recommendations for a sustainable future. In *Marine Ornamental Species: Collection, Culture and Conservation*. (Cato, J.C. and Brown, C.L., eds.), pp. 3–9. Ames, IA: Blackwell.

Gerstner, C.L., Ortega, H., Sanchez, H., et al. (2006) Effects of the freshwater aquarium trade on wild fish populations in differently-fished areas of the Peruvian Amazon. *Journal of Fish Biology* **68**: 826–875.

Hervey, G.F. and Hems, J. (1948) *The Goldfish*. London: The Batchworth Press.

Higginbotham, J. (1997) *Piscinae: Artificial Fishponds in Roman Italy*. Chapel Hill: University of North Carolina Press.

Hill, J., Roy, E., and Yanong, P.E. (2006) *UF/IFAS Circular 54 Freshwater Ornamental Fish Commonly Cultured in Florida*. http://edis.ifas.ufl.edu/pdffiles/FA/FA05400.pdf.

Klee, A.J. (2003) *The Toy Fish: A History of the Aquarium Hobby in America—The First One-Hundred Years*. Pascoag, RI: Finley Aquatic Books.

Lim, L.C., Dhert, P., and Sorgeloos, P. (2003) Recent developments and improvements in ornamental fish packing systems for air transport. *Aquaculture Research* **34**: 923–935.

Livengood, E.J. and Chapman, F.A. (2007) *UF/IFAS Circular 124 The Ornamental Fish Trade: An Introduction with Perspectives for Responsible Aquarium Fish Ownership*. http://edis.ifas.ufl.edu/FA124.

MAC (2007) Marine Aquarium Council. http://www.aquariumcouncil.org.

Miller-Morgan, T. (2006) An overview of the ornamental fish industry. Presented at the American Veterinary Medical Association Annual Conference, Honolulu, HI.

Miller-Morgan, T. and Hartman, K. (2007) Biosecurity for koi retail/wholesale facilities. Presented at the Koi Health Academy, Reno, NV, February 24–25.

Norfolk, H. (2004) *Aquariums and Public Aquariums in Mid-Victorian Times*. www.aquarticles.com/articles/literature/Norfolk_Victorian_History.html.

Oliver, K. (2001) *The Ornamental Fish Market*. FAO/GLOBEFISH Research Program, Volume 67. Rome: FAO.

Oliver, K. (2003) World trade in ornamental species. In *Marine Ornamental Species: Collection, Culture and Conservation* (Cato, J.C. and Brown, C.L., eds.), pp. 49–63. Ames, IA: Blackwell.

Taylor, J.E. (1901) *The Aquarium: Its Inhabitants, Structure and Management*. Edinburgh: John Grant Publishing.

UNEP-WCMC. (2007) *Draft Consultation Paper: International Trade in Aquatic Ornamental Species*. Cambridge, UK: United Nations Environment Program—World Conservation Monitoring Center.

Vitko, R. (2004) A history of the hobby. *Reefkeeping*. www.reefkeeping.com/issues/2004-09/rv/feature/index.php.

Wabnitz, C., Taylor, M., Green, E., et al. (2003) *From Ocean to Aquarium: The Global Trade in Ornamental Marine Species*. UNEP-WCMS Biodiversity Series No. 17. Cambridge, UK: United Nations Environment Program—World Conservation Monitoring Center.

Watson, C.A. (1999) The ornamental fish industry. In *Marketing and Shipping Live Aquatic Products, Proceedings of the Second International Conference and Exhibition* (Paust, B.C. and Rice, A.A., eds.), pp. 87–93. Fairbanks: Alaska Sea Grant College Program.

Watson, C.A. and Shireman, J.V. (1996) *UF/IFAS Circular 35 Production of Ornamental Aquarium Fish*. www.aces.edu/dept/fisheries/education/ras/publications/Update/FL%20ornamental%20production.pdf.

Whittington, R.J. and Chong, R. (2007) Global trade in ornamental fish from an Australian perspective: the case for revised import risk analysis and management strategies. *Preventive Veterinary Medicine* **81**: 91–116.

Wijesekara, R.G.S. and Yakupitiyage, A. (2000) Ornamental fish in Sri Lanka: present status and future trends. *Aquarium Science and Conservation* **3**: 241–252.

Wood, E. (2001) *Collection of Coral Reef Fish for Aquaria: Global Trade, Conservation Issues and Management*. Herfordshire, UK: Marine Conservation Society.

Chapter 3
Stress in Fish

David J. Pasnik, Joyce J. Evans, and Phillip H. Klesius

Laypeople, scientists, and fish health professionals routinely identify stress among the major contributors to fish disease and death. Whether fish are wild or captive, stress affects their health and welfare.

Introduction

Stress in fish involves a condition disruptive of physiological homeostasis that occurs in response to unfavorable external influences and is capable of adversely affecting fish. Any stimulus that provokes stress responses is known as a *stressor*, disrupting a stable condition and causing a response. While stress is an adaptive response, it can become detrimental if stressor exposure is acute or chronic in nature. Several stressors routinely encountered in fish husbandry are presented in Table 3.1 (Barton 2000; Rose 2002; Evans et al., 2006; Huntingford et al., 2006). Although stress represents a complex, dynamic process, the stages of stress are often put into basic categories for simplicity. If stressors are present or intensified, the fish may have initial behavioral changes, and then primary, secondary, or tertiary stress responses (Barton, 2000).

- Initial behavioral changes may occur within seconds to minutes of the stressor exposure. Fish presumably act to avoid harmful stimuli.
- Primary responses involve increased corticosteroid and catecholamine hormone release (e.g., cortisol, epinephrine, and norepinephrine) and may begin within seconds to hours later.
- Secondary stress responses include changes in hematological, metabolic, and hydromineral values (e.g., blood glucose and lactate, liver

and muscle glycogen, osmolality) and may begin within minutes to hours later.
- Tertiary responses involve changes in whole-fish behavior and performance (e.g., homeostasis disturbances) and may begin minutes to days after stressor exposure. This is the most apparent stage.

The central nervous system of fish must first perceive the stressor through sensations, such as discomfort or fright. Some scientists dispute if fish feel pain (Rose, 2002; Sneddon et al., 2003), precluding conclusion whether these sensations can also include pain (a conscious experience) or just nociception (an unconscious reaction). Following chromaffin tissue stimulation by the parasympathetic nervous system, the catecholamines epinephrine and norepinephrine are released. These catecholamines cause respiratory and cardiovascular effects and mobilize energy. The hypothalamic–pituitary–interrenal (HPI) axis is also activated and increases cortisol secretion, mobilizing energy reserves and maintaining ionic balance despite the presence of a stressor. These responses may help the fish maintain homeostasis and adapt to the stress. Sometimes fish can acclimate to frequent disturbances, reducing subsequent stress responses. However, if stress responses are chronically activated through repeated or excessively continuous exposure to a stressor, the effects may be detrimental and cumulative. Negative effects include decreased growth rates, immunosuppression, and increased disease susceptibility. Stress has an effect on fish metabolism, presumably because energy utilized for stress responses is no longer available for other physiological activities (Pankhurst and Van der Kraal, 1997). For example, weight gain and food conversion are reduced with chronic stress

Table 3.1 Common causes of stress in fish.

Influence	Comment
Water quality	Chemical, including ammonia, nitrite, nitrate, hardness Physical, including temperature, dissolved oxygen, pH, salinity, turbidity, suspended solids in water Pollution, including chlorine, chloramines, heavy metals
Environmental conditions	Improper substrate or lack of hiding places Light levels and photoperiod duration Excess sounds and vibrations Tank shape and construction (i.e., type of tank wall-building materials—glass, fiberglass, concrete) Lack of swimming room Harmful tank ornaments, plants Lack of/presence of water current in tank
Social environment	Improper population density according to fish species Presence of incompatible species, including predators Pain from fighting and injury Subordination in the social hierarchy Breeding behavior
Handling and transport	Overexertion due to chasing Mechanical damage due to hooking, netting, or grading Confinement and crowding in nets or during transport Handling and manipulation Prolonged exposure to air Water quality issues
Nutritional effects	Malnutrition or overfeeding Improper dietary composition and nutrients in food Diminished access to food
Therapeutics	Sedatives, antimicrobials, and chemicals can be stressors Overmedication, or incorrect medication used Use of sublethal poisons to capture fish Capture, transport, and crowding for treatment administration
Pathogen influences	Presence of bacteria, parasites, virus, fungus

following decreased feed intake, nutrient absorption, and growth hormone circulation. Genetic changes include decreased protein:DNA ratios, RNA:DNA ratios, and RNA concentration, indicating reduced protein synthesis (Prunet et al., 2008; Small et al., 2008). Stress can also increase heart rate, increase gill blood flow and breathing rate, alter gill permeability, and increase stored energy mobilization. While initial behavioral changes such as stressor avoidance may originally foster survival, chronic stress and behavioral changes may lead to negative responses such as anorexia or lethargy. Reproductive activities are also adversely changed, including gonadal steroid production, gamete quality, embryonic development, and larval survival (Pankhurst and Van der Kraal, 1997).

Immune activity may initially be enhanced with acute stress but later suppressed with chronic stress. Primary immune system barriers such as skin, scales, and mucus are compromised. Stress-related hormones can reduce macrophage, lymphocyte, and antibody activity, thus leading to increased disease susceptibility (Klesius et al., 2003). Stress has been commonly related to fish disease because disease occurrence is based on the interaction between fish health status, microbes present, and environmental conditions. All three factors can be related to or influenced by stressors. Diseases caused by nonendemic, opportunistic, secondary pathogens are frequently observed, although increased susceptibility to primary pathogens is also observed with stress.

Common stress-related diseases include bacterial (*Aeromonas* spp., *Flavobacterium columnare*, *Pseudomonas* spp., *Streptococcus* spp., *Vibrio* spp.), viral (channel catfish virus, spring viremia of carp), fungal (*Saprolegnia* spp.), and parasitic (*Ichthyophthirius multifiliis*, *Trichodina* spp.) diseases (Evans et al., 2006; Huntingford et al., 2006). Stressors commonly linked with these diseases include poor water quality (e.g., temperature changes, high ammonia, low dissolved oxygen, and turbidity), crowding and housing of different sizes of fish together, poor nutrition, and handling and transport. Exposure to these stressors can lead to the release of cortisol and other stress hormones and to the use of physiological energy to maintain homeostasis, both of which result in immunosuppression and subsequent disease caused by microbes that would not normally infect the fish.

The consequences of stress on fish are variable and not necessarily negative, and the effect and magnitude of stress responses depend on several factors: genetic makeup, stage of development, and preexisting environmental conditions (Klesius et al., 2003).

Diagnosis

Fish health professionals can determine stress levels and their impact based on a combination of history, observation, and diagnostic tests. Since a laboratory blood or hormone test diagnosis of *stress* does not distinguish the stressors involved, observation and clinical signs are often required to identify the causes (Table 3.2) (Barton, 2000; Rose, 2002; Huntingford et al., 2006). Perhaps

Table 3.2 Commonly observed clinical signs of stress in fish.

Category	Clinical signs
Behavior	Activity level (hyperactivity or lethargy) Sequestration to top or bottom of tank; seeking shelter Body positioning to protect injuries Abnormal swimming and body orientation Holding fins against body Escaping from tank Rubbing on tank Increased opercular ventilation rate (rapid gilling)
Body condition	Weight loss and change of general body shape Sloughing of scales and mucus from skin Frayed or stunted fins Changes in skin or eye color
Growth and nutrition	Reduced or no appetite Decreased food intake Prolonged low growth rate as opposed to naturally occurring short-term variability Change of general body shape Morphological changes in fry and fingerlings
Injury	Skin, scale and fin injuries (disease or fighting) Skin ulceration Slow recovery from injuries
Fertility	Lack of breeding behavior Changes in physical development required for mating display and breeding Decreased or no offspring production
Disease	Increased disease incidence, especially of nonendemic, secondary diseases Increased susceptibility to primary fish pathogens Increased gross signs of disease (e.g., skin ulceration, white spots on skin, frayed fins, exophthalmia)
Mortality	Acute mortalities with no discernable cause Delayed, chronic mortalities

the most commonly used laboratory indication of stress is the elevation of blood cortisol and/or glucose, and sometimes lactate. These may be measured by enzyme-linked immunosorbent assays (ELISA), radioimmunoassay, and/or test meters and kits. Plasma cortisol increases rapidly during stress responses, is relatively easy to measure, and has often been used to measure stress responses. Normal cortisol reference ranges have been established for numerous fish species. Plasma glucose has also received considerable attention due to the development of simple, rapid testing procedures and because normal glucose reference ranges have also been examined for different species of fish.

Automated blood analyzers can also measure other stress-associated values. Values that increase with stress include cortisol, glucose, lactate, and hematocrit, while hemoglobin decreases, and sodium, chloride, and osmolality increase or decrease according to whether the fish are salt-water or freshwater, respectively (Barton, 2000; Evans et al., 2006; Small et al., 2008). Proper diagnosis is determined by prior knowledge of fish species characteristics (e.g., normal activities, normal blood chemistry values) that are varied according with stress; certain behaviors or plasma levels may be normal for one fish species but abnormal for another. Genetics, age, and environmental factors play a role in stress, determining what values change with stressor exposure and establishing which factors and values are vital for diagnosis. Several researchers are performing genomic analysis on fish stress responses, examining genetic stress indicators and expression signatures that may help stress diagnosis.

Prevention and management

Since stressors can have a major impact on fish health, one of the most important components of a fish management plan is the prevention or management of stress in fish (Wedemeyer et al., 1990; Barton, 2000 Rose, 2002; Klesius et al., 2003; Huntingford et al., 2006). Stress can be prevented or mitigated through recommended husbandry practices that target the common causes listed in Table 3.1.

- Generate a good understanding of the biology and needs of the fish species involved. Management considerations must be tailored to the requirements and preferences of that species.
- Choose to work with species of fish that have higher stress resistance. There are often distinct genetic differences in the way individual, strains, and species of fish handle stressors.
- Use commercially available meters and kits to monitor water quality parameters, including temperature, ammonia, nitrite, nitrate, dissolved oxygen, pH, hardness, and salinity. Regular water changes, tank cleanings, and biological, mechanical, and chemical filtration can help ensure proper water quality. Poor water quality represents one of the most vital and potentially harmful concerns to fish.
- Provide a good regimen of nutrition according to the fish species involved. Food should be chosen according to plant or animal content, protein, and delivery method. Certain evidence also suggests that some dietary supplements can be used to increase stress resistance.
- Prevent overcrowding, adverse social interactions (i.e., aggression, predation), and excessive handling.
- Routinely disinfect equipment and tanks using chemical disinfectants on the tanks and husbandry paraphernalia; use water sterilization equipment (e.g., ultraviolet [UV] light).
- Minimize stressful procedures such as handling, netting, changing of the photoperiod, and all other stressful activities where feasible; limit such activities to those that are vital to the welfare of the fish. Stressors can have cumulative effect if exposure is long term or recurring, so stressful situations (e.g., handling, transportation) can be timed to give recovery time before the next stressful activity is carried out.
- Vaccinate fish for diseases endemic to the area and/or fish species, when feasible. While immersion and oral vaccination can reduce injection-associated stress due to netting and handling, these vaccination routes are usually not as effective as injection.
- Treat bacterial, viral, fungal, and parasitic diseases promptly and properly. Definitive disease

diagnosis is required to provide appropriate medical and supportive treatment and to eliminate disease as a stressor. Symptomatic treatment may also be required, including the use of salt in freshwater aquaria to correct osmoregulatory disturbances or as medication against secondary infections. Fish may be stressed when medication is used improperly (by type, duration, frequency, or dose) or used to treat healthy fish. Also, treatment may be subject to a valid veterinary–patient–client relationship and applicable laws.

- Treat fish with analgesics/anesthetics (e.g., tricaine methanesulfonate [MS-222]) if stressful procedures such as handling, transport, or surgery are required. Note that some anesthesia methods and/or anesthetics can cause stress themselves, so the utilized medication should be chosen carefully based on the procedure, fish species, and environment. Given that some anesthetics can change the water pH, buffering of the water may be required.
- Study the efficacy of over-the-counter (OTC) medications if they are to be used. Several OTC medications are marketed to prevent or treat the effects of stress. Limited supportive evidence of their efficacy exists, so the use of these medications is not necessarily recommended. These solutions are meant to reduce stress in one of two ways: (a) maintain proper water quality by neutralizing chlorine, chloramines, heavy metals and by helping develop the biological filter (*Nitrosomonas* spp., *Nitrobacter* spp.) to convert ammonia and nitrite and (b) create a replacement slime/mucus coat to help regeneration of damaged skin and to prevent osmotic imbalances.

The information in this chapter provides an initial guide to fish stress biology, stressors, diagnosis, and management. Given the numerous fish species and indefinite environmental conditions throughout the world, continual research is required to definitively understand the impact of species biology, genetics, and environment on stress. Thus, fish health professionals can deal with fish stress and welfare as a dynamic subject with continual learning experiences.

Comments

Mention of commercial products in this publication is solely for the purpose of providing specific information and does not imply recommendation by the US Department of Agriculture (USDA). Information pertaining to the practice of veterinary medicine does not replace a valid veterinary–patient–client relationship or applicable laws. The authors thank Dr. Thomas Welker (USDA/ARS, Auburn, AL), Dr. Julio Garcia (USDA/ARS, Auburn, AL), and Dr. Helen Roberts (Aquatic Veterinary Services of Western New York, Orchard Park, NY) for their editorial comments.

References

Barton, B.A. (2000) Stress. In *Encyclopedia of Aquaculture* (Stickney, R.R., ed.), pp. 892–898. New York: John Wiley & Sons.

Evans, J.J., Pasnik, D.J., Brill, G.C., et al. (2006) Un-ionized ammonia exposure in Nile tilapia: toxicity, stress response, and susceptibility to *Streptococcus agalactiae*. *North American Journal of Aquaculture* **68**: 23–33.

Huntingford, F.A., Adams, C., Braithwaite, V.A., et al. (2006) Current issues in fish welfare. *Journal of Fish Biology* **68**: 332–372.

Klesius, P.H., Shoemaker, C.A., and Evans, J.J. (2003) The disease continuum model: bi-directional responses between stress and infection linked by neuroimmune change. In *Biosecurity in Aquaculture Production Systems: Exclusion of Pathogens and Other Undesirables* (Lee, C.S. and O'Bryen, P.J., eds.), pp. 13–34. Baton Rouge, LA: The World Aquaculture Society.

Pankhurst, N.W. and Van der Kraal, G. (1997) Effects of stress on reproduction and growth of fish. In *Fish Stress and Health in Aquaculture* (Iwama, G.K., Pickering, A.D., Sumpter, J.P., et al., eds.), pp. 73–93. Cambridge, UK: Cambridge University Press.

Prunet, P., Cairns, M.T., Winberg, S., et al. (2008) Functional genomics of stress responses in fish. *Reviews in Fisheries Science* **16** (S1): 155–164.

Rose, J.D. (2002) The neurobehavioral nature of fishes and the question of awareness and pain. *Reviews in Fisheries Science* **10**: 1–38.

Small, B.C., Davis, K.B., and Peterson, B.C. (2008). Elucidating the effects of cortisol and stress on economically important traits in channel catfish. *North American Journal of Aquaculture* **70**: 223–235.

Sneddon, L.U., Braithwaite, V.A., and Gentle, M.J. (2003)
Do fishes have nociceptors? Evidence for the evolution
of a vertebrate sensory system. *Proceedings of the Royal
Society of London, Series B: Biological Sciences* **270**:
1115–1121.

Wedemeyer, G.A., Barton, B.A., and McLeay, D.J. (1990)
Stress and acclimation, In *Methods for Fish Biology*
(Schreck, C.B. and Moyle, P.B., eds.), pp. 451–489.
Bethesda, MD: American Fisheries Society.

Chapter 4

Water Quality

James L. Shelton

Introduction

Water quality in the broadest sense refers to all physical, chemical, and biological characteristics of water that regulate its suitability for a specific use (Boyd, 1979). Water quality management in fish health means regulating these parameters in order to promote fish growth—and in some cases to regulate reproduction—but mainly to make certain that fish remain disease free, exhibiting healthy appearance and behavior. Poor water quality is considered by most experts to be the most common cause of mortality and the most common stressor predisposing fish to infectious disease.

Routine water quality monitoring is essential to fish health, and fish keepers will benefit greatly from testing water quality at regular intervals and recording the data in a log book. This information can be used to establish a baseline when systems are functioning properly and fish are healthy. These data can also be useful in tracking trends over time since not all changes in water quality are sudden. A water test kit should be used to measure pH, ammonia–nitrogen, nitrite–nitrogen, and temperature frequently. Alkalinity, salinity, nitrate–nitrogen, and dissolved oxygen (DO) measurement can also be useful and kits are available for these parameters as well (Fig. 4.1). The frequency of water quality testing depends both on the specific parameter and the stocking density of the system. In addition to routine testing of established systems, there are a number of other conditions that warrant testing. All new systems should be tested frequently during start-up when conditions are likely to change rapidly. This testing should be continued until conditions stabilize. Whenever medications or additives

are applied, there is potential to impact water quality, so water quality should again be checked frequently. Water quality should also be tested anytime abnormal fish behavior (flashing, gasping for air, or lethargy) or a change in water appearance (color or clarity) is observed. Water quality should be checked during seasonal transitions (system warming in spring, onset of hot weather in summer, and cooling in fall).

First-time fish keepers should be advised to have an analytical laboratory evaluate their source water, even if it has been previously purified for human consumption. Parameters of interest include pH, phosphorus (P), potassium (K), calcium (Ca), magnesium (Mg), manganese (Mn), iron (Fe), aluminum (Al), boron (B), copper (Cu), zinc (Zn), sodium (Na), cadmium (Cd), nickel (Ni), chromium (Cr), molybdenum (Mo), silica (Si), total hardness, total alkalinity, total ammonia–nitrogen (TAN), nitrite–nitrogen, nitrate–nitrogen, and chlorine (Cl). Finally, water quality testing should be performed as part of the minimum database in every disease clinical workup.

Parameters associated with fish health

Temperature

Most fishes are ectotherms, and thus are metabolically adapted to function over a relatively wide range of temperatures (Moyle and Cech, 2004; Crockett and Londraville, 2006). It is important to know the optimum temperature range for a species of interest. Temperate species can survive in water from 0 °C (32 °F) up to 30 °C (86 °F). Most freshwater tropical fish prefer 24–27 °C (75–80 °F);

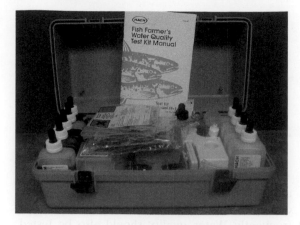

Fig. 4.1   A popular multiparameter water quality test kit (photo courtesy of Dr. Helen Roberts).

tropical marine species generally prefer 25–29°C (78–84°F); and koi and goldfish prefer 18–25°C (65–77°F). Rapid or chronic hypo/hyperthermia can result in stress and immunosuppression. Such conditions are often associated with transport of fish from one location to another, or with life-support equipment malfunction. Symptoms of hypothermia include lethargy, lying on the bottom, and anorexia in chronic cases. Symptoms of hyperthermia include hyperactivity and sudden death.

Interactions of pH, total alkalinity, and carbon dioxide

The term pH is defined as the negative logarithm ($-\log_{10}$) of the hydrogen ion (H^+) concentration. The pH required for most aquatic life is between 5.5 and 8.5. Optimal pH range varies with fish species. Marine fish prefer a pH of 8.0–8.5 (basic); temperate species prefer a pH near neutral (7.0); and some tropical species prefer a slightly acidic pH. A number of chemical and biological processes regulate pH in fish culture systems.

Respiration by submerged plants (macrophytes and algae) and animals results in the constant production of carbon dioxide (CO_2), which acts as a weak acid in water and can lower pH. Microbial decomposition of nitrogen present in all forms of organic matter also produces acidity in water lowering the pH. Conversely, photosynthesis by submerged plants consumes CO_2 during daylight hours, raising the pH. In clinical cases where pH

abnormalities are suspected, measuring the pH level in the early morning will give the lowest daily reading.

The actual degree of change in pH associated with acid-forming biochemical reactions is determined by the buffering capacity of water. A buffer resists changes in pH and results from any combination of a weak acid and one of its salts, or a weak base and one of its salts (Boyd, 1979). Total alkalinity represents the primary buffer system in most waters and is defined as the sum of all titratable bases expressed as equivalent calcium carbonate (mg/l $CaCO_3$). A total alkalinity of 50 mg/l is considered adequate, but a value above 75 mg/l is desirable for most freshwater systems (Wurts and Durborow, 1992). Values below 30 mg/l are cause for immediate concern. Alkalinity is dynamic and changes over time as buffers are "consumed" by metabolic processes that are naturally occurring in ponds and tanks.

Symptoms of suboptimal pH may include lethargy, increase in mucus production, and respiratory distress. Managing pH involves regulating alkalinity. Alkalinity can be restored to appropriate levels by adding buffers to water. Many commercial products are marketed as pH buffers, but the most common additive is sodium bicarbonate (baking soda). Limestone, crushed oyster shells, or crushed coral are used as substrates to adjust alkalinity and buffer against pH changes. Systematic partial water changes with appropriate source water will also help maintain optimal pH and alkalinity.

Clinical conditions associated with pH include a "pH crash," a sudden drop in pH, and "old tank syndrome." A crash is usually preceded by a drop in alkalinity. High fish mortalities can result suddenly. Old tank syndrome occurs in mature systems that have experienced neglect. Inadequate water changes and poor maintenance results in systems with low pH (often <5), reduced or absent alkalinity levels, elevated hardness, and elevated nitrogenous waste products. Chronic, intermittent deaths are not uncommon.

Total hardness

The carbonate minerals, which are the primary sources of alkalinity in water, are generally associated with calcium (Ca) and magnesium (Mg). Total hardness is defined as the concentration of alkaline earth metals (Ca, Mg, and other polyvalent cations) in water expressed as equivalent calcium carbonate (mg/l $CaCO_3$). While total alkalinity and total hardness levels are usually comparable for source water, a measure of one should never be used as an indicator of the other. The close relationship between alkalinity and hardness yields an alternative terminology popular among fish keepers and some water test kit manufacturers. Total hardness, as previously defined, is sometimes referred to as "general hardness." Total alkalinity (see previous section) is sometimes referred to as "carbonate hardness." A total hardness value of 30 mg/l is generally considered adequate for freshwater systems, but a value of 50–100 mg/l is more desirable. No specific symptoms have been attributed to suboptimal total hardness levels, but the use of limestone or crushed oyster shell as substrate will also adjust hardness appropriate levels. Systematic partial water changes with appropriate source water will help maintain optimal total hardness.

DO

The solubility of oxygen in water depends on water temperature, atmospheric pressure, and salinity. Table 4.1 shows solubility values of oxygen in pure water at various temperatures. Increasing temperature, increasing salinity and increasing elevation above sea level (lower atmospheric pressure) all result in decreasing the solubility of oxygen in water. Warmwater fish species (such as largemouth bass and bluegill) grow best when oxygen concentrations are 5 mg/l or greater; warmwater fish will survive, but grow poorly when oxygen concentrations are between 3 and 5 mg/l; prolonged exposure to oxygen levels below 3 mg/l result in significant physiological stress, increased disease susceptibility, and can be lethal. Coldwater fish, such as rainbow trout, are more sensitive to low oxygen concentrations. Growth of rainbow trout will be poor if oxygen levels fall below 6 mg/l on a regular basis. Trout may die at DO levels below 4 mg/l. Golden orfe, a common ornamental pond fish, are also sensitive to low oxygen levels.

Table 4.1 Solubility of oxygen in pure water at different temperatures.*

°C	mg/l	°C	mg/l	°C	mg/l
0	14.2	12	10.4	24	8.2
1	13.8	13	10.2	25	8.1
2	13.4	14	10.0	26	8.0
3	13.1	15	9.8	27	7.9
4	12.7	16	9.6	28	7.8
5	12.4	17	9.4	29	7.6
6	12.1	18	9.2	30	7.5
7	11.8	19	9.0	31	7.4
8	11.5	20	8.8	32	7.3
9	11.2	21	8.7	33	7.2
10	10.9	22	8.5	34	7.1
11	10.7	23	8.4	35	7.0

*For an atmosphere saturated with water vapor and at a pressure of 760 mmHg.

The actual DO concentration in water often depends more on biological activity (photosynthesis by plants and respiration by all aquatic organisms) than on oxygen solubility (Boyd, 2000). Photosynthesis during daylight hours means that the afternoon concentration of DO in a system with a significant plant community (algae or macrophytes) will often exceed saturation levels, yielding an oxygen surplus. At night, oxygen consumption by respiration of all living organisms (plants, fish, invertebrates, and microbes) can cause the oxygen concentration to decline to critical levels (Boyd, 1982).

Overcrowding, poor water flow, sudden plant die-offs, and certain chemical treatments (such as formalin) can result in suboptimal DO levels. Symptoms of low DO may include piping (fish gasping at water surface), respiratory distress, and lethargy. Adequate aeration is essential to maintaining appropriate levels of DO in culture systems. An effective aerator has to have key characteristics. First, it must either divide water into extremely fine particles (tiny droplets) or it must divide air into extremely fine particles (tiny bubbles). Second, but equally important, it must provide a high rate of mixing for the distribution of these tiny droplets or bubbles throughout the culture system.

Nitrogen in water

Nitrogen in water occurs in many forms, both inorganic and organic. These forms include

(1) nitrogen gas (N_2), dissolved in water, usually in equilibrium with the atmosphere;
(2) ammonia (NH_3) and ammonium (NH_4^+), in a pH- and temperature-dependent equilibrium;
(3) nitrite (NO_2^-);
(4) nitrate (NO_3^-);
(5) organic nitrogen, including amino acids, proteins, and various complex organic compounds, both particulate and dissolved.

The familiar nitrogen cycle (Fig. 4.2) is regulated by a number of biochemical reactions, and much of the nitrogen in a culture system is at least temporarily bound in living organisms and decaying organic matter. Certain forms of nitrogen are toxic to aquatic life. Excessive nitrogen in aquatic systems, even when present in nontoxic forms can lead to eutrophication. The forms most critical to aquatic life will be discussed separately, and their relationships covered.

Ammonia

Ammonia is the principal nitrogenous waste product of fish, eliminated primarily through gill tissue, and to a lesser extent via the kidney (Schwedler et al., 1985). Ammonia is also produced through the decomposition of any type of organic matter in water, such as feces, uneaten food, or dead plant material.

In water, unionized ammonia (NH_3) exists in a pH- and temperature-dependent equilibrium with ionized ammonium (NH_4^+) (Table 4.2). This is significant because NH_3 is more toxic to aquatic life than NH_4^+, so increasing pH and increasing water temperature result in more detrimental effects of ammonia present in culture systems. The term TAN refers to all nitrogen contained in NH_3 and NH_4^+ forms. Common methods for testing ammonia in water cannot distinguish between NH_3 and NH_4^+ forms, but instead provide only a measure of TAN. If a TAN value is provided, or a water quality test kit is used to determine TAN, pH, and water temperature, Table 4.2 can be used to separate NH_3 and NH_4^+ and evaluate toxicity (Durborow et al., 1997b). Volatilization (diffusion of gaseous NH_3 from water to air) can result in loss of ammonia from culture systems, but this process is also mediated by pH and temperature. Observations of behavioral and histological effects of chronic exposure to very low concentrations of NH_3 (Boyd, 1982; Masser et al., 1999) have resulted in the view among many fish health professionals that the only acceptable level of ammonia in culture systems is zero.

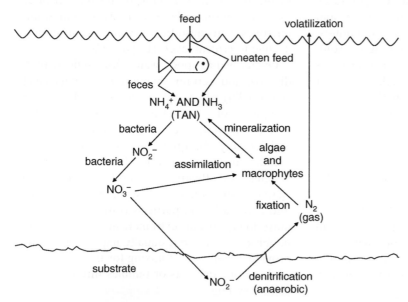

Fig. 4.2 Diagram of the nitrogen cycle. TAN, total ammonia–nitrogen.

Table 4.2 Percentage unionized ammonia in aqueous solutions of different temperatures and pH values.

pH	Temperature (°C)						
	8	12	16	20	24	28	32
7.0	0.2	0.2	0.3	0.4	0.5	0.7	1.0
7.2	0.3	0.3	0.5	0.6	0.8	1.10	1.4
7.4	0.4	0.5	0.7	1.0	1.3	1.7	2.3
7.6	0.6	0.9	1.2	1.6	2.1	2.7	3.5
7.8	1.0	1.4	1.8	2.4	3.2	1.2	5.5
8.0	1.6	2.1	2.9	3.8	5.0	6.6	8.8
8.2	2.5	3.3	4.5	5.9	7.7	10.0	13.2
8.4	3.9	5.2	6.9	9.1	11.6	15.0	19.5
8.6	6.0	7.9	10.6	13.7	17.3	21.8	27.7
8.8	9.2	12.0	15.8	20.1	24.9	30.7	37.8
9.0	13.8	17.8	22.9	28.5	34.4	41.2	49.0
9.2	20.4	25.8	32.0	38.7	45.4	52.6	60.4
9.4	30.0	35.5	42.7	50.0	56.9	63.8	70.7
9.6	39.2	46.5	54.1	61.3	67.6	73.6	79.3
9.8	50.5	58.1	65.2	71.5	76.8	81.6	85.8
10.0	61.7	68.5	74.8	79.9	84.0	87.5	90.6
10.2	71.9	77.5	82.4	86.3	89.3	91.8	93.8

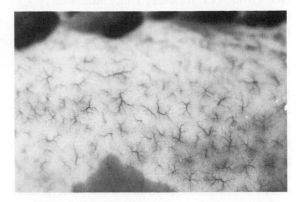

Fig. 4.3 Ammonia toxicity in fish showing capillary vessel congestion and dilation.

An immature biofilter or deleterious effects on the nitrifying bacteria caused by therapeutic or chemical additives, water quality abnormalities (low DO, pH crises, etc.), vigorous cleaning of filter units, excess feeding, and overcrowding can contribute to the development of ammonia toxicity. "New tank syndrome" is the term given to acute ammonia toxicity seen in newly established, immature filtration systems. Symptoms of ammonia toxicity in fish may include lethargy and other behavioral changes, gill abnormalities, clamped fins, and capillary vessel congestion and dilation (see Fig. 4.3). Short-term corrective measures for ammonia problems involve partial water changes, reduction or cessation of feeding, and the use of commercially marketed ammonia binders. A full review of all life-support systems should be conducted to avoid recurrence.

Nitrite

Virtually all nitrite (NO_2^-) that enters fish culture systems is a result of the direct or indirect biological conversion of ammonia, which will be discussed in a subsequent section of this chapter. Nitrite is toxic to fish at relatively low concentrations, especially in waters that are low in chloride (Cl^-). Due to similarities in the transport mechanisms for NO_2^- and Cl^- in the gills, the rate of uptake depends on the relative concentrations of NO_2^- and Cl^- in the water (Schwedler et al., 1985). Once nitrite is absorbed across the gills and enters the blood, it reacts with hemoglobin to form methemoglobin, which is not effective as an oxygen carrier (Durborow et al., 1997a). Methemoglobinemia results in a functional hypoxia. Blood containing significant levels of methemoglobin is brown, so this form of functional anemia is commonly referred to as "brown blood disease." In addition to Cl^- concentration of the water, many factors affect the toxicity of NO_2^- in fish. These include fish species, size, previous exposure of fish to NO_2^-, nutritional status, presence of infectious agents, water pH, and DO concentration (Schwedler et al., 1985). As with ammonia concentrations, the view of most fish health professionals is that the only acceptable level of nitrite in culture systems is zero. Symptoms of nitrite toxicity may include brown discoloration of gills, piping (fish gasping at water surface) and other forms of respiratory distress. Corrective measures involve partial water changes, temporary reduction or cessation of feeding, and the use of common uniodized salt (NaCl) to "treat" the problem. Because chloride competes with nitrite for absorption through the gills, maintaining at least a 10-to-1 ratio of Cl^- to

NO_2^- ($10\,mg/l\;Cl^-$ for every $1\,mg/l$ measured NO_2^-) in a culture system prevents nitrite from entering fish and accumulating to harmful levels.

Nitrate

Like nitrite (NO_2^-), nitrate (NO_3^-) enters fish culture systems as a result of the biological conversion of ammonia. Nitrate (as well as ammonia) may be removed from water by aquatic macrophytes, algae, and bacteria, which assimilate it into living tissue. Under anaerobic conditions, which can exist in aquatic substrates, some bacteria can utilize nitrate for oxidation of organic matter (Boyd, 2000). This process is known as denitrification. Despite these losses, concentrations of nitrate are generally higher than those of ammonia and nitrite. Nitrate receives far less attention than other forms of nitrogen in water that are toxic at much lower concentrations. Carmargo et al. (2005) reviewed published data on nitrate toxicity for various freshwater and marine animals, including fish, amphibians, and invertebrates.

In culture systems with high stocking densities and high feeding rates, nitrate can accumulate unless systematic partial water changes are applied. Under these conditions, excess algal growth and diminished buffering capacity may occur. These changes coupled with chronic exposure to nitrate concentrations of $50\,mg/l$ or greater are cause for concern. Negative effects associated with this syndrome include lethargy, poor growth, and increased susceptibility to infectious disease. Corrective measures include systematic partial water changes and removal of any accumulated organic debris. Feeding rates should be verified as appropriate to fish density. Plants may be employed to remove excess nitrate. Elevated nitrate levels can also be suggestive of poor maintenance and lack of water changes by the owner.

Biochemical conversion/the nitrogen cycle

All forms of nitrogen previously mentioned are related through the nitrogen cycle (Fig. 4.1). Most important among these relationships is the two-step biochemical conversion of ammonia known as nitrification. This process is carried out by highly aerobic chemoautotrophic bacteria. First, ammonia-oxidizing bacteria, including the genus *Nitrosomonas* and close relatives, act on ammonia to produce nitrite, and then nitrite-oxidizing bacteria, including the genera *Nitrobacter*, *Nitrospira*, and close relatives, act on nitrite to produce nitrate (Hovanec et al., 1998; Itoi et al., 2007). Biological conversion (commonly known as biofiltration) prevents the accumulation of ammonia and nitrite to toxic levels. Most fish culture systems depend on some sort of fixed-film biofilter, a solid substrate provided to promote the attachment, growth and function of ammonia-oxidizing and nitrite-oxidizing bacteria, for life support (Gutierrez-Wing and Malone, 2006). Various materials are used to form the substrate of a biofilter, including sand, gravel, crushed oyster shell, and specially engineered plastics.

A number of factors regulate the efficiency of the biological conversion (biofiltration) process. Nitrifying bacteria become inefficient when exposed to low DO concentrations (Masser et al., 1999). It is usually more important to provide adequate supplemental aeration to the bioconversion unit than it is to aerate the fish culture unit. Optimal conditions for rapid nitrification are temperatures of $25–35\,°C$ and pH between 7 and 8, although nitrification will occur at lower temperature and pH levels (Boyd, 2000).

Free chlorine and chloramine

Chlorine gas (Cl_2) and the hypochlorite ion (OCl^-) are highly reactive and commonly used for disinfection. Municipal water supplies are usually chlorinated to provide a residual concentration of at least $1\,mg/l$ to kill pathogenic microbes. The use of chloramine (NH_2Cl) as an alternative to chlorination is increasing because it is more stable and does not form derivatives that are toxic to humans. Chlorine and chloramine are highly toxic to fish. While the actually toxicity is dependent on a variety of factors, including fish species and chlorine form, any measurable amount is considered extremely harmful (Zillich, 1972; Heath, 1977).

Chlorine (Cl_2) and chloride (Cl^-) are the same element but have dramatically different chemical properties. Chloride is a common constituent of most water sources and is essential to fish in osmoregulation. Chloride levels of 60 mg/l are considered desirable for freshwater fish keeping. Dechlorination of free chlorine (Cl_2 or OCl^-) generally involves activated carbon filtration or water additives containing sodium thiosulfate ($Na_2S_2O_3$). Boyd (1990) recommends a rate of 7.4 mg/l $Na_2S_2O_3$ for each milligram per liter of free chlorine, but for convenience most commercial products come as a solution with instructions for use converted to drops per gallon of water to be treated. Since chloramine is a combination of chlorine and ammonia, neither activated carbon filtration nor sodium thiosulfate will be completely effective in treating chloraminated water. However, a number of commercial products are marketed for this specific purpose. Toxic effects of chlorine exposure can include piping and other forms of respiratory distress, gill abnormalities, including necrosis, and sudden death. By far, the most common source of chlorine exposure is failure to treat for chlorine in municipal water. "Forgetting" to monitor when filling or topping off a pond with a garden hose is a common cause of chlorine exposure. Treatment of chlorine exposure includes attempting to reduce the water temperature (increases DO content), vigorous aeration, and supersaturation with oxygen (when possible). The addition of sodium chloride at 1–3 gm/L can help reduce osmoregulatory effort and stress.

References

Boyd, C.E. (1979) *Water Quality in Warmwater Fish Ponds*. Opelika, AL: Auburn University Experimental Station.

Boyd, C.E. (1982) *Water Quality Managemnet for Pond Fish Culture*. Auburn, AL: Elsevier Scientific Publishing.

Boyd, C.E. (1990) *Water Quality in Pounds for Aquaculture*. Birmingham, AL: Birmingham Publishing Co.

Boyd, C.E. (2000) *Water Quality: An Introduction*. Norwell, MA: Kluwer Academic Publishers.

Carmargo, J.A., Alsonso, A., and Salamanca, A. (2005) Nitrate toxicity to aquatic animals: a review with new data for freshwater invertebrates. *Chemosphere* **58**: 1255–1267.

Crockett, E.L. and Londraville, R.L. (2006) Temperature. In *The Physiology of Fishes* (Evans, D.H. and Claiborne, J.B., eds.), pp. 231–270. Boca Raton, FL: CRC Press.

Durborow, R.M., Crosby, D.M., and Brunson, M.W. (1997a) Nitrite in fish ponds. *Southern Regional Aquaculture Center*. Fact sheet 462.

Durborow, R.M., Crosby, D.M., and Brunson, M.W. (1997b) Ammonia in fish ponds. *Southern Regional Aquaculture Center*. Fact sheet 463.

Gutierrez-Wing, M.T. and Malone, R.F. (2006) Biological filters in aquaculture: Trends and research directions for freshwater and marine applications. *Aquacultural Engineering* **34**: 163–171.

Heath, A.G. (1977) Toxicity of intermittent chlorination to freshwater fish: influence of temperature and chlorine form. *Hydrobiologia* **56**: 39–47.

Hovanec, T.A., Taylor, L.T., Blakis, A., et al. (1998) Nitrospira-like bacteria associated with nitrite oxidation in freshwater aquaria. *Applied and Environmental Microbiology* **64**: 258–264.

Itoi, S., Ebihara, N., Washio, S., et al. (2007) Nitrite-oxidizing bacteria, Nitrospira, distribution in the outer layer of the biofilm from filter materials of a recirculating water system for the goldfish, *Carassius auratus*. *Aquaculture* **264**: 297–308.

Masser, M.P., Rakocy, J., and Losordo, T.M. (1999) Recirculating aquaculture tank production systems: management of recirculating systems. *Southern Regional Aquaculture Center* Fact sheet 452.

Moyle, P.B. and Cech, J.J. (2004) *Fishes: An Introduction to Ichthyology*. Upper Saddle River, NJ: Prentice Hall.

Schwedler, T.E., Tucker, C.S., and Beleau, M.H. (1985). Non-infectious diseases. In *Channel Catfish Culture* (Tucker, C.S., ed.), pp. 497–542. Amsterdam and New York: Elsevier.

Wurts, W.A. and Durborow, R.M. (1992) Interactions of pH, carbon dioxide, alkalinity and hardness in fish ponds. *Southern Regional Aquaculture Center*. Fact sheet 464.

Zillich, J.A. (1972) Toxicity of combined chlorine residuals to freshwater fish. *Journal Water Pollution Control Federation* **44**: 212–220.

Chapter 5

Environment and Husbandry: Ponds and Aquaria

E. Scott Weber III, James L. Shelton, and Helen E. Roberts

Introduction

The water contained in any fish culture system (aquarium, pond, tank, raceway, or enclosure) should be viewed as a "biochemical broth" connecting all components and facilitating the many physical, chemical, and biological processes within. There is no such thing as equilibrium in these systems, even after they mature. A fish culture system is a *dynamic* ecological entity composed of numerous biotic and abiotic components intended to provide optimum conditions for fish health. While fish owners refer to culture units they maintain as ponds or aquaria, most are some form of a recirculating aquaculture system (RAS). Commercial fish producers may use earthen ponds, raceways (flow-through systems), or enclosures (nets or cages) for fish production, but closed-loop RAS units are also employed. The main difference between commercial and ornamental production systems is that ornamental pond and aquaria owners focus on aesthetics and the well-being of individual fish, while the commercial producer manages systems for entire populations of fish. Earthen ponds function much like natural aquatic systems, and their environmental health depends on the same biochemical processes as lake ecosystems. In raceways, a constant flow of high-quality water provides optimum conditions for life support. Dissolved oxygen (DO) and temperature are maintained, and waste products are flushed away by continuous inflow and outflow of water. In an RAS unit, optimum water quality is maintained by recycling water and utilizing various specially designed components responsible for mimicking natural ecological processes. These water treatment components must all work in conjunction and provide a healthy, aesthetically pleasing environment (Fig. 5.1). An ornamental pond or aquarium that is properly designed, constructed, and maintained will provide an appropriate means of

(1) housing fish so that they exhibit healthy appearance and behavior;
(2) recycling water throughout the system efficiently;
(3) removing solid organic waste (fecal material, dead plant and animal matter, and uneaten fish food) to prevent accumulation;
(4) facilitating bioconversion (nitrification) of dissolved organic waste (ammonia and nitrite–nitrogen); and
(5) facilitating efficient gas exchange (oxygen and carbon dioxide and others) throughout the entire system.

Some design schemes also incorporate a means of disinfection to remove pathogens and clarify water. Pond and aquarium designs range from the very simple to the highly complex. In more simple systems, the life-support components and processes described above occur in the same space where fish are housed. In more complex designs, each of these components is physically separate from the others.

Carrying capacity (stocking density)

Certain rules of thumb are commonly applied in sizing an ornamental fish pond or tank (Axelrod et al., 1992; Nash and Cook, 1999). Among

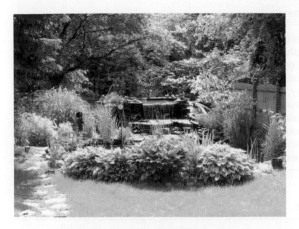

Fig. 5.1 A typical backyard ornamental pond.

these are two popular methods for determining maximum carrying capacity:

(1) For the average fish keeper, carrying capacity should not exceed 25 cm (10 in.) of total fish body length per 381 (10 gallons) of culture unit volume (25 cm [10 in.] of fish body length per 761 [20 gallons] of culture unit volume for the novice with very basic equipment, and 25 cm [10 in.] of fish body length per 191 [5 gallons] of culture unit volume for the expert with sophisticated life-support equipment).

(2) Every 155 cm^2 (24 in.^{2}) of pond surface area will accommodate 2.5 cm (1 in.) of total fish length. This measurement is based on the surface area available, which is where gas diffusion will take place. For freshwater fish aquaria, the general rule of thumb estimates 1 in. of fish body length/12 in.^{2} of surface area.

These guidelines are useful, but their misapplication can result in disaster. Many factors determine the actual carrying capacity of a culture unit, and some, such as filtration unit size and biological waste conversion efficiency, may be more important than the total length of fish per unit volume of water.

Another common method for estimating the carrying capacity of a fish culture unit is based on the size of the external filtration system being employed. As a rule of thumb, the ratio of pond size to external filter size should be 3:1 (McDowell, 1989). This guideline has been applied on either a unit area or a unit volume basis (3 m^2 of pond surface area for every square meter of filter surface area, or 3 m^3 of pond volume for every cubic meter of filter volume). As with other guidelines, this method is useful in planning and evaluating culture systems but should be used with caution.

Small water volumes can be extremely challenging when trying to manage water quality. Aquarium freshwater community tank minimum volumes of 20–55 gallons are recommended.

Marine fish will do better in larger tanks because water quality is more stable in a larger volume. In addition, most marine species grow bigger than their freshwater counterparts. The stocking density guidelines for marine aquaria depend on the type of filtration, protein skimming, use of live rock, and hiding niches available. The traditional guidelines for marine multitaxa tanks (fish and inverts) are 1 in. of fish per 4 gallons, and for fish only tanks, 1 in. of fish per 2 gallons. Using surface area calculations, recommendations for marine ornamentals are 1 in. of fish/48 in.^{2} tank surface area. A 30- to 55-gallon aquarium is an ideal starter size for most marine hobbyists.

Selecting fish

There are several aquarist references available that can aid in identifying individual species, geographical range, water quality requirements, adult size, compatibility, and captive nutritional observations. Tables 5.1 through 5.6 list several examples of fish and invertebrates (marine) for ponds, freshwater aquaria, and marine tanks.

Although freshwater fish are a great portion of the aquarium industry, a far greater variety of marine ornamental species are traded, with estimates of close to 1000 different species of marine animals (Helfman, 2007). Nearly all marine ornamentals are still wild caught as few species have been successfully bred in captivity for commercial purposes. Increasing fishing pressures on these animals has made some species extremely vulnerable, and recently, the Banggai cardinal fish become one of the first marine ornamentals to be listed on the International Union of Concerned Scientist's red list for threatened species (Vagelli,

Table 5.1 Fish commonly kept in ornamental ponds.

Common name	Scientific name	Comments
Koi	*Cyprinus carpio*	Koi need a large volume of water, at least 1000 gallons; lengths of >1 m/3 ft or more reported
Goldfish	*Carassius auratus*	Fancy goldfish with prominent eyes and delicate fins/tails should not be kept in ponds due to the high probability of injury; round-bodied goldfish should be overwintered indoors
Golden orfe ("Orfe, Ide")	*Leuciscus idus*	Sensitive to poor water quality and some medications; shoaling species, better in small groups; requires large volume of water; can be large fish (up to 1 m/3 ft reported); prohibited in some states
Mosquito fish	*Gambusia* sp.	Live-bearer, prohibited in some states

Table 5.2 Tropical freshwater fishes commonly found in Asia.

Family or grouping	Common name	Scientific name	Compatibility	Geographical range
Anabantoids	Betta	*Betta splendens*	Male bettas will kill each other; but most are good community fish	Southeast Asia
	Blue, gold, opaline gourami	*Trichogaster trichopterus*		
	Dwarf (color morphs) gourami	*Colisa lalia*		
	Honey (color morphs) gourami	*Trichogaster chuna*		
	Kissing gourami	*Helostoma temmincki*		
	Paradise fish	*Macropodus opercularis*		
	Pearl gourami	*Trichogaster leeri*		
Cobitidae: loaches	Burmese	*Botia kubotai*	Community fish that do well in small groups of three to seven animals	Southeast Asia
	Clown	*Botia macracantha*		
	Horsefaced	*Acanthopsis choirorhynchus*		
	Kuhli	*Pangio kuhlii*		
	Weather	*Misgurnus anguillicaudatus*		
	Yoyo	*Botia lohachata*		
Catfish	Algae eater	*Gyrinochelius aymonieri*	Community fish	Southeast Asia
	Flying fox	*Epalzeorhynchos kalopterus*		
	Glass catfish	*Kryptopterus bicirrhis*	Schooling fish	
Cyprinid: sharks	Iridescent shark	*Pangasius hypophthalmus*	Outgrows tanks	
	Bala shark	*Balantiocheilus melanopterus*		
	Black shark	*Labeo chrysophekadion*	Schooling fish	
	Red-fin (rainbow) shark and albino red-fin shark	*Epalzeorhynchos frenatum*	Single animal per tank	
	Red-tailed black shark	*Epalzeorhynchos bicolor*	Single animal per tank	
	Flying fox	*Epalzeorhynchos kalopterus*	Single animal per tank	
	Siamese algae eater	*Crossocheilus siamensis*	Community fish	
	Chinese algae eater	*Gyrinocheilus aymonieri*		
Cyprinidae				
Barbs	Black ruby barb	*Puntius nigrofasciatus*	Community schooling fish; some varieties are fin nippers (tiger), while others can outgrow tank (tinfoil)	Southeast Asia
	Checkered barb	*Puntius oligolepis*		
	Cherry barb	*Puntius titteya*		
	Gold barb	*Puntius sachsii*		
	Rosy barb	*Puntius conchonius*		
	Tiger barb	*Puntius tetrazona*		
	Tinfoil barb	*Barbonymus schwanenfeldii*		
Danios	Giant danio	*Danio malabaricus*	Community schooling fish	
	Glowlight danio	*Danio choprai*		
	Zebra danio	*Danio rerio*		
Rasboras	Espe's rasbora	*Trigonostigma espei*	Community schooling fish	
	Harlequin rasbora	*Trigonostigma heteromorpha*		
	Hengel's rasbora	*Trigonostigma hengeli*		

Table 5.3   Tropical freshwater fishes commonly found in Central and South America.

Family or grouping	Common name	Scientific name	Compatibility	Geographical range
Poecilidae: live-bearers	Black molly Endler's livebearer Fancy guppy Montezuma sword Platy Sailfin molly Swordtail Wild guppy	*Poecilia sphenops* *Poecilia wingei* *Poecilia reticulate* *Xiphophorus montezumae* *Xiphophorus maculates* *Poecilia latipinna* *Xiphophorus hellerii* *Poecilia reticulate*	Community fish that usually has sexual dimorphism, with males being more colorful, smaller, and have ornate fins. These animals are livebearers, but the young will be eaten in community tanks.	Central and South America
Characins Tetras	Black neon tetra Black phantom tetra Bleeding heart tetra Buenos Aires tetra Cardinal tetra Emperor tetra Glowlight tetra Lemon tetra Neon tetra Rummy-nose tetra Serpae tetra	*Hyphessobrycon herbertaxelrodi* *Hyphessobrycon megalopterus* *Hyphessobrycon erythrostigma* *Hyphessobrycon anisitsi* *Paracheirodon axelrodi* *Nematobrycon palmeri* *Hemigrammus erythrozonus* *Hyphessobrycon pulchripinnis* *Paracheirodon innesi* *Hemigrammus rhodostomus* *Hyphessobrycon eques*	All tetra and hatchet fishes are community schooling fishes. Most like soft water conditions and low pH.	South America
Hatchet fishes	Common/river hatchet fish Marbled hatchetfish	*Gasteropelecus sternicla* *Carnegiella strigata*		
Pacus/ piranhas	Black pacu Red-bellied pacu Red-bellied piranha Silver dollars	*Piaractus brachypomus* *Colossoma macropomum* *Pygocentrus nattereri* *Metynnis hypsauchen* and others	Pacu are moderate community fishes, although they can quickly overgrow the tank. Silver dollars are shy community fishes. Piranhas are not recommended for community tanks and are considered an invasive species in many states.	
Cichlidae	Agassiz's dwarf cichlid Altum angel Angelfish Blood parrot cichlid Bolivian ram Convict cichlid Discus Geophagus Festive cichlid Firemouth Flowerhorn German blue ram Green terror Jack Dempsey Oscar Severum Red devil	*Apistogramma agassizii* *Pterophyllum altum* *Pterophyllum scalare* *Amphilophus citrinellus* hybrid *Mikrogeophagus altispinosus* *Archocentrus nigrofasciatus* *Symphysodon aequifasciatus* *Geophagus jurupari* *Mesonauta festivus* *Thorichthys meeki* *Amphilophus citrinellus* × *Cichlasoma trimaculatum* *Mikrogeophagus ramirezi* *Aequidens rivulatus* *Cichlasoma octofasciatum* *Astronotus ocellatus* *Heros severus* *Amphilophus labiatus*	Angelfish, discus, rams, and geophagus are good community fish, although they can exhibit inter- and intraspecific aggression once they have lived in an established community tank. Most of the other species should be kept as individuals or with more aggressive animals. These fish prefer soft water and low pH.	Central and South America

(Continued)

Table 5.3 *Continued*

Family or grouping	Common name	Scientific name	Compatibility	Geographical range
Catfish				
Corydoras spp.	Adolfo's cory	*Corydoras adolfoi*	Corydoras catfish are a social community fish. They should be kept in schools of 4–12 animals.	Central and South America
	Albino cories	*Corydoras* spp.		
	Bronze cory	*Corydoras aeneus*		
	Leopard cory	*Corydoras julii* and *trilineatus*		
	Panda cory	*Corydoras panda*		
	Peppered cory	*Corydoras paleatus*		
	Schwartz's cory	*Corydoras schwartzi*		
	Skunk cory	*Corydoras arcuatus*		
	Sterba's cory	*Corydoras sterbai*		
Plecostomus	Bristlenose/bushynose	*Ancistrus* spp.	Plecos are excellent community fish, and some species can grow large. They are sensitive to environmental conditions.	
	Common pleco	*Hypostomus, Liposarcus* spp.		
	Gold nugget pleco (L18)	*Baryancistrus* sp.		
	Leopard sailfin pleco	*Glyptoperichthys gibbiceps*		
	Polka dot lyre tail pleco	*Acanthicus adonis*		
	Royal pleco	*Panaque nigrolineatus*		
Assorted	Spotted hypostomus	*Hypostomus punctatus*	Most of these assorted catfish make ideal community fish, with the exception of the last two species. These animals will outgrow most aquaria and will eat many of the tank inhabitants.	
	Zebra (Imperial) pleco	*Hypancistrus zebra*		
	Whiptail/twig catfish	*Farlowella acus*		
	Striped Raphael catfish	*Platydoras costatus*		
	Spotted Raphael catfish	*Agamyxis pectinifrons*		
	Banjo catfishes	*Bunocephalus/Dystichthys* spp.		
	Pim catfish	*Pimelodus pictus*		
	Colombian shark/catfish	*Hexanematichthys seemanni*		
	Red-tailed catfish	*Phractocephalus hemioliopterus*		
	Tiger shovelnose	*Pseudoplatystoma fasciatum*		
Osteoglossid	Silver arowana	*Osteoglossum bicirrhosum*	Larger community tank with fish that can hide.	South America
	Black arowana	*Osteoglossum ferreirai*		

Table 5.4 Tropical freshwater fishes commonly found in Australia and New Guinea.

Family or grouping	Common name	Scientific name	Compatibility	Geographical range
Rainbow fishes	Boeseman's rainbow fish	*Melanotaenia boesemani*	These are community fish, and many species are kept in species-specific groups that breed readily.	Australia and New Guinea
	Neon (dwarf) rainbow fish	*Melanotaenia praecox*		
	Red rainbow fish	*Glossolepis incisus*		
	Threadfin rainbow fish	*Iriatherina werneri*		
	Western rainbow fish	*Melanotaenia australis*		

Table 5.5 Tropical freshwater fishes commonly found in Africa.

Family or grouping	Common name	Scientific name	Compatibility	Geographical range
Cichlidae				Africa
Lake Tanganyika cichlids	Blue-faced duboisi Brichardi Lemon cichlid	*Tropheus duboisi* *Neolamprologus brichardi* *Neolamprologus leleupi*	African cichlids are usually kept with similar species from the same geographical location. Many species will breed readily in captivity, and the parents have a high level of investment in rearing offspring. They can exhibit intra- and interspecific aggression. They prefer hard water rocks and sandy substrate, and they and are highly evolved.	Lake Tanganyika
Lake Malawi Mbuna cichlids	Auratus Blue cobalt cichlid Electric yellow labido Kennyi Powder blue cichlid Red zebra cichlid	*Melanochromis auratus* *Maylandia callainos* *Labidochromis caeruleus* *Pseudotropheus lombardoi* *Pseudotropheus socolofi* *Pseudotropheus estherae*		Lake Malawi
Other African cichlids	Kribensis (Krib) Jewel cichlid	*Pelvicachromis pulcher* *Hemichromis bimaculatus*		Western Africa
Catfish	Cuckoo syno Decorated syno Even-spotted syno Featherfin syno Upside-down catfish	*Synodontis multipunctatus* *Synodontis decorus* *Synodontis petricola* *Synodontis eupterus* *Synodontis nigriventris*	Most are community fish, although they may eat smaller fishes such as neon and cardinal tetras.	Africa
Odds and ends	Reed fish (rope fish, snake fish)	*Erpetoichthys calabaricus*	Community fish that can jump out of the tank.	Africa

2004). This threat also includes frequently traded marine invertebrates, including corals and live rock.

Ornamental marine animals are generally more expensive to purchase and maintain than their freshwater counterparts. Many marine ornamentals may exhibit more variable behavior in the confines of a small aquarium. Some of these animals may actually be found in large schools for one part of their life, yet may pair off as adults later in life and exhibit considerable intraspecific aggression. The dietary requirements of many of these animals may also change as they mature from juveniles to adults. The greatest challenge for the marine aquarist is deciding whether to pursue a multitaxa exhibit with fish and invertebrates, fish-only tanks, or invertebrate-only tanks. There are treatments for fish diseases that will kill invertebrates, making quarantine essential for marine hobbyists. Aquarists who maintain a coral reef tank will have a less densely populated tank,

and will have to maintain better water quality, add nutritional supplements, and choose animals that will not eat the coral polyps.

Once the prospective fish owner decides on the type of fish they want, they need to identify an appropriate place to purchase aquatic livestock either directly or online. Inquiries should be made about the origin of their fish stock (pet store, wild caught, and/or captive bred). Many retailers offer limited warranties for livestock purchases that often include fish.

Options for handling organic waste

While some ornamental fish keepers strive for clear water in their ponds, the terms clear and healthy are not always synonymous. All pond and aquaria owners depend on some method of filtration to provide fish with an appropriate medium

Table 5.6 Commonly kept marine ornamental fish and invertebrates.

Family or grouping	Common name	Scientific name
Acanthuridae: surgeonfishes Larger reef fish that may have specialized dietary requirements. Many require small groups of three or more animals, such as the convict tangs. Very colorful and some can secret venom through sharp fin spines on caudal peduncle.	Achilles tang	*Acanthurus achilles*
	Atlantic blue tang	*Acanthurus coeruleus*
	Brown tang	*Acanthurus nigricans*
	Convict tang	*Acanthurus triostegus*
	Desjardin's sailfin tang	*Zebrasoma desjardinii*
	Elegant/blonde naso tang	*Naso elegans*
	Kole tang	*Ctenochaetus strigosus*
	Lined/clown tang	*Acanthurus lineatus*
	Naso tang	*Naso lituratus*
	Ocean tang	*Acanthurus bahianus*
	Pacific regal/blue tang	*Paracanthurus hepatus*
	Pacific sailfin tang	*Zebrasoma veliferum*
	Powder blue tang	*Zebrasoma flavescens*
	Purple tang	*Zebrasoma xanthurus*
	Yellow tang	*Acanthurus leucosternon*
Blennidae and Gobidae: blennies/ gobies Small bottom-dwelling community fish	Bicolor blenny	*Ecsenius bicolor*
	Lawnmower blenny	*Salarias fasciatus*
	Neon goby (Atlantic)	*Gobiosoma oceanops*
	Red-lip blenny	*Ophioblennius atlanticus*
	Yellow clown goby	*Gobiodon okinawae*
Chaetodontidae: butterfly fishes Some have very specialized diets and can exhibit intraspecific aggression in small tanks; community fish	Copperband butterfly fish	*Chelmon rostratus*
	Golden/masked butterfly fish	*Chaetodon semilarvatus*
	Longfin banner fish	*Heniochus diphreutes* and *Heniochus acuminatus*
	Raccoon butterfly fish	*Chaetodon lunula*
Pomacanthidae Larger angelfishes Good community fish but need a large aquarium. Some members of this grouping have highly specialized diets.	Blueface angelfish	*Pomacanthus xanthometapon*
	Emperor angelfish	*Pomacanthus imperator*
	French angelfish	*Pomacanthus paru*
	Koran angelfish	*Pomacanthus semicirculatus*
	Queen angelfish	*Holacanthus ciliaris*
	Rock beauty angelfish	*Holacanthus tricolor*
Dwarf/pygmy angelfishes Pygmy angels are good community fish.	Cherub fish	*Centropyge argi*
	Flame angelfish	*Centropyge loricula*
	Lemonpeel angelfish	*Centropyge flavissima*
	Potter's angelfish	*Centropyge potteri*
Pomacentridae Damsel fishes Schooling fish that are easy to care for.	Bicolor damsel	*Stegastes partitus*
	Blue velvet damsel fish	*Neoglyphidodon oxyodon*
	Domino damsel	*Dascyllus trimaculatus*
	Green chromis	*Chromis viridis*
	Dottybacks	*Pseudochromis* sp.
	Yellow-tailed blue damselfish	*Chrysiptera parasema*
Clown fishes/anemone fishes Great community fish. Many species are captive bred.	Black saddleback clown fish	*Amphiprion polymnus*
	Clark's yellowtail clown fish	*Amphiprion clarkia*
	Ocellaris clown fish	*Amphiprion ocellaris*
	Orange/yellow skunk clown fish	*Amphiprion sandaracinos*
	Pink/salmon skunk clown fish	*Amphiprion perideraion*
	Seba's brown yellowtail clown fish	*Amphiprion sebae*
	Three-stripe/three-banded clown fish	*Amphiprion tricinctus*
	Tomato clown fish	*Amphiprion frenatus*
	True percula clown fish	*Amphiprion percula*
	Two-stripe/two-banded Red Sea clown fish	*Amphiprion bicinctus*

Table 5.6 *Continued*

Family or grouping	Common name	Scientific name
Other fishes		
Apogonida	Bangaii cardinal	*Pterapogon kauderni*
	Flamefish cardinal	*Apogon maculates*
	Pajama cardinal	*Sphaeramia nematoptera*
Balistidae	Black half-moon trigger fish	*Sufflamen chrysopterum*
	Clown trigger fish	*Balistoides conspicillum*
	Huma/Picasso trigger fish	*Rhinecanthus aculeatus*
	Niger trigger fish	*Odonus niger*
	Scrawled filefish	*Aluterus scriptus*
Callionymidae	Psychedelic Mandarin fish	*Synchiropus splendidus*
	Spotted green Mandarin fish	*Synchiropus picturatus*
Labridae	Cleaner wrasse	*Labroides dimidiatus*
	Six-line wrasse	*Pseudocheilinus hexataenia*
Muraenidae	Leopard eel	*Gymnothorax* sp.
	Ribbon eel	*Rhinomuraena quaesita*
	Zebra moray eel	*Gymnomuraena zebra*
Scorpaenidae	Fuzzy dwarf lionfish	*Dendrochirus brachypterus*
Serranids	Panther grouper	*Cromilepetes altivelis*
	Royal gramma/fairy basslet	*Gramma loreto*
	Swalesi basslet	*Liopropoma swalesi*
Zanclidae	Bartlett's anthias	*Pseudanthias bartlettorum*
	Diadem anthias	*Pseudanthias parvirostris*
	Moorish idol	*Zanclus cornutus*
Invertebrates		
Crustaceans	Arrow crab	*Stenorhynchus seticornis*
	Banded coral shrimp	*Stenopus hispidus*
	Blue harlequin shrimp	*Hymenocera elegans*
	Blue-legged hermit crab	*Clibanarius tricolor*
	Fire (blood) shrimp	*Lysmata debelius*
	Peppermint shrimp	*Lysmata wurdemanni*
	Skunk cleaner shrimp	*Lysmata amboinensis*
Cnideria and echinoderms	Blue mushroom anemone	*Discosoma* spp.
	Blue starfish	*Linckia laevigata*
	Blue tuxedo (pincushion) urchin	*Mespilla globulus*
	Bubble anemone	*Heteractis dorensis*
	Chocolate chip starfish	*Protoreastor nodosus*
	Pink-tipped anemone	*Condylactis passiflora*
	Sebae anemone	*Tridacna maxima*
Mollusks	Blue/gold maxima clam	*Heteractis crispa*
	Crocea clam	*Tridacna crocea*
	Derasa clams	*Tridacna derasa*
	Flame scallop	*Lima scabra*
	Florida fighting conch	*Strombus alatus*
	Turbo snail	*Turbo* sp.
Corals	Aspera staghorn coral	*Acropora aspera*
	Efflorescens table coral	*Acropora efflorescens*
	Formosa staghorn coral	*Acropora formosa*
	Robust staghorn coral	*Acropora robusta*
	Bicolor gorgonians	*Acabaria bicolor*
	Bubble coral	*Plerogyra sinuosa*
	Common razor coral	*Fungia scutaria*
	Cap coral	*Montipora capricornis*
	Confusa coral	*Montipora confuse*
	Finger coral	*Montipora digitata*

for life, that being high-quality water. The overall function of a filtration system is twofold (Losordo et al., 1998):

(1) Mechanical filtration—to provide for the mechanical elimination of solid organic waste.
(2) Biochemical conversion—to facilitate the nitrification process, converting dissolved organic waste into nontoxic metabolites.

Many component options are available for accomplishing these objectives (Losordo et al., 1999). Some system designs utilize separate components for mechanical filtration and biological conversion, while others combine both in one unit (biomechanical filters). Filtration systems can be either internal (occupying a portion of the pond or tank volume) or discrete external units. Some systems are low pressure (gravity fed), while others have a dedicated pump for cycling water through the filter unit (high pressure). Regardless of the components chosen, mechanical filtration and biochemical conversion are very distinct and separate processes and should be treated as such, even when components designed to serve each function occupy the same physical space.

Mechanical filtration

Mechanical filtration involves the physical trapping and timely systematic removal of coarse particulate waste and debris. Sand, screens, plastic beads, pads, and brushes are all used successfully for this purpose, either singularly or in stages. The smaller the size or the tendency toward clumping of this media, the more frequently maintenance will be required to prevent channel development and clogging. However, trapping is only the first part of this process, and particulate organic material continues to decompose and contribute to the dissolved organic load of a system until completely removed. Therefore, the most critical design characteristic important to fish health is whether or not the system can operate efficiently and without failure given the level of monitoring and maintenance employed by owner.

Two additional key components of most mechanical filtration systems in ponds are the surface skimmer (designed to trap all floating particulates as they pass through the system) and the bottom drain (designed to transport all settleable coarse particulates that would otherwise accumulate in the culture unit to the mechanical filter unit).

Biological conversion of waste

Biological conversion technologies generally involve a means of providing substrate for the growth of a biofilm that utilizes oxygen to convert ammonia and nitrite to nitrate, and oxidize organic matter (Gutierrez-Wing and Malone, 2006). Porous rock and other natural materials, porous ceramics, and numerous commercially marketed plastic media are all used successfully for this purpose. From the perspective of fish health, the most critical design characteristic of a biological conversion unit is its ability to transform toxic metabolites into nontoxic forms. The factors affecting this process include

(1) the specific surface area of the substrate (the area of substrate surface per unit volume of substrate—usually expressed in square feet/cubic feet or square meter/cubic meter);
(2) the flow characteristics of the unit, which determine the rate at which biological conversion takes place; and
(3) the susceptibility of the system to clogging and channeling, and the ease with which it can be cleaned.

Biomechanical filtration

Biomechanical filters, especially those of the high-pressure variety, are becoming very popular. An example of this type of filtration system is the bubble bead filter system (Fig. 5.2). They offer the advantage of reducing the total space requirements for a filtration system since mechanical filtration and biological conversion take place in the same unit. The disadvantage of these units comes if they are the sole means of filtration; since there is no staging of the mechanical and biochemical conversation processing, system failure can be disastrous. The attachment of a prefilter "basket" can aid in reducing the entry of large particulate

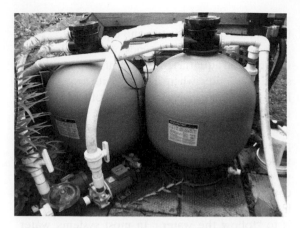

Fig. 5.2 A bubble bead filter system combines biological filtration and mechanical filtration. These two units filter 9000 gallons.

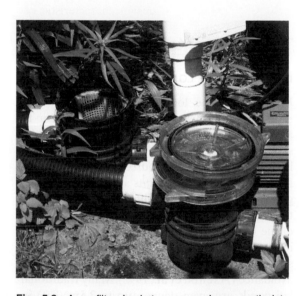

Fig. 5.3 A prefilter basket removes large particulate matter before it enters the main filter chamber, increasing the efficiency of the system.

matter and debris, such as leaves (Fig. 5.3). The trapping of waste solids generally involves some sort of expandable granular media bed through which all water passes. The solids either adhere to the medium or are trapped within the open spaces between the medium particles. On a systematic basis, filters will become clogged with solids and require cleaning or backwashing.

Gas exchange

In order to ensure fish health and efficient biological conversion of waste, culture systems should be aerated to maintain adequate DO concentrations of at least 6 mg/l and at the same time release excess carbon dioxide (CO_2). It should be noted that processes within the bioconversion system can have a higher demand for DO and higher rate of CO_2 production than the fish themselves, so both systems should be aerated. While there are many aeration systems available, the most common types used in ornamental ponds are diffused air systems. These systems utilize a regenerative blower to provide large volumes of air at low pressure. Blowers are commonly used in conjunction with diffusers placed near or on the bottom of the fish culture and biological conversion units. Diffusers that produce very small air bubbles to optimize the rate of DO and CO_2 transfer between the water and the bubbles as they rise should be selected. In addition, water movement must be sufficient to mix and redistribute aerated water.

Chemical filtration

Chemical filtration employs a more advanced media that has an ionic charge or adsorptive properties to pull chemicals, heavy metals, and toxins out of the water column using activated carbon, ammonia-adsorbing clays (zeolite), or ion-exchange resins (Gratzek, 1992).

Disinfection

Diseases can sometimes spread quickly in ponds and tanks if the fish density is high. Some chemicals used to treat diseases have a harmful effect on the nitrifying bacteria within the biochemical conversion unit. Alternatives to traditional chemical or antibiotic treatments include the continuous disinfection of the recycled water with ultraviolet (UV) irradiation. Microorganisms (including disease-causing bacteria and parasites) are killed when exposed to a sufficient amount of UV radiation. The effectiveness of UV disinfection depends on the size of the organism, the amount of UV radiation, and the level of penetration of the radiation into the water. To be effective, microorganisms must come in close proximity to the UV radiation source (0.5 cm [0.2 in.] or less). Turbidity reduces the effectiveness of UV radiation for disinfection. In order to optimize the efficiency of a UV radiation system, water should be prefiltered with some form of particulate filtration device. The main disadvantage of UV disinfection is the need for clean water with low suspended solids concentrations. Additionally, the expensive UV lamps must be replaced periodically as they age rapidly and their wattage is reduced. The main advantage of UV disinfection is that it is safe to operate and is not harmful to the cultured species. In addition to disinfection of disease agents such as viruses, bacteria, and some parasites, UV radiation can be used to control excessive planktonic algae.

Ozone (O_3) gas is a strong oxidizing agent in water. Ozone has been used for years to disinfect drinking water. It will also oxidize organic matter in water. The efficiency of the disinfecting and oxidizing action depends upon the contact time and residual concentration of O_3 in the water. Ozone must be generated on-site because it is unstable and breaks down in 10–20 minutes. Ozone is usually generated with either a UV light or a corona electric discharge source. There are many commercial ozone-generation units available. Ozone is diffused into the water from a fish culture system in an external contact basin or loop. Water must be retained in this sidestream long enough to ensure disinfection and oxidation, but also to ensure that the ozone molecules are destroyed. Residual ozone entering the culture tank can be very toxic to fish. Ozone in the air is also toxic to humans at low concentrations. Great care should be taken in venting excess ozone from the generation, delivery, and contact system to the outside of the building. Ozonation systems should be designed and installed by experienced personnel.

Filtration and fish health evaluation

Evaluating fish health requires an assessment of the equipment used in life support of the pond or tank inhabitants, in addition to water quality testing and examination of the fish. When a visit to the site is not feasible, the client should be instructed to bring pictures of the setup and equipment.

Recognizing the main types of equipment used in ponds and aquaria lends the aquatic practitioner some credibility when dealing with experienced hobbyists. Despite the knowledge of fish diagnostics, disease, and treatments, failure to recognize a trickle system or bead filter may lead to compliance issues on the part of the owner. Visiting water garden centers and local pet stores is a good way to become familiar with equipment that is commonly used in the industry. Most systems will have some equipment in place. The best approach is to "follow the water." In most systems, water flows into an intake pipe or skimmer from the pond or tank, through a series of tubing or pipes, into the main filtration system, then returns to the tank or pond.

The ornamental pond

Location and construction

Ponds should be located so that they do not receive continuous midday sunlight in order to avoid overheating or sunburned fish during the summer months. This is especially a problem in shallow ponds if no sources of shade such as floating leafed aquatic plants are provided (Wildgoose, 1998). All ponds intended to house fish throughout the year should have some portion of the total area that is at least 1–1.5 m (3.3–5 ft) in depth to serve as a refugium, ensuring a more stable temperature and providing for predator avoidance (Axelrod et al., 1992). Many traditional koi ponds are even deeper, up to 2.5 m (8 ft) in depth. In cold climates, the frost line should be considered when determining pond depth if the fish are to be overwintered in the pond.

Pond construction materials are many, each with advantages and disadvantages. The more popular choices are waterproofed concrete, fiberglass, polyvinyl chloride (PVC) liners, and butyl rubber liners. Regardless of the material used, the pond shape and design should ensure unobstructed flow (no pockets of stagnant water) and be free of sharp edges or obstructions that can impair environmental quality.

Moving water

Many of the fish kept in ornamental ponds are riverine species, physically and behaviorally adapted to flowing water. The characteristics of water movement both within the culture unit and throughout an RAS are among the most important design and operational features, yet many pond owners know little more than the flow rating of their pump and the diameter of their piping. A common method for estimating appropriate water moving capacity throughout an RAS system involves the exchange rate (the time it takes to fill or replace a volume of water equivalent to that of the fish culture unit). It is often recommended that the total volume of pond water be exchanged a minimum of once every 3 hours, with exchange once every 1–2 hours preferred, and exchange no more than once every 30 minutes (Nash and Cook, 1999).

Routine maintenance

As previously discussed (Chapter 4), water chemistry parameter testing is recommended when a pond is first constructed, opening and closing for the season, and at any time abnormalities are noted. Most outdoor ponds experience seasons requiring specific maintenance procedures.

Most of the active pond season is spent with routine maintenance. This involves visually monitoring fish health, periodic water quality testing, cleaning filters and strainer baskets, controlling algae, and keeping equipment in good working order.

In the spring, most ponds will be emerging from a winter stasis. Overwintered fish will have compromised immune systems and are at an increased risk for infectious diseases, water quality abnormalities, and the effects of stress. Life-support equipment should be thoroughly evaluated and repaired if needed before placing in use. Ponds should be cleaned of excess remaining detritus (fallen leaves, etc.). The addition of 1–3 gm/L of sodium chloride may help improve the transition from winter to spring. Feeding should begin with small amounts and gradually increase in frequency and volume as water and ambient air temperatures increase. Water changes can be performed

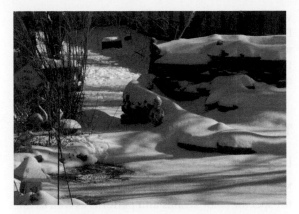

Fig. 5.4 An opening in the ice on a pond surface (lower left) made with the use of an air diffuser (airstone) placed 12 in. from the surface.

as needed. Filters need to be cleaned more often during the spring start-up.

Preparation for the fall is similar to the spring preparations, only in reverse. Netting can be placed over the pond to catch falling leaves, aquatic plants are removed or the foliage is cut back in anticipation of a dormant state, and feeding is gradually reduced. To prevent freezing of the entire pond surface, air diffusers can be moved close to the water surface to provide agitation or floating cattle trough heaters can be used. Both methods can leave a small hole in the ice; this is sufficient for gas exchange (Fig. 5.4). The heaters tend to be more expensive to run but more effective in colder climates.

Problem solving

Water quality issues are the most common problem observed in ponds but other common problems do arise. Pond owners should take advantage of feeding time to observe the animals for changes in normal behavior and for the presence of any lesions, and check equipment for proper functioning. Most pond fish are food oriented and readily appear at feeding time, making absences significant. Predation may leave visible clues (scales, fins, etc.), but often missing fish and agitation of the remaining fish are the only hints that there has been a predator appearance. Leaks are common in ponds and are most often located in the waterfalls or sidestreams. A simple way to check for a leak's location is to turn off the waterfalls and streams and see if the pond's water level continues to fall. Improperly installed bottom drains are another location that can leak.

The tropical freshwater aquarium

Introduction to tropical fish

Many species of tropical freshwater fish are bred for specific color strains and patterns as well as fin and scale variations. Breeders have created new species of fish for ornamental markets through the use of genetic selection, hybridization, and genetic engineering (e.g., the transgenic fluorescent zebra fish, Glofish®). Despite the availability of over 700 freshwater tropical species, only 30–40 species of freshwater ornamentals compose the majority of the industry (Helfman, 2007). When advising the beginning aquarist, keeping animals in similar geographic groups can often afford the best success. These groups build on similar environmental quality and husbandry requirements and on known communal relationships for local species.

Preparation of the tank

An aquarium should be set up well in advance of bringing home new fish. Biofiltration can be jump started with the use of hardy "starter" fish, or "fish free" by providing the nitrifying bacteria with a source of ammonia or by using seasoned gravel from existing disease-free tanks. Newly purchased fish should be acclimated to the established tank's temperature and water conditions. This may take 15 minutes to an hour of floating the bag on the surface of the tank or providing a drip line to slowly drip tank water into the transport container over time. Fish should be netted carefully from the transport bag after acclimation and placed directly into the established tank or a quarantine tank. Transport water in the bag should be discarded as this water may contain excess nitrogenous waste, have different physical and chemical properties, carry pathogens, or harbor unwelcome additions such as snails.

Water treatment and supply

The aquarist needs to fully understand the water quality conditions the desired fish require. Occasionally, existing water sources may preclude the owner from being able to maintain certain species of fish. For example, homes that are supplied by wells that have well-buffered and high-pH water may not accommodate water quality conditions required for South American fishes, unless some investment in pretreatment for the water source is done. See Chapter 4 on water quality for more information on testing source water.

In addition to commercial additives used to treat tap water, several methods exist to pretreat water including water softeners or reverse osmosis (RO) units/deionizing (DI) units. A water softener works by using sodium to replace calcium and magnesium ions in the water. Some disadvantages for using water softeners are that it can create more saline water and that some of the chemicals used as anticaking agents for the salt can be toxic to fish. RO/DI units require high pressure to force water through a membrane that separates pure water from its ionic components. In order for these units to work appropriately, there may be several other prefilter requirements to remove sediments, chlorine, chloramines, and heavy metals prior to passing through the unit. For some species of fish, especially African cichlids, additives may be required to optimize the water quality because all beneficial and harmful ions are removed by these units.

Tank size and placement

Tank size and design will depend on the purpose as well as the density of the animals. Although some of the unique shape designs and high tanks are more aesthetically appealing for displaying certain fish species, the aquarist will be limited by surface area for maximizing the density of plants and animals in these systems. Environmental factors such as air quality, water source, sound, light, and temperature must be considered when determining tank placement. Location of the tank can affect the maintenance required to keep optimal water quality. An aquarium requires easy access to both a water supply and electricity.

An aquarium needs to be located near ground fault interrupter-compliant electrical outlets that will be able to supply electricity for heaters, filters, lights, and air pumps safely around water.

Tanks should not be located directly on the floor, where the aquarium inhabitants can be constantly stressed by small children or other terrestrial pets. Tanks should be located out of high-traffic areas and away from loud areas of mechanical noise created from televisions, stereos, and appliances. Excess light from windows can lead to chronic algae problems, or create reproductive problems associated with inappropriate photoperiods in some fish species. Locating a tank near heating or air conditioning vents could lead to disease problems because of fluctuating water temperatures.

Commercially available stands are designed for a specific size tank and the weight of a full tank. A 30-gallon aquarium with 50 lb of gravel filled with water can weigh over 300 lb!

Filter types for freshwater aquaria

Box/corner filters are an old filtration method that was standard in 10-gallon starter aquarium kits until the early 1980s. These filters consist of a small plastic box filled with activated carbon sandwiched between cotton floss filter media. An airline enters through the top of the box attached to an airline and airstone. An air pump runs air through the hosing and airstone, creating an airlift for mechanical filtration through the filter media, and provides oxygen for the growth of beneficial bacteria in the carbon media.

A sponge filter is simply a sponge that is attached to one or two plastic tubes that rests inside the aquarium. It works using a similar principle to box filters with the creation of an airlift. The sponge provides for an increased porous surface area for increasing biological nitrification.

Undergravel filters consist of a perforated plate attached to a vertical tube. The plate is covered by the substrate, and the vertical tube is attached to a submersible power head or an air pump, airline, and airstone to provide an airlift to pass water under the gravel and create a large biological nitrification bed. Decaying waste material can also be pulled underneath the substrate, and

over time these plates will clog and can create anaerobic conditions. Some undergravel filters can operate using reverse flow pushing water up through the bottom substrate, and this method may help with long-term maintenance to decrease clogging of the plates.

The advent of outside power filters helps provide easier access for cleaning filters and decreasing equipment inside the tank to maximize exhibit space. Most of these systems hang on the back of the tank and water is siphoned into the filtration compartment. The water passes through a combination of filter media, including activated carbon and floss type media. Many newer power filters have media in preformed cartridges, and/or the carbon is held in nylon bags for convenience. Water is either returned directly into the tank via an internal pump, or water can be sprayed onto a biowheel that allows growth of nitrifying microbes in an oxygen-rich environment. The tank water level needs to be maintained to provide an adequate height for siphoning to work, and filter media needs to be changed regularly. These filters are very good at providing mechanical filtration, and systems with a biowheel also have adequate biological nitrification if functioning properly for light or medium stocking densities.

Canister filters use the same principles as power filters. Water is pumped from the tank into a canister that may have several different media compartments for mechanical, biological nitrification, and chemical filtration. Canister filters often have greater mechanical filtration and biological nitrification than power filters because of greater areas for media and stronger pumps. These filters are ideal for more heavily stocked tanks but require more maintenance for biweekly changing of the floss type media, monthly replacement of carbon media, and routine rinsing of the biomedia to prevent clogging and optimize efficiency.

Maintenance

Optimizing water quality conditions is paramount to becoming a successful aquarist, requiring regular filtration maintenance and weekly dedication for performing 25%–50% water changes using a gravel washer device. No filtration system replaces the need to do regular water changes.

Maintenance of individual filtration systems is determined by several factors, including stocking density, frequency and amount of feeding, and equipment used. Cleaning of filters and biomedia should be staggered so that biofiltration is minimally affected.

Tank substrate, furnishings, and plants

There are many options available for today's aquaria that include live and synthetic plants, stones, gravel, sand, driftwood, smoothed glass, artificial resin stones, caves and plastic figurines fashioned like shipwrecks, pirates, and so on. Some of these objects can be animated using an air pump and air curtains with specially configured airstones that can be used to provide an aesthetic quality, beneficial oxygen, and water turnover. The most important aspect of tank design is to provide adequate shelter and a diversity of safe hiding places for the future animal collection.

Most hobbyists fill their tanks with 3–5 in. of gravel (greater or equal to 3-mm diameter), sand, or a substrate mixture. The substrate should be rinsed thoroughly with freshwater before adding it to the bottom of the tank as processing and packaging the substrates can cause excess dust and sediment. The gravel will also aid in biological nitrification, provided oxygen exchange occurs in the sediments, for maintaining a healthy microbial fauna. It is critical to include substrate rinsing as a part of routine maintenance to prevent the formation of anaerobic pockets in the media. Anaerobic pockets result in hydrogen sulfide formation that is toxic to fish. This can be sometimes seen as a black cloud when siphoning gravel in a tank that has been improperly maintained. A characteristic odor will often accompany the hydrogen sulfide release. Deep gravel beds represent an increased risk factor for anaerobic pocket formation.

Sand is not recommended in freshwater aquaria because it can pack tightly and not allow water and gas flow through the substrate for many undergravel types of filtration. Although small sandy areas can be strategically placed using rock ledges for those animals that may prefer to hide in this substrate like some of the loach species. Laterite and laterite-mixed substrates are not recommended except for more advanced aquarists who may attempt to grow plants or maintain fish that require fine materials.

It is important to make sure the size of the substrate is either small enough to pass through the gastrointestinal tract of these animals or is too large for animals to ingest. Substrate sizes greater than 8–10 mm will start to decrease the surface area available to accommodate microbial organisms instrumental in establishing the microfauna for bionitrification. It is important to avoid substrates with sharp edges with bottom-dwelling animals. Quartzite or granite-type gravels are preferred in freshwater aquaria because they are least likely to leach ions into the water and alter water quality parameters, and are large enough to allow some aeration of the gravel bed.

Tank furnishings are at the discretion of the owner. Some caveats are to avoid using toys or nonaquarium items in the tanks that may be finished with unknown paint sources. Toys, metallic objects, shells, corals, or decorations purchased for other uses may contain paints that can be toxic or leach metals and ions into the aquarium that can affect water quality and in extreme cases, kill both live plants and animals. Rocks and stones can be collected for designing backdrops and caves, but avoid stones such as limestone that can leach ions into the water. Driftwood may need to be soaked prior to placing in the tank. Some driftwood will change the water color a light tea color due to tannins in the wood. All materials collected from outdoor streams, lakes, and ponds should be disinfected in a 1:10 chlorine bleach solution, and then rinsed thoroughly in fresh water before being added to the tank.

A live planted and fish-filled aquarium requires greater maintenance and restricted fish selection. Plants also carry the risk of introducing disease or disease-carrying organisms such as nematodes or snails into the home aquarium, and they require additional nutrients and maintenance.

Heating, cover, and lighting

Tropical freshwater fish prefer to stay in temperature ranges of 78–82 °F. In order to provide these animals with the proper temperature year round, a heater will be required. In warmer climates, some aquarists will actually unplug heaters for the summer and just regulate tank temperature control during the cooler months. Some heaters are actually directly built into canister-type filtration systems. Most of the submersible heaters on the market are very durable. The old immersible glass heaters are not recommended because they can easily break or crack and can lead to electrical malfunction. It is important to buy an accurate thermometer to monitor water temperature daily. A standard rule of thumb for sizing heater wattage for fish tanks is 3–5W per gallon. In cooler climates, this size will easily adjust for room temperatures, which may be 10–15 °F below the ambient tank temperature, and in warmer climates these heaters have to work less. If a heater fails, unplug the heater first. When raising the water temperature for tropical fish, it is safe to bring the temperature quickly to 65 °F. A general rule of thumb is to raise the temperature one degree F per hour. When 65 °F is obtained, gradually raise the tank temperature to its normal range by increasing the temperature by 3 °F daily. A gradual acclimation will help the animal's immune and metabolic functions to adapt while preventing pathogenic microflora and fauna from causing secondary infections.

All fish tanks need covers to prevent fish from jumping out of the aquarium, to protect fish from predators entering the tank, to decrease evaporative losses, and to help maintain temperature control. Most lids are either plastic hood-type lids, combination hoods and light fixtures, or glass/plexiglass fitted covers specified to tank dimensions that can accommodate a strip light. Some fish species such as the freshwater rope fish and eels are notorious escape artists, so a tight-fitting lid is imperative.

Lights are required to view the fish, provide light for growth of plants, and create photoperiods. A wide range of lighting is available for both incandescent and fluorescent light fixtures, including light spectrums that have been developed to enhance certain colors of fish, stimulate algae growth, and stimulate plant growth. Because of the energy and heat generated from incandescent lights, fluorescent fixtures are becoming more frequently used. More research needs to be done to better evaluate the requirements of tropical fish for UVA and UVB rays. A full spectrum light is rec-

ommended, although given that most lights have glass or plastic covers, full wavelength penetration of these spectra may not be realized in the tank.

The most common rule of thumb for providing light in aquaria is to provide 2W of energy per gallon of water in fish only tanks, and 4W of energy per gallon of water in naturally planted aquaria. It is also important to change lightbulbs every 6–8 months rather than when they burn out. The best way to manage lighting for the home aquarium is to use timer set for 10–12 hours of light per day.

Problem solving

The most obvious problems are those directly associated with poor water quality, but other problems can readily occur. Some of these problems include having animals get stuck in filter components; especially power filters and canister filters with strong pumps and greater water flow. Heaters can malfunction and either not work at all, super heat the water, or cause an electrical malfunction. Animals can get burned by heaters in the tank (Fig. 5.5), especially lethargic or very shy animals, so it is best to avoid creating hiding niches around in-tank heaters. Power outages can cause a wide array of problems, from simple to catastrophic, and the aquarist needs to develop contingency plans if this occurs during various times of the year. Filters and pumps can malfunction, underperform, or cavitate because of low water levels. Sometimes pumps can actually pump

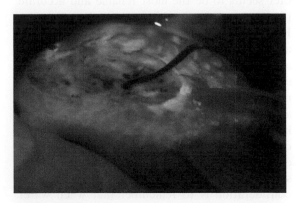

Fig. 5.5 A goldfish impaired by a buoyancy disorder badly burned by a submersible heater.

air as well as water through filters when they are not functioning properly due to mechanical problems or low water flow. This additional air can allow for a supersaturation of gases, which can be detrimental for fish. Air pumps that are not functioning properly can lead to situations where the DO levels drop too low. Because air pumps use room air, avoid using aerosolized products such as paints and cleaners in and around the air pumps or these chemical toxicants can be pumped into the tank.

The marine ornamental aquarium

Marine tank setup

Water treatment and supply

Most marine aquarists need to make artificial seawater for their aquaria and have a higher degree of knowledge regarding water treatment systems and water quality testing. Many marine hobbyists will use RO/DI units to remove all the chemical and ionic components from their tap source before making a seawater mix for their tanks. Nitrates and phosphates commonly found in freshwater supplies are particularly detrimental when setting up a reef aquarium. Seawater mixes come as a dry salt mix, wet salt mix, bottled seawater, or for those living near the coast, fresh ocean water. Before adding saltwater to an aquarium, salinity needs to be tested using a hydrometer, salinity probe, or refractometer. The refractometer seems to be the most reliable and accurate piece of equipment if it is regularly calibrated. Hydrometers can give inaccurate measurements, and salinity probes will give false readings if they are not cleaned properly. Whenever additional salt is needed in an established tank, it should never be added directly but instead diluted to an appropriate salinity. Most marine tanks will be kept at a salinity of 32–36 ppt or a specific gravity of 1.020–1.025. Reef tanks need a more narrow control and do best at salinity ranges of 34–36 or specific gravities of 1.023–1.025. One important consideration is to remember that when water evaporates from the tank, the ions contributing to specific gravity stay behind, unlike when doing actual water changes. Always measure the salinity of the tank before adding more saltwater. It is safe to top off small amounts of evaporative losses with fresh water when needed.

Tank size and placement

Many marine animals are wild caught and need a quiet, low-traffic area. Marine animals, especially invertebrates, have greater sensitivity to changing light conditions and temperature variations. Certain coral species are extremely sensitive to temperature changes, and direct light can allow unwanted types of algae to grow in reef tanks, causing destruction of certain corals and live rock, making tank maintenance exponentially more difficult.

Marine aquaria require sturdy stands because they weigh more than freshwater tanks with the addition of live rock and corals. Another important consideration is the corrosive nature of saltwater on metal and electrical components. It is best to avoid placing these tanks in areas that may be difficult to perform routine husbandry.

Filtration and maintenance

In addition to the filters discussed previously for freshwater aquaria, a few others used more commonly in marine systems will be described. Some of these filtration methods include using trickle filters, fluidized bed filters, and Berlin method filtration. Other filter components commonly used with marine aquaria are protein skimmers (Fig. 5.6), denitrators, UV sterilization, ozonizers, and power heads.

Trickle or wet/dry filters are commonly used for marine and freshwater aquaria. These filters can be purchased or easily constructed using basic plumbing and aquarium supplies. For the home aquarium, the filter is placed below the fish tank where water is gravity fed to the filter. Water is often mechanically filtered prior to entering the wet/dry sump using some type of filter floss. Water then trickles across a drip plate and flows over biomedia that has established microbial organisms necessary for bionitrification. As the water flows along the drip plate, carbon dioxide (CO_2) is released and oxygen (O_2) enters the water.

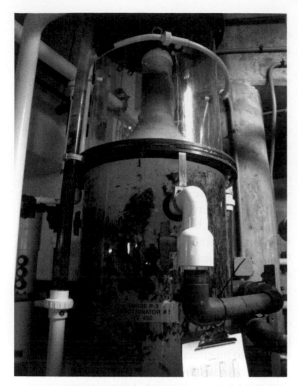

Fig. 5.6 A large protein skimmer used by a public aquarium.

Bionitrification occurs in the biomedia, and water flows through to a sump that may or may not contain additional filter media before being pumped back into the aquarium.

Fluidized beds are a more technically advanced undergravel filter design that siphons water from the aquarium into an outside receptacle that has pumps to move the water centrifugally through a sand layer before being pumped back into the tank. The sand is constantly suspended to allow oxygen to reach microbial colonies for performing bionitrification. These systems have been difficult to maintain and are limited in use but have a tremendous capacity for biological nitrification when working properly.

The Berlin method of reef aquaria involves the use of large quantities of live rock and sand. These systems require a lot of space but can provide both bionitrification and denitrification because they have areas that are aerobic and anaerobic to promote microbial colonies beneficial for these biological processes. Organisms growing on the live rock also use waste material as nutrients for growth.

Protein skimmers/foam fractionators take advantage of the ionic affinity of organic chemicals for bubbles. A protein skimmer is simply a fractionating column to create fine air bubbles where water and air are mixed. Organic compounds stick to these bubbles and the fractionating device serves to skim these bubbles out off the water into a collection cup for disposal. Although foam fractionators are being developed for freshwater systems, they work much better in marine systems because of the available ions in seawater that help organic ions to bind to these bubbles.

Denitrators are a recent addition for home aquarists. These systems have water flow through anaerobic boxes that contain a specialized biological media to remove nitrate from the water via anaerobic denitrification.

UV sterilizers are commonly used by more advanced aquarists to help control water quality. This component uses the UVC or UV light spectrum for germicidal properties. Unfortunately, unless the aquarists has a working understanding of the principles of UV sterilization, these systems often have water flowing through them but often are not working properly. Some problems frequently encountered with these systems are improper water flow, biofouling of the bulb, inadequate light replacement, inappropriate positioning in the filter schematic, and salt corrosion of electrical components.

Ozonators are also new products for home aquarists that use ozone to disinfect aquarium water by oxidation using a similar mechanism as chlorine. These can be complicated systems and require an advanced understanding of water chemistry, as mistakes in monitoring ozone levels can lead to the death of aquarium inhabitants.

Marine animals are accustomed to tide and wave action. An easy and effective way to simulate this in the tank is by submerging a few power heads positioned in different locations. If positioned correctly, the pumps will aid in circulating food near invertebrates when the animals are fed. A rippling of the tank surface water by the power heads will help exchanges of oxygen and carbon dioxide more efficiently. There are also wave machines commercially available for the home marine aquarium.

All these filters require regular maintenance and replacement of filter media for mechanical and chemical filtration. During routine water changes, excess algae should be removed and all the glass should be cleaned. The biggest difference with marine aquarium is the rapid buildup of "salt creep," a white crust that develops wherever water splashes or seeps. This needs to be removed weekly as well. If sand is used as a substrate, it will often pack tightly and waste can be gently filtered off the surface, while gravel substrates should be vacuumed. Weekly water changes of 25% should help remove a substantial amount of this biological waste. Home water quality test kits are limited in the ranges for detecting certain parameters and having an extensive panel run in an established tank every 6 months is highly recommended. Reef aquaria will require testing a larger number of parameters to determine if adequate building blocks for coral growth are present. Filters should be checked weekly, filter floss changed biweekly, and carbons and other chemical filtration should be changed monthly.

Tank substrate, furnishings, live rock, and corals

In marine aquaria, the most common substrates are either crushed corals or aragonite sands, with the former being used for fish-only tanks. Aragonite sands are more commonly used in reef tanks and release stores of calcium carbonates and strontium for coral growth. These include shell grit, crushed limestone, crushed dolomite, crushed marble, crushed coral skeletons, coral sand, and other calcite/aragonite substrates.

Many aquarists will purchase some live rock for their tanks to create a naturalistic underwater environment of caves, rocky shelves, tunnels, seamounts, and overhangs. Live rock may be directly harvested or a few companies actually seed their own rock for commercial harvest. Live rock is rock that has been conditioned for a period of time in the ocean to promote growth on macro- and microorganisms. Some organisms found in live rock are beneficial for bionitrification.

The complexity and husbandry requirements of a marine aquarium will increase greatly if the home aquarist wishes to maintain a live reef tank with fish and other invertebrates. Corals are marine invertebrates from the class Anthozoa. They appear as polyps on a hard calcium carbonate skeleton. Although individual polyps can be distinguished on a piece of coral, the coral reef is made of a few to billions of polyps that are genetically identical, working in concert as a single organism connected by a complex gastrovascular system. There are both hard and soft corals. The hard corals are responsible for secreting calcium carbonate, which forms the coral exoskeleton, which is the foundational scaffolding for reefs. Certain varieties of corals can use nematocysts or stinging cells to capture a wide variety of prey, from plankton to small vertebrate fishes. Most corals gain nutrients through symbiosis with unicellular algae known as zooxanthellae to convert plankton into nutrients. For this symbiotic relationship to be effective, corals must be located in a place to have regular water flow to bring plankton, they must have appropriate temperatures to optimize metabolic activity of both polyps and algae, and they must receive adequate light intensity and wavelength for photosynthesis. When planning a reef tank, coral type and coral acquisition are one of the most important factors. The ornamental marine industry is directly responsible for causing the destruction of pristine reef areas in certain geographical locations. Marine ornamentals, live rock, and corals should be purchased from places that acquire them from sustainable resources. Many corals can be propagated, and pieces of coral called "frags" are available for sale or trade from collections established in captivity decades ago. One of the other important considerations in maintaining live reef aquaria is that these live polyps are extremely sensitive to water quality conditions and additives. Many of the chemical treatments we use to treat fish diseases will kill live coral and other invertebrates.

Heating, chilling, cover, and lighting

Many of the same principles for heating and covering the freshwater aquaria apply to marine exhibits. Two exceptions are chilling and lighting requirements. When heating an aquarium, most tanks will require at least 3W/gallon. The ranges for most marine ornamentals will be from 78 to 84°F. Since many saltwater aquaria use wet/dry or trickle filters, the heater usually is placed in the sump areas of these filters rather than in the fish tank itself, and heaters can also be placed in line with canister filter setups. Although the thermostats are very accurate on many of these heaters, a thermometer is required to check water temperature at least once daily. Digital thermometers can be used to offer continuous temperature reads.

Because of the sensitivity of corals to changes in temperature, a chiller may be required in an unairconditioned home located in warmer climates to keep the aquarium temperature in the narrow range preferred by the specimens in the tank below 86°F. Chillers can be expensive to operate, require regular maintenance, and may contain hazardous coolants that need disposal periodically.

Lighting is much more challenging for the marine aquarium. Unlike most freshwater systems, one light system does not fit all, and there is a fine balance for providing lighting for both exhibiting animals and providing health benefits.

Lighting can be evaluated at several levels. The first is wavelength. Aquatic invertebrates in captivity require UVA for metabolic and reproductive activity and UVB spectrum lighting for stimulating vitamin D synthesis (Fig. 5.7). The ratio of red to blue light waves is measured in Kelvin (K). Many commercial bulbs are measured in Kelvin ranging from 5500 to 20,000K, with the ratio of red to blue being equal around 6000K and having an increasing blue spectrum as K increases from 6000K. The higher the K, the deeper the blue spectrum can penetrate into the water, providing fixed corals and invertebrates a healthy source of light.

In order to achieve this lighting balance in the marine aquarium, a variety of bulb and lighting options exist that include fluorescent lighting, actinic lighting (blue spectrum), full-spectrum lighting, 50/50 bulbs, metal halide lights, compact fluorescents, mercury vapor, and lunar lighting. Even though a bulb may appear to be working properly, the spectrum on many of these bulbs changes over time. Specialized bulbs will have to be replaced every 6–8 months. Aquaria that are deeper than 20 in. will require additional lighting to penetrate to the bottom of the tank. Also, many aquaria glass tops filter out 90%–95% of beneficial UVB rays, unless they have been manufactured with specialized glass to allow penetration. Timers should be set up to maintain a 12-hour day/night light cycle. Lunar lighting is provided to help stimulate reproduction in a variety of fish, coral, and other invertebrate species.

Problem solving

Common problems in marine tanks are similar to those in freshwater tanks (see previous section), with a few additional problems. In marine aquaria, salinity must also be measured periodically as evaporation can lead to hypersaline conditions, and topping of sumps regularly with freshwater can also cause hyposalinity.

Other specific problems associated with marine aquaria include red acro bug, bristle worms, hair algae, cyanobacteria causing red slime, and coral bleaching. The first two are parasite problems of the reef brought in on live rock or coral fragments, while the remaining factors are related to environmental quality. Red bug, *Tegastes acroporanus*, is a copepod found on coral reefs. They eat the soft portions of *Acropora* sp. corals and detrimentally affect the health of corals in the reef aquarium. Prevention is the best control. Red

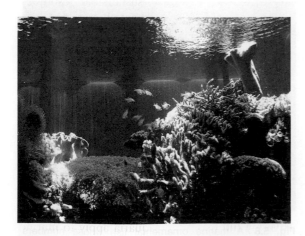

Fig. 5.7 Lighting is crucial to marine invertebrate tanks.

acro bugs have been controlled in reef aquaria using Interceptor®, milbemycin oxime. The pills for large dog breeds (51–100 lb) are used, and a 1-g tablet (23 mg of active milbemycin oxime) ground up can treat 380 gallons. Once ground, the dosage is 25 mg of the entire tablet per 10 gallons of actual tank water. Before treatment, all arthropod invertebrates should be removed from the aquarium. When treating any aquarium system, the entire volume of water in the tank and all life-support systems needs to be included. UV sterilization, ozone, and protein filters should be turned off during treatment as they will filter out or degrade the medication. After treatment, a 25% or greater water change is done after 6 hours, and the treatment should be repeated every 7 days for a total of four treatments. Bristle worms or fire worms are polychaete marine worms of the Amphinomidae family. They can sting and are extremely destructive due to a voracious appetite for invertebrates in the marine aquarium. They are best controlled through prevention, manual removal, and certain predatory fish and larger invertebrate species. Inspect all live rock carefully for fire worms before adding to the aquarium and remove any hitchhikers using tweezers. There are other marine polychaetes that are beneficial to the aquarium, so the aquarist may want to have a reef specialist or advanced reef hobbyists identify potential problem species. Hair algae are green macro algae that form hairlike strands all over the aquarium, especially adhering to the live rock and corals. Hair algae are caused by high nutrient loads in the water, especially elevated nitrates, total carbon, and phosphates. These conditions, when coupled with direct light, can allow for hair algae to grow excessively throughout the tank, making control difficult. When all these factors are optimally controlled, beneficial algae will be able to grow. Red slime algae are caused by cyanobacteria and are a consequence of high nutrient loads and inappropriate lighting. These blooms can be prevented with methods similar to that described for hair algae. There are many over-the-counter treatments for controlling red slime algae. Many of these products contain erythromycin, an antibiotic that if dosed incorrectly could destroy bionitrifying bacteria. If treatment with an antibiotic or other chemicals is used, water quality should be monitored for bionitrification. Coral bleaching can be caused by a variety of factors in the aquarium related to predation from parasitic organisms, improper temperature control, misplacement of specimens in the tank for height or water circulation, predation by certain invertebrates or fish purchased for the aquarium, improper lighting, changes in bulb spectrum over time and sudden replacement, medications and chemical additives, and a host of bacterial, fungal, viral, and protozoan infections.

Conclusion

Keeping fish is similar to maintaining any other living animal. Preventive medicine is the key. Proactive aquatic animal health management includes reading and researching aquatic animals, creating and preparing an appropriate habitat, understanding and performing proper husbandry and regular maintenance, testing the environment and environmental parameters, and providing appropriate nutrition. Recognizing problems of both the collection and equipment by being familiar with the normal behavior and appearance and remediating problems quickly and effectively when they occur can aid in avoiding further complications. By simply using consistent husbandry practices and exercising common sense, an aquarium or pond can provide years of enjoyment for all levels of hobbyists (Fig. 5.8).

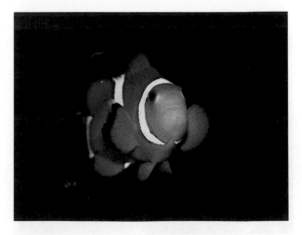

Fig. 5.8 A marine ornamental fish whose numbers soared after a popular movie release.

References and further reading

Axelrod, H.R., Benoist, A.S., Kelsey-Wood, D., et al. (1992) *Garden Ponds*. Neptune City, NJ: T.F.H.

Gratzek, J.B. (1992) *Aquariology: The Science of Fish Health Management*. Morris Plains, NJ: Tetra Press.

Gutierrez-Wing, M.T. and Malone, R.F. (2006) Biological filters in aquaculture: trends and research directions for freshwater and marine applications. *Aquacultural Engineering* **34**: 163–171.

Helfman, G.S. (2007) *Fish Conservation: A Guide to Understanding and Restoring Global Aquatic Biodiversity and Fishery Resources*. Chicago, IL: Island Press.

Losordo, T., Masser, M.P., and Rakocy J. (1998) Recirculating aquaculture tank production systems: an overview of critical considerations. *Southern Regional Aquaculture Center* Factsheet 451.

Losordo, T., Masser, M.P., and Rakocy, J. (1999) Recirculating aquaculture tank production systems: a review of component options. *Southern Regional Aquaculture Center* Factsheet 453.

McDowell, A. (1989) *The Tetra Encyclopedia of Koi*. Blacksburg, VA: Tetra Press.

Nash, H. and Cook, M.M. (1999) *Water Gardening Basics*. New York: Sterling Publishing.

Simon and Schuster Inc. (1976) *Simon and Schuster's Guide to Freshwater and Marine Aquarium Fishes*. New York: Simon and Schuster.

Vagelli, A.A. (2004). Significant increase in survival of captive-bred juvenile Banggai cardinalfish, *Pterapogon kauderni*, with am essential fatty acid enriched diet. *Journal of the World Aquaculture Society* **35** (1): 61–69.

Wildgoose, W. (1998). Skin disease in ornammental fish: identifying common problems. *In Practice* **20**: 226–243.

Wildgoose, W.H. (2001). *BSAVA Manual of Ornamental Fish*: 2nd Edition. Gloucester: BSAVA.

Fish Health

Chapter 6

Biosecurity and Ornamental Fish

Timothy J. Miller-Morgan and Jerry R. Heidel

Introduction

Biosecurity is a common topic in discussions of fish health and well-being. Definitions may vary, but all focus around this basic concept: Biosecurity consists of the practices and procedures used to prevent the introduction, emergence, spread, and persistence of infectious agents and disease within and around fish production and holding facilities. Furthermore, these practices help eliminate conditions that can enhance disease susceptibility among the fish. In short, biosecurity precautions are put in place to exclude and contain fish pathogens. Biosecurity practices are applicable to all levels of the ornamental fish industry: producers, exporters, importers, wholesalers, retailers, and hobbyists. Proper use of biosecurity measures will help prevent the introduction of infectious disease in a fish facility and will also help minimize the risk of diseases being passed from producer to hobbyist.

Infectious disease is a constant threat to ornamental fish, whether as individuals or as a group. An infectious disease outbreak in a group of fish can, and will, occur at any time. Prompt diagnosis and treatment are means of controlling these infections. The preventive measures found in a facility's biosecurity program complement this by stopping the spread of the disease within the facility. But as important, the biosecurity measures will minimize the likelihood of introduction and spread of the pathogen and eliminate the conditions that enhance disease susceptibility among fish.

While more often associated with intensive types of animal production, the principles of biosecurity are applicable to any level of animal husbandry, from high-density, high-volume production units to backyard ponds and aquaria. While specific features of a biosecurity program may vary between a fish aquaculture facility and a hobbyist's aquarium, the basic principles of biosecurity apply to any unit under consideration.

It is crucial that those charged with the care and handling of animals understand, implement, and adhere to the policies and procedures of a sound biosecurity program. The success or failure of an animal-related business will depend on the attention to basic biosecurity concepts. Biosecurity is not to be feared or avoided. It is an essential component of a facility's business plan. It requires effort and action by management and employees, including planning, implementation, training, auditing, and revision as circumstances change. A good biosecurity program does not have to be burdensome or confusing. It will result in greater success for an ornamental fish business and increased satisfaction for aquarium and pond fish owners.

Space limits this chapter to only a brief review of the basic principles of biosecurity and related husbandry practices. The reader is encouraged to consult more detailed references devoted to biosecurity standards for aquaculture (Lee and O'Bryen, 2003; Scarfe et al., 2006).

Biosecurity practices

Important and consistent biosecurity methods and protocols help protect a fish-holding facility against pathogen entry and spread. Basic biosecurity procedures are uniform across the industry, but the biosecurity plan will be customized to meet the special needs of each business. Each facility manager will modify and adjust biosecurity measures as needs change and finances allow.

Designing and implementing biosecurity practices can be simplified if you consider some basic themes: pathogen exclusion, pathogen containment, and basic best health practices.

Pathogen exclusion

The goal of pathogen exclusion is to prevent the entrance of an infectious agent into a facility, thereby preventing infection and possibly disease in a group of fish. Recognizing and understanding the various routes by which an infectious agent can enter a pristine fish tank or pond allows you to plan defensive measures that will block that entry.

Fish-associated entry

An obvious route of entry of pathogens into a facility is via the incoming fish. These animals may be asymptomatic carriers of a pathogen or may have frank disease. It can be very difficult to determine if one is receiving healthy fish, and rarely can a manager be totally confident that the fish he has received are in fact healthy. To help minimize opportunities for diseased fish to enter a facility, consider the following as you select a supplier:

- Is there a long business relationship with this supplier? Have there been any health problems among the purchased fish? A long track record of providing healthy fish is an obvious step toward preventing the entrance of unwanted and undetected pathogens.
- Can the supplier provide references from satisfied customers? Is there a history of selling quality products? As with any business, a list of satisfied customers goes a long way to build and validate consumer confidence.
- Does the supplier receive fish from multiple sources? Are fish from the same source in separate containment systems, or do they mix fish from multiple sources? The optimal approach would be to use a limited number of trusted fish sources and to hold the fish from each source separately.
- Does the supplier conduct disease screening? For which diseases? What tests do they use?

Screening is essential to assess disease prevalence in a group of fish and helps identify silent carriers of disease. Be aware that not all test techniques are equal, and some tests will not pick up asymptomatic carriers of disease.
- Does the supplier work with a veterinarian or fish health professional? In what capacity? Does the veterinarian come in only when health problems arise, or are they present or available to assist with health screening of new shipments as well as conduct reviews of husbandry and biosecurity practices? The latter indicates a high priority placed on healthy fish.
- Does the supplier keep species separate? Again, species in separate systems prior to shipment allows for easy identification, isolation, or removal of sick animals.
- Does the supplier have a biosecurity program? Are they willing to share the details with their clients? Be extremely cautious if the answer is "no." Such a lack of transparency may indicate that the supplier has no biosecurity program or may have significant disease problems within the facility.
- Are the fish "certified" to be free of disease? Customers need to be very careful if they hear this statement or receive a document attesting to such a fact. Typically, fish farms or fish lots are certified free of specific diseases. They are not certified or guaranteed to be healthy. In order to be certified as being free of a specific disease, fish must be sampled and tested in accordance with specific protocols established and accepted by state, national, or international authorities. For a fish farm to be certified free of a specific disease, multiple years of highly regulated testing under specified environmental conditions are required. And in some cases, no disease free certification exists (Yanong, 2001a; OIE, The World Animal Health Organization, 2006).

Water-associated entry

The presence and persistence of pathogens in water makes this medium a potential source of pathogen entry into a fish facility. Water supply is a major consideration when designing a biosecurity program based on pathogen exclusion.

Many facilities utilize municipal water. This is generally one of the safest sources of pathogen-free water as it is treated to minimize the chances of contamination. The primary concern with municipal water is water quality; facility managers must ensure that the water is properly treated to eliminate chlorine or chloramines before use in the holding systems. Another potential problem with municipal water is that it may come from multiple sources during the course of the year. Water may come from a reservoir during part of the year and from wells at other times. This can result in some dramatic water quality shifts that may compromise fish and predispose them to disease.

Wells are another good source of water for many facilities. Wells may be periodically treated with chlorine to eliminate bacterial contamination. However, the water should be regularly tested for bacterial contamination as well as heavy metals and chlorine. Be aware that well water often contains high levels of dissolved gasses, which can lead to supersaturation that can compromise fish. Installation of degassing towers will generally eliminate this problem.

Surface water runs a high risk of containing pathogens. These water sources can be home to fish, invertebrates, birds, and mammals that might be carrying pathogens or possibly toxins. The potential for contamination by sewage overflow must be considered as well. If a facility relies upon surface water, assessing and treating the water source is recommended. This would include a visual assessment of the source and the animals living in it, testing the water for bacterial or chemical contamination, and potentially treating the incoming water with prefiltration and ultraviolet light, ozone, or chlorine (Strange, 2008).

Shipping water presents a great risk. It comes from an unknown source, perhaps already contaminated by pathogens. Fish have been sealed in the water, in some cases for 12–36 hours, contaminating it with fecal material that may promote pathogen growth. Diseased fish or carriers release pathogens into the water. Water chemistry deteriorates during shipping, with high ammonia, high carbon dioxide, and low pH. Shipping water should not mix with water of any holding system except that of quarantine.

Food-associated entry

Fish food cannot only serve as a source of pathogens, but poor or contaminated diets can also compromise the fish and make them more susceptible to infection by pathogens. In most cases, good-quality commercial diets will satisfy the basic nutritional requirements of ornamental fish and are unlikely to host infectious agents. As with fish suppliers, one should consider reputation and history of service when selecting food suppliers. The food should be carefully inspected to ensure that there is no spoilage. Live foods deserve special consideration as there is a higher potential for harboring pathogens, and caution is warranted. Pretreatment or quarantine of the live food animals may be considered.

Contamination and spoilage of poor-quality feeds, before or after purchase, are valid concerns. Precautions can be taken to minimize these hazards. Commercial food should be purchased in quantities that will be used within 6 months. Once food is purchased, it should be divided into airtight containers that contain only a few days worth of food. This food should be stored in a freezer unless instructions specify otherwise. Individual bags may then be thawed in a refrigerator and fed as appropriate. If large quantities of food are being used quickly (e.g., in a large retail facility), the food should be stored in airtight moisture-proof containers in a cool, dry location free of vermin. Damp or moldy food should be immediately discarded (Crissey, 1998).

Person-associated entry

The people that enter a facility, whether staff or customers, should be considered in a biosecurity plan as they can be a source of pathogen introduction as well as pathogen persistence. Obviously, these people cannot be excluded from the facility, but the risks they pose should be managed.

Staff members have continual close contact with the facility and fish. They will be working with all components of the operation, from fish to tanks to equipment. If a worker handles an infected fish, pathogens can adhere to their skin or clothes, and as that worker moves through the facility during the course of their work, they can spread organisms to other fish, water, feed, and equipment, contaminating them and providing opportunity for further dissemination. Workers who maintain fish at their homes, participate in aquarium service activities, or work at other fish facilities could carry potentially pathogenic organisms from one facility to another if protective measures are not taken.

Customers must also be considered a potential source of pathogen introduction. It is impossible to identify those who may be coming from a visit to a facility experiencing a disease outbreak or who are having health issues in their home aquarium or pond. In either case, contamination of their skin or clothing is a real possibility, and entry into another facility without proper decontamination poses a serious threat to the health of your animals.

There are strategies that will reduce the risk of pathogens entering and spreading within a facility due to the traffic of staff, customers, and visitors, and specifics may differ depending upon whether they target staff or customers (Wolfgang, 2001).

Staff:

- Hands should be washed regularly using alcohol-based hand cleaners or soaps and hot water. This is especially important upon entering and leaving the facility, and when working from one tank to another.
- Footwear should be disinfected upon entering and leaving a facility; disinfectant footbaths should be at all entrances. The disinfectants should be changed regularly according to label directions. If the solutions become heavily contaminated with organic material (soil, feed, etc.), they should be changed as this can inactivate the chemicals. In lieu of disinfection, disposable shoe covers should be available for use upon entry and discarded upon exit from a work area. Boots can be assigned to specific work areas, being donned upon entry and removed and left at that work area upon exit.
- Uniforms or clothing specific for certain work areas will help prevent the entry and spread of contaminants into and between different areas of a facility. Individual sets of coveralls should be available at each facility site.

- Limit access to the quarantine area. Ideally, quarantine staff should only work in that area and not in the retail portion of the facility. For further protection, the quarantine area could have coveralls available that do not leave the site.
- If staff has their own ponds or tanks, do not allow them to bring fish or equipment used in their ponds into the facility.
- Staff should notify the facility manager immediately if they are having a disease outbreak in their home pond or aquarium. During that period of time, or until the nature of the outbreak is resolved, managers may not want them to work directly with fish in the facility.
- Many retail operations also encompass pond or aquarium maintenance businesses. Facility managers may want to keep maintenance staff and equipment separate from the retail facility.

Customers/visitors:

- Encourage customers to wash hands regularly, and provide wash stations with alcohol-based hand cleaners or soaps and hot water. This should be required upon entering and leaving the facility, and also when moving between tanks. In lieu of sinks, waterless hand washing stations can be provided at multiple sites throughout the facility.
- Consider utilizing a disinfectant footbath at all entrances to the facility. Ensure that disinfectant solutions are changed regularly and when contaminated with organic materials.
- Ensure that staff monitors customer activity and can see all fish tanks and customers in the facility at all times.
- Discourage customers from putting their hands in any tanks, aquaria, or ponds. If they do, ensure that they disinfect their hands afterwards.
- Do not allow customers or visitors in the quarantine facility.
- Limit entry to all restricted area and record all entries. Those entering restricted areas must follow all biosecurity guidelines appropriate for those areas.
- Restrict visitor parking to the periphery of the facility (Wolfgang, 2001).

Equipment/instrument-associated entry

Equipment and instruments brought into a facility can harbor pathogens. It is important to recognize this potential and to take precautions to neutralize this threat.

- Unless purchased new and contained in original packaging, all equipment or instruments brought into a facility from outside the building should be appropriately cleaned and disinfected. This is particularly important if they have been delivered from an unrelated fish holding facility.
- Vehicles, instruments, and equipment owned by the facility that is used for pond or aquarium maintenance at other sites should be maintained at the periphery of the facility. They too should be properly cleaned and disinfected after each visit away from the facility. Vehicle wheels and other areas that contact pond water at away sites should be a special focus of disinfection.

Quarantine to prevent pathogen entry

Quarantine is critical to preventing the introduction of pathogens into a facility. Quarantine also provides for the important process of acclimation of fish to new water conditions, new husbandry protocols, and new feeds. Furthermore, the quarantine system and quarantine period allows time for the fish immune system to recuperate from the stresses of transport and handling.

All new fish that arrive at a facility should be quarantined. Fish from separate sources should be quarantined separately. Additionally, any fish that have had contact with fish or water from other facilities, that are wild caught or farm raised, or have been returned to the facility by customers should also be quarantined before they are mixed with holding or display stock. Finally, many plants and invertebrates are capable of carrying potential fish disease agents, including intermediate stages of many common fish parasites. Therefore, it is wise to quarantine all plants and invertebrates in separate quarantine systems (Gratzek and Matthews, 1992; Yanong, 2003b; Peeler and Thrush, 2004).

Quarantine facilities and systems

A quarantine facility should be distinct from the retail or wholesale facility, either located in a separate building or within a room adjacent to the main fish holding area, physically separated by a closed door and footbath. Access to this facility is restricted to those employees assigned to this work area. The restricted access to the quarantine area should be clearly emphasized by appropriate and well-placed signage, limiting access to those properly trained and authorized to be in that area (Fig. 6.1).

Holding systems in the quarantine area are generally smaller and less extensive than retail holding or display facilities, making it easier to monitor, capture, and treat fish, remove mortalities, and more efficiently and economically heat or cool the water (Fig. 6.2). Multiple tank and life-support systems are often needed to accommodate different lots of fish. Optimally, individual life-support systems should be provided for each tank. Each setup should have a separate filtration system designed to handle fluctuating bioloads and to be easily maintained. Interconnected tanks (those that share the same water) are suitable *only* for housing fish from the same source. As water-based treatments may be necessary in quarantine tanks to address disease problems, the biological filter assembly should be designed to allow easy bypass. Poorly designed or complicated quarantine systems that are difficult to access tend to suffer from poor maintenance.

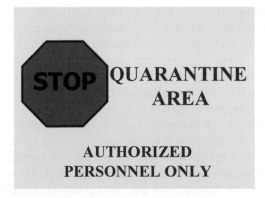

Fig. 6.1 This sign is an example of signage that might be used at the entrance to a quarantine facility.

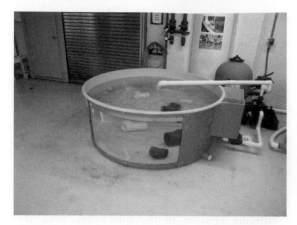

Fig. 6.2 Example of an isolated quarantine tank in a dedicated quarantine facility. Note the window for easy viewing of the fish and the life-support system that serves only this tank, thus reducing the risk of potential disease agents spreading to multiple interconnected systems.

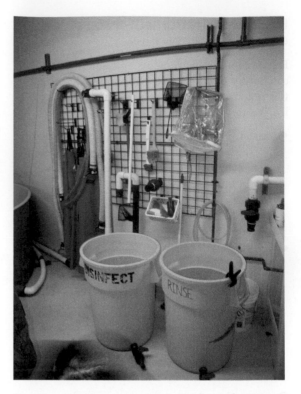

Fig. 6.3 Example of dedicated equipment for servicing a quarantine facility or system. Note the easily accessible disinfectant and rinse containers, drying racks for cleaned and disinfected equipment, and dedicated coveralls for the quarantine facility.

Water quality and husbandry for the quarantine system should be equal to or better than that of the display systems. The biofilter should be fully cycled before new fish are added, and water quality parameters should be optimal and stable. New fish are always stressed postshipping, and it is essential that they be placed in a stable environment while they undergo quarantine and acclimation.

The system should be able to comfortably accommodate the largest fish size and numbers commonly received. Habitat and hiding places in the tank should be simply constructed, easy to clean and disinfect, and should not have parts that could injure the fish. Each quarantine tank should have its own set of equipment (nets, totes, bowls, and siphons) and disinfectant baths (Fig. 6.3). Some facilities may also want to consider appropriately sized ultraviolet or ozone systems to reduce pathogen loads in the water column of the quarantine tank.

Figure 6.4 illustrates the features of a quarantine system as well as the recommended movement of fish through the ornamental fish facility.

The duration of quarantine is generally based upon the life cycle of the most common disease organisms found in the fish species of interest. A quarantine period of 2–4 weeks at the optimal

temperature is often recommended. The authors generally recommend a 4-week quarantine as a minimum for most species of fish, although many veterinarians would recommend 60–90 days of quarantine for many cool-water pond fish (Saint-Erne, 2003; Yanong, 2003a). This duration may not be practical for many businesses. If a retailer is unable to complete recommended quarantine periods, they should strongly urge their customers to establish their own quarantine in the above fashion for the recommended period of time.

Whenever possible, ornamental fish facilities should practice "all-in-all-out" stocking of the quarantine facility, that is, when a shipment of fish arrives and is placed in a system in the quarantine facility, no new fish are added to that system during the quarantine period. At the completion of the quarantine period, all fish in a quarantine system are moved out, and all tanks and associ-

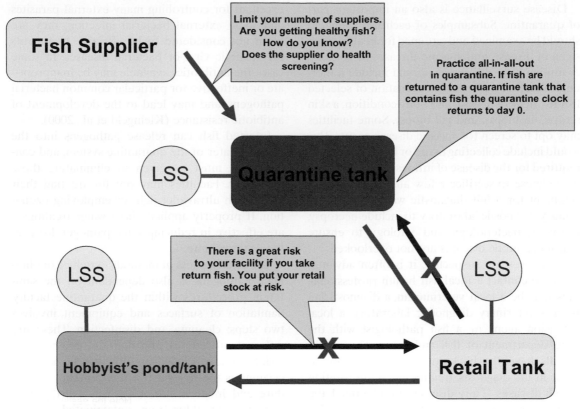

LSS = Life support system

Fig. 6.4 This diagram illustrates the recommended flow of fish through a quarantine facility at an ornamental fish retail establishment. The figure also reiterates some of the important questions and issues a facility manager must consider in order to prevent disease introduction and propagation within a facility. These same considerations would be generally applicable within any ornamental fish enterprise. LSS, life-support system.

ated life-support systems are disinfected before being used for a new lot of fish.

Fish from each supplier should be quarantined in separate systems and *not* mixed with fish from other suppliers. In the event that a group of quarantined fish breaks with disease, these precautions allow an accurate determination of the source of the diseased fish.

Ideally, a single group of fish would come into the quarantine facility, and all of the tanks would start and complete quarantine simultaneously, with the fish moving out to the retail space as a cohort. Realistically, a tank-by-tank approach is more often used due to the staggered arrival of new fish lots. But in this situation, be sure that each delivery is assigned to its own tank system

and quarantine schedule. If new fish are added to a system before the quarantine is completed, the quarantine period resets to day 0, and this combined cohort of fish are quarantined together for the entire quarantine interval.

Quarantine requires regular, periodic observation and feeding of the fish, with detailed record keeping of behavior, feeding, signs of disease, mortalities, and system maintenance. These records should be maintained by trained staff and should be easily accessible. Record keeping is important because it allows the facility manager to ensure that the fish are being observed regularly, the system is being properly maintained, and disease problems are tracked and reported in a timely manner.

Disease surveillance is also an important part of quarantine. Subsamples of each fish shipment should be examined and screened for health status, signs of disease, and specific diseases of concern. A minimum health screen should include a thorough visual and physical examination of selected fish for signs of disease and body condition, a skin scrape, fin biopsy, and gill biopsy. Some facilities may opt to screen for specific disease agents. This would include collecting tissue or blood samples as required for the disease of interest. Some facilities may choose to sacrifice a few animals from each shipment for a full diagnostic workup by a veterinary diagnostic laboratory to include necropsy, histology, bacteriology, and virology to ensure that more subtle diseases are not overlooked.

If diseases are suspected, it is often advantageous to contact a local fish health professional. This may be a local veterinarian, a diagnostician from a veterinary diagnostic laboratory, a local extension agent, or a fish pathologist with the state department of fish and game. These individuals have the background and expertise to assist in the diagnosis, treatment, and prevention of fish diseases. If any diseases are identified, the facility manager, in consultation with the fish health professional, must decide whether to treat the affected fish and/or the entire population, cull the entire population, or accept diseased fish.

Reduction and elimination of pathogens within the quarantine system

As the fish progress through the quarantine period, diseases may emerge, and treatment rather than culling of the affected fish may be considered. Prophylactic treatments may be useful, especially if there is a disease history with a particular supplier and health managers are familiar with common disease agents that might arrive with those fish. Remember that arriving fish are stressed and many of the common broad-spectrum treatments may further compromise the fish.

Some of the typical prophylactic treatments for ornamental fish include salt dips/baths, formalin bath or prolonged immersion, and copper, potassium permanganate, and various antibiotics added to the water. While these treatments are excellent for controlling many external parasites and some external bacterial infection, they are often not considered to be effective treatments for systemic viral or bacterial diseases. In some cases, the antibiotics available may be inappropriate or ineffective for particular common bacterial pathogens, and may lead to the development of antibiotic resistance (Kleingeld et al., 2000).

Infected fish can release pathogens into the holding water of the quarantine system, and consideration must be given to eliminating those pathogens. Facilities may opt for treating their water with ultraviolet light or employing ozonation. If properly applied, these water treatments are effective in reducing some pathogen loads in the water column.

The effectiveness of methods to reduce or eliminate pathogens is also dependent on the sanitation procedures within the quarantine facility. Sanitation of surfaces and equipment involves two steps: cleaning and disinfection. These are different procedures, and both are essential. As disinfectants are inactivated by organic material, cleaning is the first part of the sanitation procedure and involves removing heavy dirt, debris, and organic buildup from contaminated surfaces. Once clean, disinfectants are applied in the second part of the sanitation procedure, eliminating pathogenic organisms from the surface or rendering them inert. It is important to use an appropriate disinfectant, at the proper concentration, and allow the recommended contact time with all equipment and surfaces to assure efficacy. Table 6.1 lists some of the common disinfectants that may be used in ornamental fish facilities. Always follow the label directions on these disinfectants to ensure that they are being applied correctly (Dvorak, 2005).

Equipment should be cleaned and placed in a disinfection solution for the appropriate amount of time after each use. Buckets of disinfectants should be placed by each quarantine tank.

Ensure that all dead and moribund fish are removed promptly from the quarantine tanks as they may serve as amplification sites for pathogens, increasing their load in the water. Similarly, tanks should be kept free of fish waste and uneaten food. All can serve as sites for potential pathogens to multiply, and they will foul the water.

Table 6.1 Common disinfectants and their effectiveness.

Disinfectant	Gram-positive bacteria	Gram-negative bacteria	Acid-fast bacteria	Bacterial spores	Enveloped viruses	Nonenveloped viruses	Fungal spores
Acids	+	+	+	±	+	–	±
Alcohols	++	++	+	–	+	–	±
Aldehydes	++	++	+	+	++	+	+
Alkalis	+	+	+	±	+	±	+
Biquanides	++	++	–	–	±	–	±
Halogens—hypochlorite	+	+	+	+	+	+	+
Halogens—iodine	+	+	+	±	+	±	+
Oxidizing agents	+	+	±	+	+	±	±
Phenolic compounds	++	++	±	–	±	–	+
Quaternary ammonium compounds	++	+	–	–	±	–	±
Ozone	++	++	+	±	++	++	+
Ultraviolet light	++	++	+	±	++	++	+

Note: Removal of organic material must always precede the use of any chemical disinfectant.
Sources: Adapted from Dvorak (2005) and Opitz (1994).
++, highly effective; +, effective; ±, limited activity; –, information not available.

After fish leave the quarantine system, all tanks should be sanitized, and if possible, allowed to air-dry. If no disease outbreaks have occurred, it is probably safe to leave the biofilter functioning. If an infectious disease outbreak occurs in quarantine, all fish in that system may need to be culled and discarded, and the tanks and the biofilter should be cleaned and sanitized using the appropriate disinfectant procedures; if the biofilter cannot be sanitized easily, it should be discarded. The tanks should be allowed to air-dry after disinfection.

Pathogen containment

The quarantine system is only as strong as its physical components and the management and husbandry protocols in use. It is an accepted means to prevent the introduction of infectious disease into a fish holding facility. Quarantine, coupled with purchasing from reliable sources, provides a strong level of security from the introduction of infectious disease. But despite the best precautions, it is possible for disease to emerge in a facility. Breaks in biosecurity do occur. Quarantine failures, contaminated materials, failure to adhere to biosecurity, and simple accidents may result in the delivery of pathogens or infected fish

into a pristine tank. Managers must be prepared to deal with this situation, working to contain and eliminate the disease from the operation, and conducting a trace back investigation to determine the cause of the biosecurity break.

The methods of containment and elimination of pathogens in a facility are entwined with concepts and procedures that promote fish health and well-being. It is important to promote procedures that will assure the highest level of health in the fish, offering them the best chance to resist infection and disease by pathogens that have entered or persisted in the holding system.

Factors influencing disease resistance

A healthy, closed aquatic system, whether a pond or an aquarium, is dynamic and requires constant monitoring by the facility staff to ensure that the environment is safe and stable and fish can remain healthy and able to resist disease. Environmental fluctuations in these systems beyond normal operating parameters may compromise the fish and the environment. This can set up a situation in which pathogens may be able to infect the fish or multiply in the environment.

Fish have optimal, and often species-specific, water quality and environmental parameters required to maintain homeostasis, grow, and reproduce. If these requirements are not met, the result can be stress and its attendant deleterious effects. Fish can tolerate stressors for a time by utilizing extra energy to compensate. However, this comes at a cost as the energy to resist the stressors is taken from other important bodily functions such as osmoregulation, growth, and disease resistance. After a period of time, energy reserves are exhausted and the fish may die or become immunocompromised and susceptible to disease. For more information on stress, refer to Chapter 3 of this book.

Dramatic fluctuations in water quality can also affect biofiltration in the aquarium or pond. Water quality changes can result in the death of the bacteria in the biofilter. If not caught early through regular water quality testing, the loss of the biological filter can exacerbate the situation, resulting in further deterioration of water quality parameters.

When systems are not cleaned regularly, including removal of dead or sick fish, or if there is slow water turnover, an environment may be created conducive to pathogen growth. Pathogens will accumulate in decaying fish, food, and other organic material. The increased pathogen concentration in the fouled tank or pond will favor infection of susceptible or even healthy fish.

Overcrowding of a tank or pond, particularly if attention is not paid to proper cleaning, can quickly lead to the buildup of uneaten food, fecal matter, and subsequent pathogen overgrowth. The overcrowding not only contributes to water fouling but will also cause stress, as well as favor horizontal transmission of pathogens between fish (Wedemeyer, 1996).

Multiple aquarium or pond systems connected in a continuous water circulation loop are often used, and can be a good means of housing fish. The design of these systems requires that careful attention be paid to their proper upkeep. Accelerated pathogen growth in a contaminated unit of a recirculating loop system will rapidly progress to contamination of the entire loop by the simple flow of water from tank to tank. Poor water quality and other adverse environmental conditions can similarly propagate rapidly throughout the system. An interconnected aquarium or pond

system does not provide the same level of security that isolated or individual tank systems offer. Furthermore, while a disease outbreak in an isolated system can be easily controlled by depopulation, cleaning, and disinfection with no deleterious effect on other tank systems, all tanks comprising the contaminated loop system must be broken down and treated (Fig. 6.5). Even if there is only one tank of sick fish in a loop, there is no assurance that a disease has not spread throughout the system and/or that the other fish in the system are not compromised.

Pathogen persistence within the facility

Pathogen containment must address the persistence of pathogens within the facility. There are places in a fish holding system in which introduced pathogens may survive and perhaps even multiply. If not recognized and addressed, these persistent organisms will continue to deliver infectious agents throughout a tank or facility.

Fish can be asymptomatic carriers of disease and be capable of shedding pathogens. This is a particular problem with certain fish viruses, as survivors may be infected for life and under the right conditions will shed virus yet not show any signs of the disease themselves.

Dead and diseased fish may also serve as pathogen reservoirs. Pathogens multiply in decomposing dead fish as well as those that are ill. These pathogen reservoirs release these agents into the water, infecting tank mates and compromising water quality.

Invertebrates can serve as pathogen reservoirs (Noga, 1996; Yanong, 2003b). Invertebrates may harbor intermediate stages of certain parasites. Often the risk is rather low since these parasites require specific species of invertebrates and fish to be present for them to complete their life cycle, and not all of these are often present in typical ornamental aquariums and ponds.

Plants can also serve as pathogen reservoirs; root balls and wet leaves may harbor intermediate or resting stages of many parasites, bacteria, and viruses (Prince-Lles, 2001; Saint-Erne, 2003; Peeler and Thrush, 2004). This is the reason why a separate quarantine of pond plants, as well as

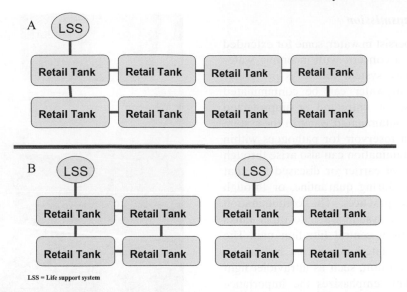

Fig. 6.5 This diagram compares two types of fish holding systems in a retail facility. Facility A represents a fish holding system that is fully interconnected (the red lines represent plumping connections between tanks) and shares one life-support system (LSS). Facility B represents two systems that are isolated from one another, each connected to their own LSS. A disease outbreak in a single tank in diagram A could easily spread throughout the whole system, while a diseases outbreak in the diagram B system would be isolated to only one of the systems. Such an outbreak might require complete depopulation and disinfection of system A, while system B would only require depopulation and disinfection of the affected system.

invertebrates, is recommended before they are mixed with fish.

The water and the life-support system can also harbor pathogens. When water quality is poor, some pathogens can multiply in the water column and, if the systems are interconnected, can spread throughout multiple tanks or ponds. The life-support system itself can, and frequently does, harbor pathogens. This includes the sumps, filtration materials, tank and pipe walls, pumps, and aeration devices. This emphasizes the importance of proper cleaning and disinfection of equipment and tank surfaces after lots of fish have moved out of a system, and certainly after a serious disease outbreak.

Other surfaces besides tank walls can be the site of pathogen persistence and proliferation. Porous materials are particularly good at offering hiding places to contaminating organisms. Pathogens can accumulate in the areas where water and dirt can accumulate and that are not easy to clean, disinfect, and dry. These would include uncoated or cracked concrete, wooden tank supports, covers and tabletops, gravel pathways, and low spots

in the floor that are poorly drained. The use of nonporous surfaces, or waterproof epoxy coatings of porous surfaces, may help eliminate such risks.

Pathogens can also accumulate on equipment that is not properly cleaned and disinfected between uses. Nets, totes, buckets, siphon hoses, scrub pads, brushes, and feeding implements should be routinely cleaned after use to prevent contamination. This includes boots and clothing of staff as well.

Routes of pathogen transmission

Once established in a tank, pathogens can be moved to other tanks, systems, or facilities in several ways. These mirror the mechanisms that allowed the entry of the organism into the facility. This movement can be even more pronounced during a disease outbreak. It is important to consider these routes of pathogen dispersal and some approaches to mitigate these risks. Additional discussion is found in the "Pathogen exclusion" section in this chapter.

Waterborne transmission

Pathogens can persist in water, some for extended periods. This is a concern with incoming water as well as in-place system water. As previously described, system water can be contaminated through the use of untreated or unprotected water sources. Contaminated water in the system then serves as a reservoir for pathogens within the facility. Contamination can also arise through the introduction of carrier or diseased fish that were not culled during quarantine, or through poor husbandry practices. The contamination can spread via the system water to other tanks interconnected by a central filtration unit. The problem is accentuated in systems lacking an in-line disinfection unit, such as ultraviolet light or ozonation. This emphasizes the importance of having isolated individual holding systems with their own life support, or individual banks of holding systems with all-in-all-out stocking in order to prevent multiunit contamination by the system water (Fig. 6.4).

Unprotected or untreated groundwater can also carry pathogens that can contaminate tank systems. Water from streams holding fish upstream from intakes can carry disease-causing agents into a facility, where design elements already described may precipitate rapid spread from tank to tank. Again, proper treatment of this water, through mechanical filtration, chlorination/dechlorination, ultraviolet light, or ozone treatment, can destroy those pathogens carried in the groundwater.

Airborne transmission

Airborne transmission of fish pathogens has significant potential for the spread of fish diseases, especially in facilities where holding tanks or ponds are in close proximity without the benefit of solid covers or substantial dividers. Water splashing, whether from cascading water, moving equipment, or surface agitation from pumps or aeration, produces water droplets that can be contaminated with pathogens, forming mists that settle over adjacent surfaces, contaminating adjacent tanks or ponds. Drafts or ventilation airflow from open windows, doors, or fans can exacerbate

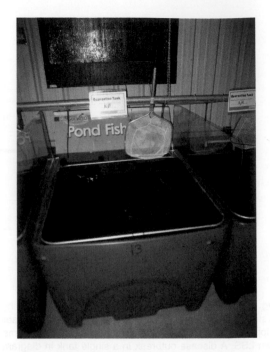

Fig. 6.6 Quarantine tank with a clear acrylic top and splash guards to reduce splash and aerosol cross-contamination between adjacent systems. Note the dedicated net for this tank hanging above the tank cover.

the problem, pushing these water droplets even further. Recent laboratory studies have shown that three common fish pathogens, *Aeromonas salmonicida*, *Ichthyophtherius multifilis*, and *Amylodinium ocellatum* could be transferred to tanks over 3 ft away through air droplets moved by a small ventilation fan (Wooster and Bowser, 1996; Bishop et al., 2003; Roberts-Thompson et al., 2006).

The risks of airborne transmission can be greatly reduced through the use of solid, preferably transparent, tank covers and/or splash guards between tanks (Fig. 6.6). In addition, careful attention to splash reduction from pumps or cascades, or when installing or moving equipment or fish, will further reduce the risk of aerosol transmission.

Vector transmission

Vectors are living organisms that may harbor and transmit pathogens from one fish to another. Examples in the aquatic environment include the crustacean parasite *Argulus* sp. and some species of leeches. Pathogens harbored by these vectors can be deposited on or within fish, and disease may follow. Vectors often cause disease in their own right. Heavy infestations of *Argulus* or leeches are capable of inflicting serious damage to fish skin and gills. Prevention of vector transmission is best achieved through the control of the vectors themselves, either during quarantine or via prompt identification and control in the display or holding system. Control measures include bath treatments of formalin, organophosphates, and chelated copper, or manual removal (Noga, 1996; Yanong, 2003c).

Fomite transmission

Fomites are inanimate objects on which pathogens can be transmitted from location to location. This can include equipment used in a facility as well as staff and visitors. Pathogen transmission via fomites usually occurs by sharing equipment between tanks or systems without proper cleaning and disinfection after each use. To prevent this, they must be properly handled and disinfected. Each tank, isolated system, quarantine facility, and site should have its own set of equipment and instruments, including nets, totes, buckets, brushes, scrapers, siphons, and pumps. In addition, each area should have its own cleaning, disinfection, and drying station. Disinfection of equipment between uses is an industry standard to prevent cross contamination and to eliminate persistence of pathogens on equipment and instruments. Anything that is exposed to fish, holding water, or potentially contaminated surfaces should be cleaned and disinfected before the next use. None of these should contact or move to other work areas. All materials should be dried on a drying rack or hanger. Laying equipment on the ground or draping over the side of a tank is not recommended, as there is the potential to pick up contaminants and move them to another site. Workstations (tables and counters) where fish, water, or equipment is used should likewise be cleaned and disinfected. Facilities that provide on-site pond and aquarium construction or maintenance should also consider the cleaning and disinfection of work vehicles, especially in the face of potential serious disease outbreaks.

Pathogen transmission in the feed

Fish foods, whether live, fresh, or frozen, carry the potential for disease transmission if contaminated by pathogens or toxins. All foods must be of the highest quality and obtained from reputable sources that understand the importance of proper animal food manufacture and storage. Just as with newly arrived fish, live foods should be quarantined, examined, and treated for any identified diseases before they are used. Fresh and frozen food should be of high quality and not show any signs of spoilage or decay. Commercial feeds should be purchased in lots that can typically be fed in 6 months, broken up into small packages for weekly or daily use, and properly stored. Feeds should not be fed if they are damp, moldy, or have a foul odor (Tacon, 1992; Crissey, 1998; Yanong, 2001a).

Best health practices that support biosecurity

There are husbandry practices that promote fish health and well-being, and in so doing help support the principles and goals of a biosecurity program. These help assure healthy stock that are free of stress and are in optimal condition to resist infection.

Routine and reliable visual assessment of the fish is essential. This may be the first line of defense against disease outbreaks within the tanks. Staff should constantly be scanning the fish populations and looking for signs of outright disease, as well as signs of distress or abnormal behavior, both of which may be the first signs of an impending disease outbreak. Affected animals should be moved to a hospital tank for observation and treatment.

Fish holding systems should be designed so that fish can be easily viewed and captured, yet still have adequate hiding spaces. There should be no edges or objects within the tanks or ponds that might injure the fish. Furthermore, all tanks and life-support systems should be easy to maintain and service. If systems are difficult to access and clean, then it is likely that staff will tend to avoid the optimal level of maintenance and cleaning.

Staff should also be encouraged to frequently wash their hands, particularly when moving from work areas in one fish holding system to another. Hand washing stations and footbaths, soap or other appropriate disinfectants, and paper towels should be easily accessible so that they will be used regularly.

Equipment cleaning and disinfection stations must also be easily accessible to ensure regular use. A schedule for regular changes of disinfectants must also be initiated.

Ensure that the staff adheres to the principles of isolation and independence of systems. Reducing the number of systems connected to a single central filtration unit, limiting the movement of fish from tank to tank, and striving to prevent cross contamination via waterborne, airborne, and fomite transmission will enhance the isolation of fish holding systems.

Anything that might stress fish should be eliminated or minimized. It is the responsibility of the staff to be vigilant for any signs of stress in the fish, as well as any aspect of the husbandry or system design that might contribute to stress. Fish density, water quality, water flow, and tank/pond sanitation should be continually monitored to assure that they remain in optimal ranges or conditions. Fish should be handled as little as possible, and when handled, all precautions must be taken to assure that the fish are minimally stressed and not injured.

Nutrition must not be ignored. Foods should not only provide a balanced diet, but they also must be handled and stored appropriately to assure their continued quality. Nutritional diseases, whether due to nutrient deficiencies or food contamination, can impact immune function in fish, reducing their resistance to infection, and impacting the success of your biosecurity plan. Care must be taken to assure that all fish are receiving an adequate and complete diet. Items to consider are as follows:

- Insufficient quantity or intake of food will lead to starvation, causing poor growth, poor survival, increased susceptibility to disease, and a loss of reproductive capacity.
- An imbalanced diet due to the feeding of one particular food type to the exclusion of all

others may lead to deficiencies of certain essential nutrients, with diminished survival.
- Many diets may not meet the needs of certain fish species that have specific nutritional needs or feeding behaviors. Special diets or supplementation of commercial diets may be necessary. Seek guidance from those familiar with husbandry of the species or from the literature.
- Be wary of poorly formulated diets. This is rare when good-quality, commercially prepared diets are used.
- Outdated, spoiled, or improperly stored diets will lose nutritional value, and dietary deficits may occur. These foods should be discarded (Winfree, 1992; Roberts, 2001; Yanong, 2001a).

Dead or sick fish should be promptly culled and examined by trained staff or veterinarians to identify the cause of death or illness so that corrective and preventative measures and treatments can be started. Routine health monitoring of apparently healthy fish may be considered to identify emerging disease issues within a facility before they become a serious problem.

During the daily work routine, the staff should address the needs of the most susceptible fish and their holding facilities first, moving to the fish with the highest probability of carrying disease last. Typically, this means that the display fish are cared for first, starting with the youngest and moving to the oldest fish. Then the staff goes to systems holding fish under quarantine. Finally, any hospitalized fish or fish undergoing treatment are attended to. These workers should not go back and work with display fish until the next day. If not possible, that individual should wash well and perhaps change clothes after working with quarantine and hospitalized fish. Alternatively, facilities may opt to designate one individual that only works with animals under quarantine and treatment and never works with display or holding fish.

Quality management

A quality management program (aka quality assurance, quality control) is an integral part of any biosecurity plan. It will help assure that the biosecurity practices that are established for a facility are actually put into place and followed. It is essential that biosecurity practices are used consistently and accurately and are not just brought out when they are remembered or might help control a problem. The quality program will instill a sense of routine to the biosecurity procedures and will assure that employees use the procedures correctly. It also provides a means of checking and verifying. Quality management concepts should permeate all aspects of the biosecurity protocols. Quality management is the key to a successful biosecurity program.

The basic components of the quality program include written standard operating procedures (SOPs), training, record keeping, accountability, and audits. All are important, and none can be neglected.

SOPs

SOPs are documents that detail the daily practices a facility employs to ensure that disease agents are not introduced and do not spread within a fish facility, and these are the tools that will help keep those fish healthy. The SOPs provide specific, step-by-step instructions for performing each of the procedures that form the biosecurity system, and help ensure that employees correctly and consistently perform these tasks. SOPs provide information about the reason for a task, the materials needed to complete the task, the actions taken to complete the task, reference information, and the date the SOP was approved or revised.

Controlled copies of SOPs are kept in each work area, or minimally, in a central location accessible to workers. If questions arise regarding a particular procedure, the SOPs are readily available to the employees in that area and will provide the necessary guidance.

Employees must read and understand each of the SOPs used in their work area or that apply to their position. It does no good to have SOPs if they are not read and followed. Training in the SOPs should be part of the training for all employees.

A standard format for SOPs is recommended. This makes them readily recognizable within a facility or business and provides a routine pattern for their composition. Using a standard format also makes it less likely to leave out important components.

SOPs are not static; they undergo continual evolution. New information is continually being generated regarding fish husbandry, and the SOPs must keep pace, assuring they provide accurate information regarding procedures. Revision of SOPs is part of the quality process, and SOPs should be reviewed on a regular basis for relevance and accuracy. Changes can be made and revised SOPs can be issued. Any new procedures require matching new SOPs. Employee training on new or revised SOPs is essential to assure that proper procedures are being used.

Staff training

The success of a biosecurity program is dependent on making it a part of routine operations. Its components must be employed on a regular basis. Implementation of the program requires that all of those entrusted with the care and handling of the animals receive thorough training in the biosecurity protocols selected for the operation. This also requires that those employees understand the importance of the program, not only for the health of the fish but also for the security of their jobs. Employee buy-in is essential for the beneficial effects of the biosecurity program to be realized.

New employees should receive standardized training on all biosecurity policies and procedures used in their facility. Training should include instruction by the trainer on the security procedures in use in the work area, followed by the employee demonstrating their ability to conduct the procedures in a competent manner with continued support through peer-to-peer training and evaluation. Details of the policies and procedures should be found in the appropriate SOPs. It is essential that facility management demonstrate the commitment to biosecurity through their own example in facility operations by providing regular continuing education opportunities, providing regular positive and negative feedback, and ensuring that employees have the necessary resources to practice effective biosecurity (Delabbio, 2006).

Employee training should be documented, and training records should be maintained either in work areas or employee files. These records can take the form of simple checklists showing training activities and dates of successful completion for each employee. This provides a readily available means to verify that all employees have been instructed in the proper use of biosecurity measures within their work area.

Periodic review of biosecurity protocols for all employees should be conducted. This can be individual or group instruction. This is an opportunity to reinforce the importance of the program and review procedures, helping assure that all employees are adhering to the security protocols and implementing them in the same manner. Periodic reviews will reduce the likelihood of breaks in compliance.

Retraining should be considered for any employee who fails to comply with biosecurity protocols. Noncompliance may be determined through direct observation or follow-up investigations following breaks in biosecurity. It is crucial for the success of the operation that these security breaks be addressed quickly and effectively.

Training must be timely. This should be one of the first activities provided to new employees. Training must also reflect changes in SOPs. As new biosecurity protocols are evaluated and employed, the SOPs must reflect these changes, and employees must be trained in the new methods.

Record keeping

Written records are essential in order to maintain a performance history for a facility. A record system that documents and archives information on all aspects of the operation will be an invaluable tool for demonstrating the effectiveness of a biosecurity program, the performance of the equipment and instruments, and the health of the animals. It provides a documented history of performance that can assist in determining where weaknesses may exist. These records can also be a useful tool to convince customers of the quality of the products.

Some types of records are considered standard for aquatic systems: water temperature and water chemistry values, cumulative mortalities, production statistics, and feed consumption and conversion are routinely used in aquaculture facilities.

But there are additional records that should be considered. Performance, calibration, and maintenance records for instruments and equipment should be developed and archived. For example, daily temperatures readings for refrigerators and freezers, and periodic calibration reports for oxygen meters or water chemistry units help verify that on any given day, the equipment was operating within specifications and is doing so consistently. It also helps highlight trends that may indicate equipment failure.

These records can take the form of simple checklists, set up for entry on a daily basis, or any other time frame that is appropriate. Or they can consist of logbooks assigned to an instrument. No matter the format, it is important to retain these records for a selected period of time. These archives provide performance tracking and can be a tool to troubleshoot biosecurity failures. Archived records can be kept for a time period that suits specific needs, but in some facilities, records may be retained for years.

Record keeping should extend to the training of employees. Training records are a means to quickly verify that an employee has received the information needed to perform their job correctly and consistently. And it is the means to verify that time for retraining has arrived.

Accountability

All recorded information should be accompanied by notation that includes identification of the person entering the information and the date/time of entry. This provides accountability within the operation. For any given recorded activity of record, one can identify not only the result but also the employee responsible for the activity on that date and time. This provides a valuable and reliable means of trace back when trying to determine the cause of a system malfunction or failure. It can also provide a cross-check of the facility training program, verifying that employees continue to follow the expected procedures.

Audits

In order to verify that the components of the quality management system are fully implemented, and likewise that the biosecurity program is protected by that quality system, it is necessary to perform periodic performance evaluations, or audits. The audit is a careful review of all components of the quality system to assure each is in place, each is in use, and each is being used in the correct fashion. The audit can be conducted by a designated person from within the operation or by an individual from outside, such as a veterinarian. Audits should be done periodically, on a timetable to meet your individual needs, and certain components of the quality system may be audited more frequently than others.

The audit should include a review of SOPs. SOPs should be available for all important activities. Employee training documents for the SOPs should be part of this review as well.

Records should be examined. They should be complete, dated, and signed by the employee responsible for the activity of record. Training records should be verified for completeness for all employees.

A review of equipment and supplies is an important part of the audit. Expiration dates on feeds, medications, and chemicals should be verified, and outdated materials should be discarded and replaced. Equipment records should be reviewed to assure that they are being serviced and calibrated appropriately and that they are performing within specifications. This not only assures that the biosecurity program is not weakened in these areas but may also help identify sources of business inefficiency and economic waste.

Worker safety issues are typically included in quality audits. It is an opportunity to evaluate safety training programs as well as safety equipment (e.g., ground fault indicators, fire extinguishers, nonslip floor coverings), enhancing the work environment for employees.

The results of audits should be documented, and records of audits should be retained as with other quality documents. Deficiencies identified during audits must be corrected, and those corrections verified.

While audits of SOPs or training records may occur annually or semiannually, some components of the quality system are reviewed more often or continually. As entries are made for temperature and water quality reading from holding facilities or refrigeration and heating units, previous readings on that record are easily reviewed and the data can be assessed for trends or abrupt transitions that indicate reduced or erratic performance. Corrective actions can be implemented immediately before complete system failure occurs.

Audits of the biosecurity program may reveal weaknesses that need to be corrected. Those corrections will result in modified or new procedural SOPs. All employees must therefore be trained on those new methods (Delabbio, 2006).

Quality management is important to the success of the biosecurity program, and hence to the success of the operation. Implementing a quality management program is well worth the time and effort. It is an integral part of biosecurity—providing a means to verify and validate the strength of your biosecurity program.

Summary

A biosecurity program is essential to successful fish production and husbandry. The components of the program address exclusion of pathogens, control of pathogens, and good health practices, and assemble to provide a security system that will help minimize the impact of disease on a fish facility. A successful biosecurity program requires commitment by the management and staff to follow operational policies and procedures and to continually assess, and modify as necessary, those practices. A good biosecurity program protects the business by protecting the animals and the customers.

References and further reading

Bishop, T.M., Smalls, A., Wooster, G.A., et al. (2003) Aerobiological (airborne) dissemination of fish pathogen *Ichthyophtherius multifilis* and the implications in fish health management. In *Biosecurity in Aquaculture Production Systems: Exclusion of Pathogens and Other Undesirables* (Lee, C-S. and O'Bryen, P.J., eds.), pp. 43–61. Baton Rouge, LA: World Aquaculture Society.

Crissey, S.D. (1998) *Handling Fish Fed to Fish-Eating Animals, A Manual of Standard Operating Procedures.* Beltsville, MD: US Department of Agriculture, National Agricultural Research Service, National Agricultural Library.

Delabbio, J. (2006) How farm workers learn to use and practice biosecurity. *Journal of Extension* **44** (6). http://www.joe.org/joe/2006December/a1.ph (accessed June 19, 2009).

Dvorak, G. (2005) *Disinfection 101*. Center for Food Security and Public Health. www.cfsph.iastate.edu/BRM/resources/Disinfectants/Disinfection101Feb2005.pdf.

Gratzek, J.B. and Matthews, J.R. (1992) *The Science of Fish Health Management*. Morris Plains, NJ: Tetra Press.

Kleingeld, D.W., Braune, S., Schotfeldt, H-J., et al. (2000) Bacterial isolations, resistance development and risk analysis in the ornamental fish trade. Paper presented at the 5th International Aquarium Congress, Monaco Oceanographic Institute. http://intaquaforum.org/PROC%20MONACO%20I/.

Lee, C-S. and O'Bryen, P.J., eds. (2003) *Biosecurity in Aquaculture Production Systems: Exclusion of Pathogens and Other Undesirables*. Baton Rouge, LA: World Aquaculture Society.

Miller-Morgan, T.J. and Hartman, K. (2007) Koi herpes virus (KHV) biosecurity for ornamental pond fish retailers. Paper presented at the Koi Health Academy, University of Nevada—Reno, Reno, Nevada, February 24–25.

Noga, E.J. (1996) *Fish Disease: Diagnosis and Treatment*. New York: Mosby.

OIE, The World Animal Health Organization. (2006) *Manual of Diagnostic Tests for Aquatic Animals 2006*. www.oie.int/eng/normes/fmanual/A_summry.htm.

Opitz, H.M. (1994) *Biosecurity in Aquaculture: Practical Steps for Healthy Fish (VHS tape and circular)*. Orono: University of Maine Cooperative Extension.

Ornamental Aquatic Trade Organization. (2004) *Biosecurity and the Ornamental Fish Industry—Future Proofing the Industry*. Westbury, Wiltshire: Ornamental Aquatic Trade Association.

Peeler, E.J. and Thrush, M.A. (2004) Qualitative analysis of the risk of introducing *Gyrodactylus salaris* into the United Kingdom. *Diseases of Aquatic Organisms* **62**: 103–113.

Prince-Lles, F. (2001) Pond fish keeping. In *British Small Animal Veterinary Association Manual of Ornamental Fish*, 2nd Edition (Wildgoose, W.H., ed.), pp. 25–36. Gloucester: British Small Animal Veterinary Association.

Roberts, R.J. (2001) The nutritional pathology of teleosts. In *Fish Pathology*, 3rd Edition (Roberts, R.J., ed.), pp. 347–366. New York: W.B. Saunders.

Roberts-Thompson, A., Barnes, A., Fielder, D.S., et al. (2006) Aerosol dispersal of the fish pathogen, *Amyloodinium ocellatum*. *Aquaculture* **257**: 118–123.

Saint-Erne, N. (2002) *Advanced Koi Care for Veterinarians and Professional Pond Keepers*. Glendale, AZ: Erne Enterprises.

Scarfe, A.D., Lee, C.S., and O'Bryen, P.J. (2006) *Aquaculture Biosecurity: Prevention, Control and Eradication of Aquatic Animal Disease*. Ames, IA: Blackwell.

Strange, R. (2008) Facility design considerations for healthy fish. Paper presented at the Koi Health Academy, University of Nevada—Reno, Reno, Nevada, February 24–25.

Tacon, A.G.J. (1992) Nutritional Fish Pathology, Morphological Signs of Nutrient Deficiency and Toxicity in Farmed Fish. *FAO Fisheries Technical Paper 330*.

Wedemeyer, G.A. (1996) *Physiology of Fish in Intensive Culture Systems*. New York: Chapman and Hall.

Winfree, R.A. (1992) Nutrition and feeding of tropical fish. In *Aquariology: The Science of Fish Health Management* (Gratzek, J.B. and Matthews, J.R., eds.), pp. 186–206. Morris Plains, NJ: Tetra Press.

Wolfgang, D.R. (2001) *Biosecurity: A Practical Approach*. Pennsylvania State University, College of Agricultural Sciences, Cooperative Extension. http://vetextension.psu.edu/resources/pdf/biosecurity/BiosecurityIRS.pdf.

Wooster, G.A. and Bowser, P.R. (1996) The aerobiological pathway of a fish pathogen: survival and dissemination of *Aeromonas salmonicida* in aerosols and its implications in fish health management. *Journal of the World Aquaculture Society* **27**: 7–14.

Yanong, R.P.E. (2001a) US legislation. In *British Small Animal Veterinary Association Manual of Ornamental Fish*, 2nd Edition (Wildgoose, W.H., ed.), pp. 281–283. Gloucester: British Small Animal Veterinary Association.

Yanong, R.P.E. (2001b) Nutritional disorders. In *British Small Animal Veterinary Association Manual of Ornamental Fish*, 2nd Edition (Wildgoose, W.H., ed.), pp. 225–229. Gloucester: British Small Animal Veterinary Association.

Yanong, R.P.E. (2003a) *UF/IFAS Circular 120 Fish Health Management Considerations in Recirculating Aquaculture Systems—Part 1: Introduction and General Principles*. http://edis.ifas.ufl.edu/FA099.

Yanong, R.P.E. (2003b) *UF/IFAS Circular 121 Fish Health Management Considerations in Recirculating Aquaculture Systems—Part 2: Pathogens*. http://edis.ifas.ufl.edu/FA100.

Yanong, R.P.E. (2003c) *UF/IFAS Circular 122 Fish Health Management Considerations in Recirculating Aquaculture Systems—Part 3: General Recommendations and Problem-Solving Approaches*. http://edis.ifas.ufl.edu/FA101.

Chapter 7
Nutrition in Fish

Richard Strange

Introduction

Nutrition impacts every life stage of an animal. Failure to provide optimal nutrition can directly result in disease outbreaks or in a weakened immune system that can predispose fish to disease. The specific dietary requirements have not been identified for every species of fish held in captivity so careful attention to the variety, quality, and freshness of ingredients is important when attempting to duplicate a natural diet in aquatic pets.

Constraints of the aquatic environment

The aquatic environment differs greatly from the terrestrial environment. In the terrestrial environment, ambient temperature rapidly changes; in the aquatic environment, there are slower changes and temperature changes are buffered by the high specific heat of water. Additionally, the aquatic environment may suffer from a lack of oxygen availability (see Chapter 1 for a full discussion of the temperature and oxygen constraints). These two environmental traits favored poikilothermy over homeothermy in the dominant aquatic vertebrates, that is, fish.

Essentially, poikilotherms need less food than similarly sized homeotherms for maintenance of body weight. Young, rapidly growing animals of both types need more food for weight gain than mature animals; however, fish tend to have somewhat indeterminate growth. The fact that fish need less food to live is part of the reason why overfeeding is such a problem with begin-

ning fish hobbyists. The other reason is that when one overfeeds their dog, the uneaten food sits in the bowl with little consequence. Not so in the water; the ignored food soon disperses and begins contributing to the organic load of the pond or aquarium, which results in a decline in dissolved oxygen and an increase in ammonia.

Another big difference in the aquatic and terrestrial environments that has determined the nutritional requirements of fish is the food chain. Consider that while the terrestrial ecosystem is well represented by large herbivores, including many ruminants that have the ability to digest cellulose, the aquatic environment, conversely, is almost entirely populated by carnivorous, or at most omnivorous, vertebrates. Even the marine mammals, with the sole exception of the manatee, are meat eaters. The only truly herbivorous fish that comes to mind is the white amur or "grass carp," and it is not a ruminant.

The reason for this vast difference in fauna is the source of plant production, and that relates to the effects of gravity. Along with temperature and oxygen, the aquatic environment differs from the terrestrial one in the lack of effective gravity (technically, aquatic organisms are under a $1g$ gravitational pull like terrestrial organisms, but as a practical matter, gravity is offset by buoyancy). On earth, plants compete for sunlight by growing upward toward the sun against gravity using the structural carbohydrate cellulose, that is, woody matter, for support. This means that all plants, from grasses to redwoods, are sizeable and contain lots of cellulose, which many terrestrial animals exploit as a food source. In the aquatic realm, plants also compete for light, but they do not have to fight gravity to do so; they simply float up to the top of the water column and the smaller they are, the easier it is to float above their competitors. Thus, plant production in water is dominated not by large woody plants but by microscopic phytoplankton. Animals must have appropriate-sized food particles to effectively feed themselves. The smallest vertebrate animal is, in fact, a fish and is just over an inch in length at maturity. This is still much too large to efficiently graze on microscopic phytoplankton. So, what ecologists call the "primary consumer" or herbivore in the food chain is not a fish but microscopic invertebrate predators known as zooplankton. Zooplankton are much larger than the phytoplankton and can be used as food by fish fry and adult fish if they are specialized planktivores. Thus, by the time we get up the food chain to vertebrates (fish) in aquatic habitats, we find that they are, by necessity, carnivores. There are, of course, vascular plants, "water weeds," and large algae (e.g., kelp) in aquatic environments, but they provide little food for fish. Also, in some freshwater aquatic environments (e.g., streams), plant material imported from the terrestrial environment (e.g., leaf litter) brings a lot of energy into the aquatic system, but the components that are easily digestible are soon leached and decomposed leaving only the cellulose, which insects can utilize, but not fish. This explains why many pet fish (e.g., koi), while not as strictly carnivorous as trout, still require a sizable percentage of their diet as protein and have other requirements that reflect the animal food-based nature of the aquatic food chain.

One more effect of habitat on nutrition is the way fish metabolize protein differently from terrestrial animals. All animals create ammonia during the catabolism of the amino acids that make up proteins. Ammonia is toxic, and its accumulation in the body cannot be tolerated. Mammals turn ammonia into urea in the liver. Urea is water soluble and less toxic than ammonia, and mammals excrete it in the urine. In order to reduce water weight for flight, birds create a solid nitrogenous waste product, uric acid, which is excreted with the feces. Since fish have constant exchange with water at the gill, they can continuously excrete ammonia directly, without conversion, as soon as it is produced. Mammals and birds pay a caloric penalty for eating protein.

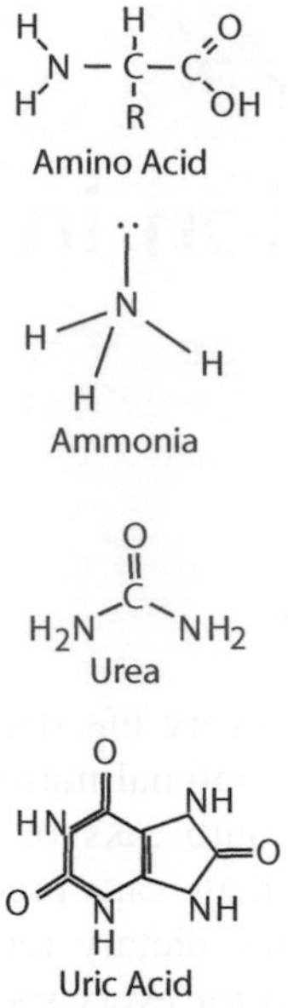

Fig. 7.1 Typical amino acid and waste forms of nitrogen used in different vertebrates (ammonia, fish; urea, mammals; uric acid, birds).

When carbohydrate or fat is metabolized, about 5% of the assimilated energy is used for changing the structure of the food molecules into forms the body can use, and the remaining 95% can be used for maintenance and growth. When mammals and birds metabolize protein, however, the metabolic cost increases to about 15% because of the energy used to build urea or uric acid (see Fig. 7.1). Since fish do not have to expend energy to change ammonia to urea or uric acid, they do not have to pay the energy expense to use protein for food as birds or mammals do. Fish have about a 5% metabolic cost of digestion whether protein is part of the meal or not. Since fish do not have an additional metabolic cost associated with feeding on protein, they can direct more of the energy in food toward production and maintenance. This is another reason why fish need less food than birds and mammals. The fact that fish excrete ammonia directly is the reason why high-protein feeds, whether eaten or not (aquatic, decomposing bacteria also directly excrete ammonia), cause an ammonia spike in the pond or aquarium. In crowded conditions, ammonia may build up to toxic levels. This is rarely a problem in nature, where fish are fewer and available food is less.

Different species of fish vary with respect to nutritional requirements just as different homeotherms do. Scientific determination of nutritional requirements is a slow, expensive endeavor, and the few fish that have been thoroughly researched are the common production aquaculture species: trout, salmon, channel catfish, tilapia, and common carp. While a variety of fish are kept as pets, the only pet fish for which there is a systematic scientific information of nutritional requirements is the colorful variant of the common carp, the koi. So, while much of this chapter is generally applicable to all pet fish, specific recommendations can only be given for koi.

Proteins and amino acids

While all living things require protein for enzymes, plants and animals differ somewhat beyond that in their use of protein. In plants, the carbohydrate cellulose serves as the primary structural element in forming the body of the plant, and therefore they are rich in carbohydrates. Animals, on the other hand, contain very little carbohydrate and depend primarily on protein to form the body (along with calcium for bone in vertebrates). So, fish, like all animals, consist mainly of protein, although some individuals may also contain a significant portion of fat. Given the importance of protein in enzymes and structure of fish and the fact that over 50% of the dry matter in a typical fish diet is protein, the importance of protein is clear.

Proteins are made up of a series of amino acids connected to each other by strong covalent chemical bonds. Amino acids themselves, of course, are small organic molecules characterized by having an amino group (NH_2). When this amino group is cleaved during deamination, ammonia is formed. Proteins are significant in that they are the only organic compounds containing significant amounts of nitrogen. While the primary structure of proteins is the linear "bead on a string" form, most proteins assume secondary, three-dimensional (3-D) structures that are held together by hydrogen bonds. This 3-D version is usually required for

proper function of enzymes and occurs after the basic backbone is formed.

Essential amino acids

There are about 20 different amino acids commonly found in life forms. Of those, some are termed essential (or indispensible) in animal nutrition because they cannot be synthesized in the animal from other amino acids and must occur at some minimal level in the diet or malnutrition and death will occur. Different animals have different essential amino acids. For example, humans have eight (or nine depending on how they are counted) essential amino acids, while all the fish that have been tested require 10 (arginine, histidine, isoleucine, leucine, lysine, methionine, phenylalanine, threonine, tryptophan, and valine).

Moreover, the exact minimum requirement as a percentage of the diet for any essential amino acid is different for each species. This can only be determined by painstaking experimentation; therefore, the exact requirement of the essential amino acids is only known for a few fish. Of the common pet fish, the exact amino acid requirement is known for carp (koi) only.

Animal versus plant proteins

Vegetarians sometimes insist that there is no difference between animal and plant protein; however, the distinction is valid one. While it is true that all essential amino acids occur in both plant and animal sources, there tends to be a significant difference between the amino acid profiles found in plants and animals. The percentage of the different amino acids in human protein are much more similar to a cow than to, say, a soybean plant. So, an animal can consume less total protein and still meet its amino acid requirements if it consumes an animal source. As mentioned previously, plant protein comes along with a lot of carbohydrate, both digestible (sugars, starch) and indigestible (cellulose, i.e., fiber). For omnivores such as humans, consuming plenty of carbohydrates with our protein is no problem; but for fish, which tend toward carnivory, it can be a serious problem, as we shall see in a later section.

Table 7.1 Total protein requirements of humans and common domestic animals as % of diet (dry).

	%
Humans	10–15
Dogs	15–27
Cats	30
Tilapia	32
Channel catfish	32
Common carp	35
Rainbow trout	38
Pacific salmon	38

Note: A source of confusion when studying nutrient requirements is the basis of comparison. There is no real standard, and different sources report nutritional information in different ways. For example, protein requirements can be reported as mg protein/kg body weight/day or as a percent of the total diet. Amino acid requirements are reported both as a percentage of the total diet and as a percentage of the protein portion of the diet. A percentage of the diet may be on an "as fed" basis (with a dry diet, that would be about 10% moisture) or, a similar but slightly different, absolute dry weight basis (0% moisture), or even on the basis of energy (kCal).

Table 7.2 Amino acid requirements of juvenile common carp.

Amino acid	Requirement as % protein	Requirement as % of dry diet
Arginine	4.3	1.6
Histidine	2.1	0.8
Isoleucine	2.5	0.9
Leucine	3.3	1.3
Lysine	5.7	2.2
Methionine*	3.1	1.2
Phenylalanine†	6.5	2.5
Threonine	3.9	1.5
Tryptophan	0.8	0.3
Valine	3.6	1.4

Source: Committee on Animal Nutrition, Board on Agriculture, National Research Council (1993).
*In the absence of dietary cystine.
†In the absence of tyrosine, with 1% tyrosine in the diet, phenylalanine requirement was 3.4% of protein or 1.3% of dry matter.

Total protein requirement of koi

Since the complete dietary requirements are known for one pet fish (koi), it will be the focus of this chapter. It should be understood that other captive fish may have slightly different, but probably unknown, requirements; however, the generalizations in this chapter will hold for almost any fish. In Table 7.1 are the protein requirements of the five fish species for which dietary requirements are well established, compared with three common terrestrial animals. The fishes needing the least protein in the diet (tilapia and channel catfish) have higher protein requirements than one of the most carnivorous domestic terrestrial animals, the house cat.

Table 7.2 shows the essential amino acid requirements for koi. Simply adding the individual amino acid requirements will not yield the total protein requirement, of course. Much more protein must be provided for normal growth and health.

Protein, especially animal protein, tends to be an expensive ration component compared with fats and carbohydrates. Therefore, in production rations developed for food animals, great

effort is made to keep protein content close to the minimum required. The cost of feed is of a lesser concern to the koi owner, and feeds with higher protein content are commonly available. All animals, especially fish, easily use protein in excess of the amount necessary for maintenance and growth as an energy source. It should also be mentioned that the 35% requirement for koi is a minimum for normal growth. During periods of slow growth, such as cold water conditions, the percentage protein can be reduced with no ill effects. However, this author does not believe that lower protein would be advantageous in the winter, although some feed manufacturers recommend seasonal changes in diet. One caveat: When protein content is reduced, the energy of the diet is almost always made up with more carbohydrate. As we will see later, carbohydrate needs to be used cautiously in fish foods.

Proteins and water quality

The two water quality characteristics most likely to cause a crisis in a koi pond are oxygen and ammonia, and both are heavily influenced by feeding. Oxygen is used by koi and decomposing bacteria to break down all feed components (proteins, fats, and carbohydrates). When protein is digested by fish or bacteria, ammonia is produced. More feed, or higher-protein feed, will produce more ammonia. Fasted fish produce relatively little ammonia. The vast majority of ammonia production in a koi pond occurs in the 2 hours immediately after feeding; therefore, biofilters must manage large pulses of ammonia, and it is impossible to keep enough nitrifiers alive between spikes to completely eliminate the pulses when they occur. Moreover, the nitrifiers themselves consume large amounts of oxygen as they oxidize ammonia to nitrate. So, the pond owner must be aware that feeding the fish will always produce an increase in ammonia and a decrease in oxygen. Overfeeding can cause the spike to be deadly.

Fats (lipids) and carbohydrates

Saturated versus unsaturated fats

Not surprisingly, fish use fats differently than homeothermic terrestrial animals. The primary difference is that temperate fish have almost no saturated fat compared with birds and mammals, which contain primarily saturated fats. That difference relates to the environment, just like all the nutritional differences do.

All fats consist of a three-carbon backbone derived from glycerol (i.e., glycerin). Attached to these three carbons are additional strings of carbons (fatty acids). Combined, the glycerol and the three fatty acids are termed triglycerides or, simply, fats. As you can see from Figure 7.2, fats contain little oxygen; therefore, they are fully reduced carbon compounds. This is why they contain twice the energy (about 9 kCal/g or 240 kCal/oz) compared with carbohydrates and proteins (4 kCal/g or 110 kCal/oz), which contain significant oxygen, making them about half reduced. Fully reduced carbon compounds, such as fats, or gasoline for that matter, contain more energy because all the carbons can be oxidized to carbon dioxide, while half-reduced compounds such as sugars, or wood, already have the carbons partially oxidized.

Both saturated and unsaturated fats contain little oxygen, but they differ in that all the carbon in the strings of saturated fats has every possi-

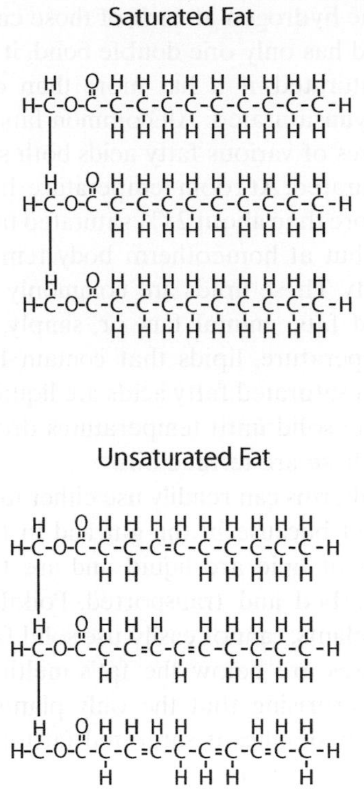

Saturated Fat

Unsaturated Fat

Fig. 7.2 Examples of structure of saturated and unsaturated fats (triglycerides).

Table 7.3 Lipids in order of saturation.

Lipid origin	% saturated	% unsaturated
Coconut	90	9
Butter	61	33
Aji-aji*	46	42
Beef	37	61
Carp	31	68
Chicken	29	65
Brook trout	26	72
Salmon	18	80
Peanut	16	79
Soybean	14	81
Olive	12	86
Canola	6	92

*Tropical fish.

ble bond of the fatty acids filled with hydrogen (they are saturated with hydrogen) (Table 7.3). Unsaturated fats have one or more carbons that are double bonded to their neighbor, and so are lacking one hydrogen at each of those carbons. If a fatty acid has only one double bond, it is called monounsaturated; if it has more than one, it is called polyunsaturated. All common fats and oils are mixtures of various fatty acids both saturated and unsaturated. At room temperature, lipids that contain more than about 25% saturated fatty acids are solid, but at homeotherm body temperature they liquefy. These lipids are commonly referred to as solid fats, animal fats or, simply, fats. At room temperature, lipids that contain less than about 25% saturated fatty acids are liquid and do not become solid until temperatures drop below freezing. These are termed oils.

Homeotherms can readily use either fats or oils in their diet because in the gut and in the body, both types of lipid are liquid and are therefore easily absorbed and transported. Poikilotherms, including plants, cannot easily use solid fats when temperatures are below the fat's melting point. It is not surprising that the only plants or fish that contain significant saturated fatty acids are tropical ones such as coconut or aji-aji that live in climates where those fats are always liquid. Temperate plants and fish contain only oils that remain liquid at ambient temperatures. While saturated fats are sometimes called "animal fats," they are really homeotherm fats since temperate fish oils contain less saturated fatty acids than homeotherms, and temperate fish get almost no solid fat in their natural diet.

In conclusion, temperate fish get no solid fat in their natural diet and have difficulty digesting and metabolizing it, especially at cooler temperatures. In fact, when fish are fed significant solid fats at cool temperatures, the fat remains in their gut as a mass. It is best to avoid highly saturated fat in fish diets, but that is not so easy. As was discussed earlier, fish are best fed animal protein. The cheapest and most ready source of animal protein for feeds is slaughterhouse by-products derived from terrestrial animals, and these are high in saturated fats. The best source of protein for fish is fish meal as it has an ideal amino acid profile and no solid fat. Fish meal, however, is expensive and getting more so as humans overfish our oceans. Fortunately, for the hobbyist, the cost of the ration is not an important criterion. This is not true in commercial production aquaculture, where substitutes for fish meal are actively being sought.

Essential fatty acids

All vertebrates require some fatty acids they cannot synthesize; these must come from the diet. Koi have two essential fatty acids: linolenic (18:3 omega-3) and linoleic (18:2 omega-6), and both are required at about 1% of the diet (dry). In the case of linolenic, the 18 indicates that there are 18 carbons in the fatty acid chain and the first 3 means there are three double bonds, and the omega-3 means that the first double bond occurs between the third and fourth carbon from the oxygen-containing end of the string. As an aside, the "omega 3" lipids (linolenic) have gained recognition as important in the human diet in preventing heart disease. Fish are a prime source of these nutrients for people.

Lipids and protein are the most important major constituents of a good fish diet. Fish readily use unsaturated fatty acids for energy and growth. In fact, if a diet is rich in quality lipids, the protein content can be reduced without affecting growth.

Carbohydrates

Carbohydrates (sugars and starches, which are digestible by nonruminants, and cellulose, which is not) are typically not found to any great extent in a fish's natural diet. So, they have little need for them and little capacity to use them. This stands in contrast to the huge importance that carbohydrates play in the diets of terrestrial homeotherms. If readily assimilated carbohydrates such as sugar and cooked starch are fed to fish in quantity, they can cause serious problems because the fish absorb them into the body but have difficulty efficiently metabolizing them. For example, insulin occurs in fish, but since fish have evolved without carbohydrates in their diet, insulin does not play the same role in stimulating the cellular uptake and metabolism of sugar as it does in us. When the blood sugar of fish on an artificial diet is compared with that of fish on a natural diet it is typically twice as high. The carbohydrate that almost always comes along with an artificial ration makes fish seriously hyperglycemic. We should think of pet fish, such as koi, as type 2 diabetics and feed them the same way. When fish consume a typical ration, they use the protein and lipid components for maintenance energy and growth, but they store the carbohydrate calories as body fat because it is difficult for them to use it as energy.

Koi and carbohydrates

It is a common perception that carp are omnivorous fish that need, or at least tolerate, carbohydrates. In examining that assumption, let us begin by looking at the natural diet of carp. A study examining the gut contents of carp in the wild has shown three main categories of food items: algae, insects, and "other." A partial proximate analysis of these contents showed they contained 30%–50% ash (dry weight basis). Ash is the noncombustible portion of the food and is essentially mineral. This remarkably high level of ash is attributable to sand that is incidentally consumed along with the organic material. After the ash content of the diet is subtracted, the remainder contained 30%–50% protein (dry weight basis) and a little over 4 Kcal/g energy (dry weight basis). Analyses for lipids and carbohydrates were not performed. What about all that algae that was seen in the carp? Filamentous algae, the kind that would be retrieved from a carp's gut are a notoriously poor food that contributes little energy to the aquatic food chain. Algae are the foundation of the food chain in ponds, lakes, and oceans. These algae, however, are microscopic phytoplankton, not the filamentous type. Then why are the carp eating this filamentous algae? Two reasons: First, just like the sand, it comes along with the valuable food (insects), and like the sand, it is simply passed through. Second, the algae may provide some food value, not so much from the plant itself but from the slippery coat of microscopic organisms (biofilm) that grow on the algae (and any other underwater substrate).

A common homily regarding fish digestion is that more carnivorous fish have a large stomach and short digestive tract and that more omnivorous fish have a smaller stomach (or none in the case of carp) and a longer gut. If you compare the digestive anatomy of a trout and that of a koi, you will certainly see the differences in stomach and gut length. In my opinion, however, we should not attribute these differences so much to the nutrient content of the respective diets, but instead more to the method of feeding. Trout are predators adapted to feeding on whole live organisms (insects, fish, crayfish, and salamanders) and little else, while carp, as was seen in the study above, are benthic grazers that take in a complex mix of organic and inorganic matter. Since trout eat "meals" that may contain large single items, they need a stomach. The trout's highly digestible food stream of whole creatures is easily absorbed in a short gut passage. Carp, however, constantly graze and consume small amounts almost continuously (the study mentioned above found round-the-clock feeding in wild carp). The complex mix they eat must pass through a relatively long gut to sort out the food from the chaff. As for a "long gut," that is relative. A trout's gut is one body length and a carp's is two; humans, on the other hand, are true omnivores and have a gut five or six times their body length.

Consider the high-protein natural diet of the carp. Consider also the fact that koi are in the middle of the pack in terms of the protein requirement of fishes, just below the highly carnivorous salmonids (refer to the protein requirements list provided earlier). The conclusion will be that koi display a high degree of carnivory, defined as the need for animal food. Carp and goldfish feeds have traditionally contained significant carbohydrate, and some ration manufacturers offer higher-carbohydrate diets for winter feeding of koi. This is not a good idea given what we know about the nutritional requirements of koi. As in trout rations, carbohydrate is something to avoid in a healthy koi food. This is not so easy because almost any plant material (e.g., soybean meal) used in a ration brings along a lot of carbohydrate along with the desirable protein, making feed formulation challenging.

Fiber

So far, we have considered only the digestible carbohydrates. Cellulose, and related compounds such as hemicellulose and lignin, are a large component of terrestrial plants and enter the diet with the plant-based feedstuffs. These compounds are very similar in atomic composition to starch, but a different chemical bond makes them indigestible to vertebrates, except for ruminants. Fiber does play a nutritional role in moving the bolus and absorbing toxins. Fiber is not typically found in natural fish diets because structural carbohydrates are not as abundant in aquatic plants that need little support "skeleton" in their buoyant environment. Besides playing a role as a "binder" that holds the pellet together, fiber is considered an unnecessary part of a fish ration. Moreover, in excess, fiber can prevent absorption of some nutrients and is best kept below 5%.

Vitamins and minerals

Vitamins

Vitamins and minerals are nutrients that organisms cannot synthesize and are required only in small quantities. The need for micronutrients was not fully understood until the 20th century. We now recognize 15 vitamins and almost as many minerals that are important in the diet of fish. Vitamins are categorized as two types: oil soluble and water soluble.

Oil-soluble vitamins

There are four oil-soluble vitamins commonly required in the diet of fish: A, D, E, and K. The exact requirements of D and K, however, have not been determined for carp. Oil-soluble vitamins, as the name implies, may be dissolved in lipids but not in water. This has two important consequences. One, since the vitamins are stored in the fish's fat, they cannot be lost in the urine (freshwater fish) or through passive water loss at the gill (saltwater fish); therefore, the fish can store them in its body for long periods and does not necessarily need to eat them on a daily basis. The other side of the coin is that if the animal is overfed these vitamins, it cannot easily rid itself of the excess and toxicity can occur. The requirements for oil soluble vitamins are reported in international units (IU) rather than in milligrams. The IU is a unit of measurement for the amount

of a substance based on measured biological activity (or effect) rather than on weight. The precise definition of one IU differs from substance to substance and is established by an international agreement.

Water-soluble vitamins

There are 11 water-soluble vitamins commonly required in fish: thiamine (B_1), riboflavin (B_2), niacin (B_3), pantothenic acid (B_5), pyridoxine (B_6), folic acid (B_9), B_{12} (cyanocobalamin), vitamin C, biotin, choline, and inositol (myoinositol). Testing has not revealed a need for folic acid or B_{12} in carp. The opposite of oil-soluble vitamins, the water-soluble ones pose no threat of toxicity if overfed, but they must be fed regularly since they "wash out" of the fish and cannot be stored. Interestingly, only primates, fish, and guinea pigs have a requirement for vitamin C; all other animals can synthesize it themselves. Often, koi feeds are advertised as containing "stabilized vitamin C." Simple vitamin C is ascorbic acid and breaks down through oxidation and becomes ineffective over time, especially when exposed to heat. Various derivatives that are more stabile and longer lasting yet retain vitamin potency have been developed. One such product that is used in fish feeds is L-ascorbyl-2-polyphosphate. Stabilized vitamin C in a feed is good idea in that it extends shelf life, although not absolutely necessary, if feed is kept fresh and protected from heat.

All vitamins must be in adequate amounts in the fish's diet or deleterious signs of deficiency will occur. Unfortunately, these signs of deficiency are often the same for several vitamins and, moreover, are easily confused with signs of pathogen-caused disease (e.g., hemorrhagic fins and skin). Vitamins are typically added to a fish diet in the form of a "vitamin premix," essentially a powdered vitamin pill. Addition of vitamins should be done after any heat treatment (e.g., steam extrusion to form a floating pellet) has been done since vitamins are sensitive to heat.

Minerals

Fish are different from terrestrial animals in that they easily obtain required minerals from the water they swim in, as well as from the diet. In order to maintain sufficient blood osmotic pressure while swimming in a hypoosmotic solution, freshwater fish have developed an excellent ability to scavenge ions from the water around them. This is done by specialized cells in the gills (chloride cells). Most required minerals occur as soluble salts and so are found dissolved in most surface water, albeit sometimes in very small amounts. A terrestrial animal might drink from a pond that contained low levels of a required mineral in solution and not be able to drink enough water to meet its requirement. A fish swimming in that same pond could easily obtain enough of the mineral from the endless pumping of salts into the fish. In fact, it is quite difficult to determine the mineral requirements of fish because not only is a purified, mineral-free diet required but also the fish must be kept in highly distilled water. Despite this, the dietary requirement of six minerals has been determined for carp: magnesium, phosphorous, copper, iron, manganese, and zinc. It is likely that other minerals (e.g., iodine) are also required, but the necessary research has not been done. The good news for koi keepers is that since koi are excellent at getting the minerals they need from the water, mineral deficiency is seldom a problem. Minerals should never be overfed as many are toxic at higher concentrations.

Color enhancers, immune stimulants, and egg binding

Color enhancers

Color in fish is imparted by two types of cells: biochromes, which contain pigment, and schematochromes, which produce color by reflection and refraction of light. Chromatophores can contain three pigments: melanin (black), carotenoids (red and yellow), and guanine (white). When these are combined they can produce a range of color, but clearly, koi colors are dominated by black, red, and white. Fish, including koi, are able to change color quite rapidly. These changes are under both neural and hormonal control and are caused by the movement of pigments within the chromatophore. When the pigment is tightly aggregated,

the fish is pale, and when the pigment is dispersed throughout the cell, the fish is vivid. Blanching of fish is often caused by fright (adrenaline is a melanin aggregator) or when light reaches the fish's eyes from both above and below. This commonly occurs in the scattered light in muddy water or when a fish is swimming over a light-colored bottom in clear water. Calm fish and those in clear water with a dark bottom will tend to be more vivid.

People keep koi for their beautiful color and many koi rations are sold as "color enhancing." Animals can synthesize melanin and guanine, so there is no need to enrich a ration with those. Carotenoids, however, are only produced by plants, and therefore, a dietary deficiency could result in a reduction in red and yellow colors. Koi foods sold as "color enhancing" contain components rich in carotenoids, primarily astaxanthin, such as krill or spirulina algae; however, something as pedestrian as paprika would work as well. While a good-quality koi ration should contain enough marine-based foods to provide all the carotenoids necessary for full color development, carotenoids may be degraded by heat and oxygen and so there is an argument for adding them back.

Immune stimulants

Some koi rations are advertised to contain immune stimulants, compounds that are said to increase disease resistance. These are just beginning to receive scientific evaluation of their value. Furthermore, they are proprietary, so their exact composition is not available and so it is hard to even speculate how they might work. This author has a colleague that has recently conducted a series of experiments on such a compound. The results are unpublished at this writing, but here is what he found.

A proprietary probiotic was fed to golden shiners as part of a complete ration. According to its manufacturer, active components of this product include yeast and dairy fractions, as well as dried fermentation products. Golden shiners are widely raised for bait and are in the minnow family Cyprinidae, like koi. The shiners were then exposed to columnaris bacteria. The control group experienced about 50% mortality to columnaris.

The group fed the diet containing the probiotic had less than 10%. This author cannot speak to all immune stimulants, but there is evidence that this one, at least, does work.

Egg binding

A discussion of egg binding is included in a chapter on nutrition because, while no solid research exists on egg binding, my informed speculation is that egg binding tends to occur in abundantly fed, fatty koi. Koi, like most temperate organisms, reproduce at a specific time of the year. The primary spawning time for koi, of course, is spring; although repeat spawning in the warm months can occur. Both photoperiod (day length) and temperature are important cues for koi to reproduce. Photoperiod times spawning and temperature triggers spawning. Beginning in the fall, first the shortening of the photoperiod and then, after the solstice, the lengthening of the photoperiod are perceived by the koi and the release of gonadotropin hormones stimulates the growth of the ovaries. As the water begins to warm in the spring, the ovaries are almost fully developed. When a triggering temperature is reached, about 70 °F for koi, spawning behavior, including ovulation that releases the eggs, occurs. If something happens that does not allow the normal release of eggs, such as failure of the water to reach and hold the triggering temperature at an appropriate time in the spring, the koi may not ovulate and carry her eggs into the summer.

A female that is still full of mature eggs after spawning time passes is termed egg bound. Egg binding can become a problem if the eggs are not reabsorbed in a timely manner. It is considered stressful for a female to remain egg bound for months at a time and, in extreme cases, the ovaries can become necrotic and threaten the fish's life. Ovaries mature as a consequence of vitellogenesis, and a vast quantity of energy in the form of lipids is stored in the eggs. This energy, of course, is what will feed the embryo during development. All fishes miss spawning opportunities rather regularly; however, egg binding is not considered a problem in wild fish. In fish on a spare diet, the energy required to fuel the eggs comes at the expense of mesenteric fat stores and even muscle protein. Simply, the female sacrifices her own energy reserves for that of her future offspring. After spawning, a fish is typically in poor condition and must feed vigorously to gain back those reserves. If she fails to spawn, she readily reabsorbs the energy in the eggs and puts it back into her own body. A typical koi female, however, enters egg development with unusually abundant stores of energy and is getting well fed daily as well. Consequently, she "eats for 2000" and adds egg yolk to her already fatty body cavity. If the koi fails to shed her eggs, she not only carries all that egg yolk and mesenteric fat but is receiving as much daily feed as she can eat. No wonder, then, there is no physiological need to reabsorb the eggs and egg binding occurs. If this speculation is correct, then egg binding would be greatly reduced if koi were fed a restricted ration and kept lean.

Ration selection and feeding

Koi digestion

As mentioned earlier, koi are grazing feeders that feed almost continually in nature on a rather complex mix of inorganic and organic matter, only part of which is digestible. Koi have molariform pharyngeal teeth that reside on the fifth, nonrespiratory, gill arch deep in the fish's throat. These teeth are quite functional, and the first step in digestion is the mastication of the food for more complete digestion. When food is swallowed, it passes to the anterior gut since there is no stomach. Early in its gut transit, the bolus passes by the liver (see Fig. 7.3).

In recent years, it has been recognized that in many fish, including carp, the liver is best termed hepatopancreas. Liver cells have a blood side served by sinusoids and a bile side served by bile ducts. Hepatocytes store blood sugar as glycogen and break down certain wastes and toxins. The wastes, as well as fat-emulsifying compounds from the hepatocytes, flow down the bile ducts and into the gall bladder, where they are stored until dispensed into the intestine. The pancreatic cells produce the digestive enzymes (proteases, lipases, and carbohydrases) that presumably flow

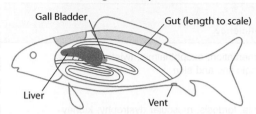

Koi Digestive Syestem

Fig. 7.3 Schematic of koi (carp) digestive system showing the major components.

from the pancreatic islands to the gut via the bile ducts.

Digestive enzymes are proteins that break foodstuffs into simpler molecular pieces so that they are more easily absorbed from the intestine. Protein-digesting enzymes are called proteases and include trypsin and chymotrypsin. Lipid-digesting enzymes are called lipases. Carbohydrate-digesting enzymes are called carbohydrases and include amylase, which breaks starch into sugar units. As the enzyme-treated bolus moves down the gut, the nutrients are absorbed both passively by diffusion and actively, which requires energy, by membrane transport proteins.

Scientific ration formulation

It is almost impossible to keep fish in captivity and feed them a natural diet. The size of the pond needed would be prohibitive. The necessary data for scientific ration formulation has been gathered for several commonly cultured species, including carp. Most scientific ration formulation is based on a least-cost assumption; in other words, the goal is to determine the cheapest combination of ingredients that meets the minimum requirements for normal growth and reproduction (complete ration). In the pet market, however, least cost is not usually an important consideration, and the feeds may contain expensive ingredients intended to have some additional benefits beyond normal growth.

Selecting a koi diet

Any "treats" or other food fed koi dilute the carefully calculated nutrient balance in the primary complete ration. Some ration makers caution not to feed incomplete supplements over 10% of the total diet because of the danger of diluting the necessary nutrients too far. This is sound advice. There is no problem in mixing two or more rations if they are all complete.

The US Food and Drug Administration (FDA) regulation of pet food requires that pet food must be pure and wholesome, contain no harmful or deleterious substances, and be truthfully labeled. Also, anything added to food that is not simply nutritive but is intended to improve "performance or function" is considered a "drug" and must be shown to be safe and effective through a controlled scientific study. Beyond "foods" and "drugs," there is a third category, "additive." Any additives that are not "generally regarded as safe" must have a petition on file with the FDA. The petition must state the chemical identity, safety data, and more. Since evaluating petitions is time consuming, the FDA allows additives that do not raise safety concerns to forgo an expensive petition process that drugs require.

A diet should be labeled with a proximate analysis and a list of ingredients in the order of their predominance in the ration. The diet should exceed the crude protein minimum we have discussed (35%). In my opinion, there should be less than 25% digestible carbohydrate. The ingredients should be dominated by feedstuffs of fish origin (e.g., fish meal and oil). Slaughterhouse by-products (e.g., meat and bone meal) and plant foods (e.g., soybean meal) should be further down the ingredient list (meaning they are more minor ration components). A reputable manufacturer would provide nonproprietary information such as percentage of the essential amino acids (see Table 7.2 for minimum requirements), linolenic and linoleic fatty acid content (minimum 1%), and vitamin content (see Table 7.4 for minimum requirements), if not with the food or on a Web site, at least upon inquiry.

Fish foods are made in two different forms, floating and sinking. Most koi hobbyists prefer a floating diet since the koi can easily be seen feeding. This helps the hobbyist to more closely evaluate the condition of their fish and allows them to see if they are eating and how much. However, sinking feed is as good and is usually

Table 7.4 Required vitamins of koi.

Vitamin	Requirement in koi (per kilogram diet, as fed)	Sign of deficiency
A	4000 IU	Skin depigmentation, exophthalmia, twisted opercula, hemorrhagic fins and skin
D	Not tested	Not tested
E	100 IU	Exophthalmia, lordosis, muscular dystrophy, kidney degeneration, pancreatic degeneration
K	Not tested	Not tested
Thiamine	0.5 mg	Nervousness, skin depigmentation, subcutaneous hemorrhage
Riboflavin	7 mg	Emaciation, photophobia, nervousness, hemorrhagic fins and skin, kidney necrosis
Niacin	Required	Skin hemorrhage, mortality
Pantothenic acid	30 mg	Poor growth, lethargy, exophthalmia, skin hemorrhage
Pyridoxine	6 mg	Nervousness, anemia
Folic acid	No requirement	None detected
B_{12}	No requirement	None detected
C	Required	Poor growth
Biotin	Required	Lethargy, increased mucus
Choline	500 mg	Fatty liver, liver damage
Inositol	400 mg	Loss of mucus

cheaper. Feed is made to float by steam extruding the mix of feedstuffs, which puffs it up and makes it buoyant. Sinking feed is cold extruded. Steam extruding heats the ration and partially cooks the starch, making it more digestible (not particularly good in my opinion) and damages the vitamins which are typically heat labile. For this reason, the vitamin premix is added after steam extrusion, typically by spraying on an oil/vitamin mixture.

Feeding and fasting

Koi need <1%–10% of their body weight per day in feed (based on dry ration and live fish weights) for normal maintenance and growth with 2%–3% being typical. Larger fish need less food than smaller fish (on a body weight basis), and fish in warmer water need more than fish in colder water. There are widespread recommendations that koi not be fed in cold water (below 50°F). In the early days of catfish farming, the farmers would not feed their catfish below 50°F either. It was then learned that while the fish did not grow in that cold water, a little food helped them come into spring in better condition and more able to fend off the bacterial infections that are common in warming water. So, the recommendation is to offer koi food even in cold water but not expect them to eat much or to grow.

As discussed earlier, carp are "grazers" that lack a stomach and feed around the clock in the wild. Best food assimilation and growth will occur if koi are allowed to follow this way of feeding as much as possible. Multiple smaller daily feedings are preferable to one or two larger ones (Fig. 7.4). Frequent feeding means more constant ammonia production and oxygen demand and minimizes these problems. Therefore, an automatic feeder has advantages. An automatic feeder should dispense a large number of small feedings a day. There are problems with automatic feeders such as clumping of feed and other malfunctions, as well as a tendency for the feed to get damp. The

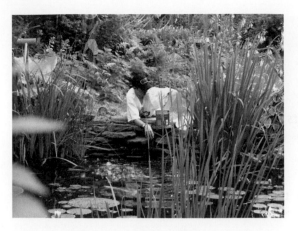

Fig. 7.4 A pond owner feeding his fish.

feeders are best not used to feed more than 1 day at a time where fresh food is loaded daily.

Another routine recommendation for feeding koi, for which there is often no scientific basis, is a type of "phase feeding," where in cool water (say, 50–60 °F) koi are to be fed a low-protein, high-carbohydrate diet; such things as bread, breakfast cereal, squash, and lettuce are recommended. Lettuce, certainly, and even squash, are low enough in energy to be harmless aside from diluting the primary complete ration, but this author would never recommend feeding any fish foods as rich in simple carbohydrate as bread and breakfast cereal. It is interesting that the extremely carnivorous trout, when raised in captivity, develop a "taste" for carbohydrates, such as canned corn, which their wild counterparts would never eat. Presumably, this develops when they are offered no alternative but to eat a formulated ration that is overly rich in carbohydrate. Compared with wild trout, these captive trout are hyperglycemic, have a lot of mesenteric fat, and have large pale livers due to accumulation of glycogen and lipids.

Pushing growth of koi

Larger koi are more desirable and valuable than smaller ones, so people who raise koi like to see fast growth that results in large koi. Interestingly, the largest koi seem to top out at about 1 m and about 50 lb. Wild carp, on the other hand, grow to 80 lb; this is very rare but does occur. Koi do not reach this size even though they have more abundant food than their wild cousins. We can speculate that this is due to genetics, nutrition, or both. Over the many generations koi have been kept, there has been intense selection for certain traits. Consciously, koi keepers have linebred for color and markings, but perhaps less consciously, there has also been strong selection for fish that do well in captivity. This tolerance of captivity always includes tameness (essentially an attenuation of the fight-or-flight reaction) that is the hallmark of domesticated animals, but that in koi may also include smaller body size that "fits" better in koi ponds. Also, genes for smaller growth may be linked to obviously desirable traits such as color. As for the role of nutrition, the food of koi may be more abundant than that of a wild carp, but it may not be as good at promoting health and growth.

Abundantly feeding koi to push growth and achieve the plump condition demanded by judges in show-quality koi, almost certainly, is unhealthy for the animal and shortens its life. It is firmly established in both human and veterinary medicine that excess fat hurts health in myriad of ways. This is one area in which fish and mammals are not different, in this author's opinion. Anecdotally, most of these 1-m prize-winning koi live very short lives.

References and further reading

Cerrutti, L.M.G. (1982) Monthly Differences in Food Consumption and Diet of Common Carp (*Cyprinus carpio*) and the Effects of Temperature and Ration Size on Their Growth. MS Thesis, University of Minnesota.

Committee on Animal Nutrition, Board on Agriculture, National Research Council. (1993) *Nutrient Requirements of Fish*. Washington, DC: National Academy Press.

Halver, J.E. and Hardy, R.W., eds. (2002) *Fish Nutrition*. San Diego, CA: Academic Press.

Chapter 8

Parasites of Fish

Stephen A. Smith and Helen E. Roberts

Introduction

Probably the most common problems of tropical and ornamental fishes are those associated with parasites. Parasites come in all sizes and shapes and include single-celled protozoans, and multicellular trematodes (flatworms), cestodes (tapeworms), nematodes (roundworms), acanthocephalans (spiny-headed worms), crustaceans, and arthropods (Lom and Dyková, 1992; Smith and Noga, 1992; Hoffman, 1999; Woo, 2006). Some of these parasites are host specific, parasitizing only a single genus or even species of fish, while others are cosmopolitan, crossing over species lines. Fish parasites can infest the outer surfaces, inhabit the lumen of any organ, or penetrate the parenchyma of almost any tissue of the host. Fish can serve as an intermediate, paratenic (transport), and/or definitive host for the various stages of parasites.

Parasitic infections in fish are diagnosed by wet mount cytology preparations of skin scrapes, gill biopsies, and fecal samples, and by direct observation (macroscopic parasites). Intestinal squash preps, organ biopsy, blood film evaluation, and histopathology are also used on occasion for diagnosis. See Chapter 17 for a more complete discussion of diagnostic techniques.

Protozoan parasites

For purposes of this chapter, the protozoan parasites will be subjectively divided into those that parasitize the external surface of the fish and those that invade the internal tissues of the fish. This simplifies the ensuing discussion on therapeutics as almost all external parasites can be treated with the same compounds, whereas the internal parasites have very limited treatment possibilities.

External protozoan parasites

Numerous species of protozoan parasites inhabit the surface of the skin of fish. Most of these do not actually invade the tissues but instead feed off the mucus and the bacterial and sloughed epithelial cells on the surface, or have attachment organs that anchor the parasite in place on the surface of the skin and feed on bacterial, protozoan, and other materials in the passing water.

In the assemblage of protozoans that inhabit the skin of the fish is a group of flattened, discoid scrub brush-like ciliates that belong to a number of genera, including *Trichodina*, *Trichodinella*, and *Tripartiella*. These are readily identified by their internal circular denticular ring that has both an inward- and outward-facing ring of tooth-like projections (Fig. 8.1). Numerous species of trichodinids parasitize freshwater, brackish, and marine species of fish. Certain species are more destructive than others, with those inhabiting the gill being generally the most pathogenic where they cause significant tissue irritation, hyperplasia of epithelial tissues, and respiratory problems. In general, *Trichodina* infestation causes pruritis and increased mucus, giving a whitish cast to the skin (Gratzek, 1993). Trichodinosis is often associated with overcrowding and poor water quality conditions such as high organic loads. Several species of *Trichodina* also infest the urinary bladder and oviducts of some freshwater and marine fish. These parasites invade the luminal surfaces by retrograde migration up the tubular tracts and generally do not cause significant pathology.

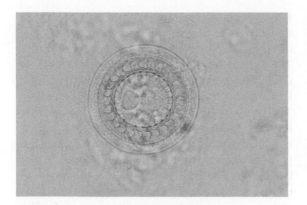

Fig. 8.1 *Trichodina* sp. at 100× magnification.

Chilodonella sp. is a dorsoventrally flattened, oval protozoan that has cilia located in distinct bands along the surface of the body. This freshwater ciliate causes irritation to gills and fins by its feeding activity, which results in hyperplasia and fusion of gill lamellae and hyperplasia of fin tissue. This parasite is common on freshwater fish, such as catfish, goldfish, and koi, that frequent the bottom of ponds or pools. Clinical signs include respiratory distress, clamped fins, excess mucus production, and death. Infection can occur in a wide range of water temperatures. The marine counterpart of this parasite is the *Brooklynella* sp., which has the same distinctive bands of cilia and similar pathology.

Ichthyobodo sp. (sometimes referred to by its older name of *Costia* sp.) is an extremely small (about the size of a red blood cell) oval to pyriform-shaped flagellate parasite of freshwater, and occasionally marine, fishes. This parasite can be found either attached by one of its two flagella to the skin and gill tissues or motile in the water displaying a characteristic spiraling swimming behavior. The parasite's characteristic movement has been described as a "flickering flame" of a candle. Clinical signs include depression, anorexia, respiratory distress, and death. Hyperirritation of the skin leads to increased mucus production, resulting in a cloudy appearance to the skin. This parasite can be very pathogenic and is often overlooked because of its small size.

There is a diverse group of sessile parasites that attach directly to the skin of the fish and do not actually feed on the fish but obtain food from the water as it passes by the fish. *Ambiphyra* sp. (previously known as *Scyphidia* sp.) is a small urn-shaped protozoan with a distal oral ring of cilia. These are common on pond-raised fish, especially catfish, carp, and goldfish, and sometimes even on coldwater species of fish such as trout. This parasite has a broad, flat disk for attaching to the surface epithelial cells of the skin or gill, which probably hinders the diffusion of oxygen and carbon dioxide across this area. Although this parasite does not normally cause a problem in small numbers, the health of the fish can be affected if large numbers of the parasite are present on the gills, where they can block a significant amount of diffusion of respiratory gasses and excretory products. *Trichophyra* sp. is a pincushion-like ciliate parasite of the gills of pond-raised fish, especially carp, goldfish, and ornamentals. Similar to *Ambiphyra* sp., *Trichophyra* sp. does not normally cause fish health problems in small numbers, but large numbers of the parasite can impede the natural diffusion of respiratory gasses and excretory products. Two additional sessile protozoans found on goldfish, ornamental fishes, and pond fishes are *Epistylis* sp. and *Heteropolaria* sp. These parasites are often found on fish in ponds with high organic loads. Both are peritrichous ciliates that have a rounded, contractile oral disk and a rigid, noncontractual stalk that is attached to the skin of the fish. These parasites often form a branching colony of organisms and cause damage to the host in a manner similar to other sessile fish parasites. Both of these colonial ciliates have been associated with secondary bacterial infections of *Aeromonas hydrophila* or *Flavobacterium columnare* causing a syndrome know as "red sore disease."

Dinoflagellates of the genera *Piscinoodinium* (*Oodinium*), *Amyloodinium*, and *Crepidoodinium* are parasitic on freshwater and marine species of fish. These parasites cause a disease commonly called "velvet disease" or "rust disease" in the aquarium industry due to the yellow to red coloration the parasites impart to the affected body, fins, or gills. These parasites may also be found in the gastrointestinal tract. The parasite has three distinct life stages of development: an attached trophozoite stage on the host, an encysted stage in the environment, and a free-swimming infectious dinospore stage. In the trophozoite stage, the parasite has fingerlike projections, or rhizoids, that penetrate into the epithelial cell as holdfast organs and also for obtaining nutrients from the cell. Infestations of the gill tissue cause epithelial hyperplasia and fusion of the lamellae, resulting in secondary hypoxia and osmoregulatory compromise. Infestation of the skin causes a yellowish red coloration of the mucus and hyperplasia of the surface epithelial layers, causing osmoregulatory problems. Shining a flashlight in a darkened room on the affected fish can enhance the dusty color change seen with infestation (Gratzek, 1993).

Internal protozoan parasites

A number of protozoan parasites penetrate the epithelial tissues of the skin and invade the deeper tissues of the fish. Perhaps the most widely recognized protozoan parasite of fish is *Ichthyophthirius multifiliis*, commonly referred to as "Ich" or "white spot disease." The name is derived from the multiple small, raised, white lesions that develop as a result of the parasite in the skin, fins, and gill tissue of the host. Heavily parasitized fish often "flash" and twitch fins trying to dislodge the parasite. This parasite affects cultured and wild species of freshwater fish worldwide. This large holotrich ciliate can measure up to 1.0 mm in size and is entirely covered with an external surface layer of cilia. The parasite is easily identified by the presence of a relatively large horseshoe-shaped or C-shaped macronucleus (Fig. 8.2).

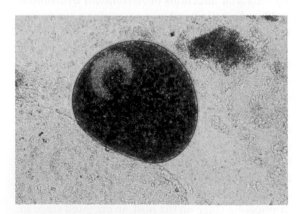

Fig. 8.2 *Ichthyophthirius multifiliis* at 100× magnification.

However, the rolling motion of the parasite within the cyst in the host or when freed into the water often makes observation of the C-shape difficult. The parasite has three developmental stages in its direct life cycle that are associated with specific locations on the host or within the environment. The trophozoite or trophont, or feeding stage, is typically located within a cyst in the superficial epithelial tissues of the host. When mature, the parasite excysts from the host and forms a cyst (tomont stage), the dividing stage, in the substrate or on surfaces of objects in the water (such as plants, aquarium tubing, or filter material). The parasite undergoes multiple divisions, forming up to 256 theront stages. These small free-swimming ciliated theronts are then released into the water, where they have a short time (up to 48 hours) to find and infect a fish host. The theront penetrates the epithelium of the fish and continues the life cycle. The time required for the development of the complete life cycle is primarily dependent on environmental temperature, with the life cycle being completed in as short as 5–7 days at an optimal temperature of 70–75 °F (23 °C) or as long as 30+ days at colder temperatures. There is a limited production of host immunity to this parasite, which can cause fish to become nonsymptomatic chronic carriers of this parasite. Numerous treatments have been suggested, including raising the water temperature a few degrees and various chemotherapeutics; however, the encysted trophozoite/trophont stage buried in the epithelium of the host and the cyst (tomont) stage in the environment are resistant to waterborne chemical treatments. Only the unprotected free-swimming stage (theront) is affected by waterborne chemical treatments. Raising the water temperature does not kill the parasite but hastens the life cycle so that tomonts are released sooner from the host, and ultimately, the subsequent theront stages are exposed to the chemical-treated water.

Cryptocaryon irritans is the saltwater equivalent of the freshwater *Ichthyophthirius* organism. It is also sometimes referred to as "white spot disease" since the parasite causes similar clinical signs of raised, white lesions on the skin, fin, and gill tissue of the marine fish. The parasite is another relatively large holotrich ciliate, but it does not have the large C-shaped nucleus that is characteristic of *Ichthyophthirius*. Its life cycle and pathology are similar to that of *Ichthyophthirius*.

Another ciliate that occasionally causes problems by invading the tissues of the host is *Tetrahymena pyriformis*. This particular parasite causes "tet" or "guppy disease" in a number of species of tropical aquarium fishes, especially guppies, neon tetras, and mollies. The organism is a small, cylindrical to pyriform-shaped ciliate that is normally free living in the environment. However, under certain conditions, the organism becomes parasitic and penetrates the skin and/or gills. Initially, the organism penetrates the epithelial tissues and burrows under the scales. This skin damage may lead to secondary bacterial or fungal infections. The parasite may then continue migrating along the fascial planes of the underlying muscles and invade many of the internal organs, including the liver, intestinal tract, and even gonads. As long as the organism is confined to only the external surfaces of the fish, treatment can be attempted; once the organism invades the internal tissues of the fish, treatment is unrewarding and the infected fish usually dies. Similar histophagus protozoans have been described in numerous food fish species, including *Tetrahymena* sp. in freshwater trout, yellow perch, and striped bass, and *Uronema* sp. in marine fish such as salmonids and flounder.

Flagellates, microsporidians, coccidia, and hemoprotozoans

Spironucleus sp. and *Hexamita* sp. are relatively small flagellate parasites that are bilaterally symmetrical and contain two nuclei. Both are frequently found in the lumen of the intestinal tract of freshwater and marine tropical fish, especially various species of freshwater cichlids. Light infestations of the intestinal tract are generally asymptomatic, while heavy infestations can be pathogenic causing necrosis and sloughing of the intestinal epithelium and coelomitis. The resulting clinical signs include inappetence, unthriftiness, mucoid or pale stool, poor condition, emaciation, and death. *Hexamita* sp. have also occasionally been found in skin lesions of various freshwater cichlids, where they have been reported to be one of the proposed etiologies of the "hole-in-

the-head" (HITH) syndrome. See Chapter 21 for a discussion of HITH.

Numerous microsporidians use freshwater and marine species of fish as hosts. These sporozoan parasites produce a whitish cyst within almost any tissue of the host that contains the vegetative or spore stages. The intracellular spores are very small and contain no polar capsule with a polar filament that is not normally visible. Transmission is by rupture of the cyst to the outside environment or death of the host, which similarly releases the spores into the water. These are most commonly ingested by the fish, transformed into an amoebula stage, which then migrate to various tissue sites in the fish and eventually develop a spore-filled cyst. As the disease progresses and the cysts gets larger, infected muscle tissue becomes displaced and turns white in color, the function of infected digestive organs can cause the fish to become emaciated, or infected gonads can result in decreased fecundity. One of the more commonly observed microsporidians, *Pleistophora hyphessobryconis*, causes a syndrome called "neon tetra disease." Although originally described in neon tetras, this parasite can infect many different species of fish, including zebra danios, cichlids, cyprinids, and even goldfish. Damage to the muscles can cause a lumpy appearance to the body as the cysts deform the muscles or result in the curvature of the spine, both of which may result in the fish having difficulty swimming. This parasitic disease in neon tetras is invariably fatal.

Coccidial (*Eimeria* and *Goussia* sp.) infections of the intestinal tract are a common occurrence in young fish with immature immune systems where infection can cause poor growth, emaciation, and death. Mucoid, yellow stool casts may also be observed in affected fish. Infections can also be found in adult fish, but the resulting pathology is generally less severe. Coccidia have a direct life cycle and can rapidly increase in numbers in aquaria or closed recirculation systems. Diagnosis can be made by finding oocysts in a fecal sample, by intestinal scraping, or by histopathology.

Freshwater and marine fish also have a number of species of flagellated hemoprotozoans that can cause health problems. These are easily identified in blood smears by their well-developed undulating membrane. *Trypanosoma* sp. has been described in the blue-eyed plecostomus (*Panaque suttoni*) imported from South America (Khoo et al., 2006), while *Cryptobia iubilans* has been described as causing a granulomatous disease in African cichlids and discus (Yanong et al., 2004).

Myxozoan parasites

Myxosporidians are common sporozoan parasites of fishes. To date, all described myxosporidians of fish have an indirect life cycle that involves an aquatic oligochaete worm as an intermediate host. Otherwise, the life cycle is similar to the microsporidian and results in a spore-filled tissue cyst that displaces or disrupts the function of the infected tissue. The oval or sperm-shaped spore has a large sporoplasm and two polar capsules, each with an associated coiled filament. Spores are released when the spore ruptures to the outside environment or the death of the host releases the spores into the water. Several species of this parasite are important parasites of cultured fishes, such as *Myxobolus cerebralis* and *Ceratomyxa shasta* in salmonids, and *Henneguya ictaluri* and *Aurantiactinomyxon ictaluri* in channel catfish. Other species have been described from various bottom-dweller tropical fish such as *Corydoras* and *Leporinus*. Figure 8.3 shows a cutaneous myxosporidian infection in a koi.

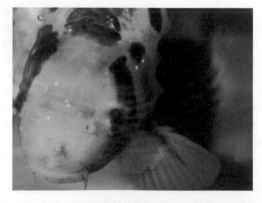

Fig. 8.3 Cutaneous *Myxobolus* sp. infection in a koi, *Cyprinus carpio*. Note the small circular white lesions on the head and proximal body.

Helminth parasites

Monogeneans are parasitic flatworms or flukes with a direct life cycle that infest the external surfaces of almost any species of fresh, brackish, or marine fish. The monogeneans have an anterior oral sucker used for feeding on mucus and sloughed epithelial cells, while the posterior end has a holdfast organ for attaching to the host. Depending on the species, the attachment (or opisthaptor) organ is composed of a variety of hooks, hooklets, clamps, or adhesive suckers. Monogeneans cause direct pathology by two methods: one by physical attachment to the tissues of the host with the holdfast organ, and the other by abrasive feeding activity. Thus, it is common to see small circles of denuded tissue as a result of the feeding activity around the central attachment point of the monogenean. These parasites cause focal irritation, increased mucus production, and hyperplasia of the epithelial tissues, and open a portal for secondary bacterial and fungal infections. Severe infections can cause erratic swimming behavior, "flashing," increased respiratory activity, scattered hemorrhages with epithelial ulceration, and frayed fins. Some monogeneans have a predilection for parasitizing only the body and fins, or only the gills; others show no preference. Monogeneans have a direct one-host life cycle and replicate by either producing larval monogeneans or eggs that are released into the water. Common genera found in pet fish include *Neobenedenia* sp. (oviparous), *Dactylogyrus* sp. (oviparous), and *Gyrodactylus* sp. (viviparous) (Figs. 8.4 and 8.5). Fancy goldfish are commonly infected with "gill" flukes, dactylogyrids, while gyrodactylid fluke infestations are more often observed in koi. *Neobenedenia* sp. are marine flukes. Treatment regimens for oviparous species require longer intervals of treatment, making identification of the fluke species important for the effective resolution of the problem.

Many species of digenetic trematodes, cestodes, nematodes, and acanthocephalans use fish as an intermediate host for the developing parasites. These larval stages generally cause minimal pathology in the host fish, but heavy infestations can result in tissue or organ displacement, stunted growth, and emaciation. In addition, migration of

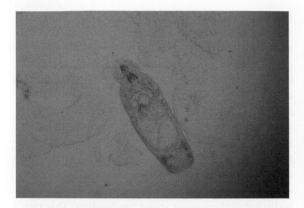

Fig. 8.4 *Gyrodactylus* sp. fluke found on a skin scrape of a koi, *Cyprinus carpio.*

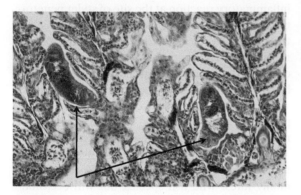

Fig. 8.5 Monogenean fluke (arrows) in gills of a koi, *Cyprinus carpio*, at 40x magnification (histology section).

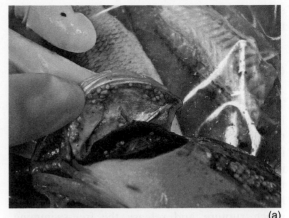

(a)

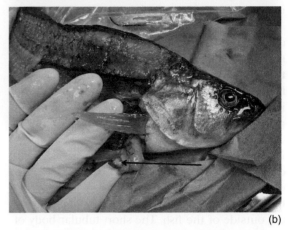

(b)

Fig. 8.6 Digenetic trematode infestation, *Clinostomum* sp., in a perch. (a) "Yellow grub" encysted on the gills, fins, and inside the operculum of a perch. (b) The intermediate host of *Clinostomum* sp., a snail, found in the stomach of a yellow perch clinically affected by "yellow grub" (arrow).

larval parasites through the tissues can sometimes also cause pathology. There are many examples of larval digenetic trematodes described in wild and pond-raised fishes, which include *Clinostomum* sp. (the "yellow grub") (Fig. 8.6), *Neascus* sp. ("black spot"), and *Diplostomulum* sp. (the "eye fluke"). In pond-reared tropical fish, the encysted metacercarial stage has been reported to cause respiratory problems when heavy burdens are located in the gill tissue. Larval cestodes can sometimes be observed encysted in the mesenteric tissues of the coelomic cavity of fish, and encysted immature nematodes can occur in the mesenteric tissue or internal organs of fish. Examples of intestinal nematodes commonly found in pet fish include *Camillanus* sp., a nematode often diagnosed in live-bearers may be seen protruding from the vent

of affected fish, and *Capillaria* sp., diagnosed by the appearance of oval, double operculated eggs shed in the stool, and is often found in some cichlid species and angelfish.

Fish also can act as a definitive host and can harbor a variety of adult digenetic trematodes, cestodes, nematodes, and acanthocephalan parasites in the lumen of their intestinal tracts. In the fish, the parasite completes its life cycle to the adult stage and produces eggs. As in mammals, these helminthes generally cause minimal pathology in the host fish, although heavy infestations can cause poor growth and emaciation. Diagnosis of these parasites is generally made by examining a fecal sample by standard techniques (i.e., direct smear, fecal flotation, or sedimentation) or post-mortem at necropsy (Smith, 2006).

Crustacean parasites

There are a number of crustacean parasites that infect the skin and gills of tropical and ornamental fishes. These parasites have a free-swimming immature stage that matures over time into an infectious larval stage, of which only the female then develops into an adult parasite on the fish host. The female produces a pair of egg sacs, which rupture and release the free-swimming immature stages to complete the life cycle.

Lernaea sp., or "anchor worm," is a copepod crustacean of pond-reared fish, especially goldfish, carp, and koi. The infectious larval stage of this particular parasite penetrates the skin of the fish and continues to develop. There is usually an intense focal inflammatory reaction at the site of penetration, which often results in hyperplasia of tissue around the site of parasite development. Eventually, the mature adult female parasite will develop an anchor-shaped anterior end that is embedded in the muscle of the fish, while the posterior portion of the female's body hangs along the outside of the fish. The short tubular body of the female with a pair of eggs sacs trailing from the body of the fish into the water column is the most commonly observed stage of this parasite. A similar parasitic copepod, *Lernaeocera* sp., is common on the gills of marine fishes. The life cycle of this parasite is similar to that of *Lernaea* sp. Treatment of anchor worms includes the gentle, manual removal of the parasite and various chemotherapeutic agents (see Table 8.1). Treatment also includes managing secondary infections and cutaneous wounds caused by the parasite.

Ergasilus sp. is a species of another type of copepod parasite, in which the second antennae are modified into specialized prehensile pincers used to grasp onto the host (Figs. 8.7 and 8.8). These parasites are most commonly found attached to the gill filaments of many species of pond and ornamental fish. The life cycle is similar to *Lernaea* sp., where the immature stages are free swimming, the adult males are nonparasitic, and the adult females are parasitic on fish. Eggs are produced in a pair of egg sacs, which rupture and release free-swimming stages that after several molts become infectious to the host.

The "fish louse," *Argulus* sp., is a common branchiurid crustacean parasite of many species of pond and ornamental fish. Although not a true insect but more closely related to shrimp, this oval, dorsoventrally flattened parasite has eight short legs and a dorsal carapace covering the body (Fig. 8.9). Other readily visible characteristics include two ventrally located prominent circular sucking disks, two dark compound eyespots, and a ventrally located piercing stylet for feeding. This parasite crawls over the surface of the fish and uses its stylet to pierce the outer epithelial cells of the fish and ingest the cell's contents. There is a severe inflammatory reaction at the site of stylet penetration, suggesting that a substance is released by the parasite to facilitate feeding. Because of this feeding activity, this parasite has also been implicated in the mechanical transmission of several bacterial, viral, and hemoprotozoal diseases. As with other aquatic crustaceans, the adult female produces two posterior egg sacs that rupture and release free-swimming infectious stages.

Leeches are external parasites of fish belonging to the annelid subclass Hirudinea. Leeches commonly infest wild fish species, but will occasionally infest ornamental and pond species of fish. These segmented worms have rasping, sucking mouthparts that allow them to attach to the body, fins, or gills of the fish. Although generally not associated with any significant pathology, large numbers of leeches on an individual can sometimes cause severe anemia and death. Leeches feed on blood and tissue fluids of the fish and have been reported to transmit some bacterial and hemoparasitic diseases. In addition, the site of leech attachment may also allow secondary bacterial and fungal infections to invade the host. Leeches are hermaphroditic and can rapidly increase population numbers, causing numerous fish to become infected in a short time.

Treatment

In addition to the use of chemotherapeutic agents for the treatment of parasites, attention to good

Table 8.1 Parasite treatments used in pet fish.

Antiparasitic agent	Dosage	Parasite treated	Comments
2-amino-5-nitrothiazol	4.4 mg/g of food oral treatment[3] 10 mg/l × 24 h × 3 days[3]	*Cryptobia iubilans* *C. iubilans*	Not 100% effective; may only reduce infestation Immersion for anorexic fish
Chloroquine	10 mg/l prolonged immersion[2]	Dinoflagellates	—
Closantel/mebendazole (Supaverm®, Janssen Animal Health, High Wycombe, Buckinghamshire, U.K.)	1 ml/400 liters[2]	Monogeneans in koi	Toxic to goldfish, and possibly to other species; efficacy increased by the addition of sodium chloride (0.1%–0.3%) in water
Copper	0.2 mg/l free copper ion prolonged immersion[2] 100 mg/l bath[2]	Protozoan ectoparasites and dinoflagellates in marine fish	Not recommended for freshwater systems; bound to inorganic compounds; toxic to invertebrates; elasmobranchs may react adversely; copper levels should be monitored daily; solubility affected by pH and alkalinity; immunosuppressive and toxic to gill tissue
Diflubenzuron (Dimilin®, Chemtura, Middlebury, CT)	0.4 mg/l prolonged immersion 0.01 mg/l prolonged immersion[1,2]	Crustacean ectoparasites	Chitin inhibitor; may affect nontarget invertebrates; EPA regulations apply
Dimetridazole	20 mg/g of food; oral treatment[3] 150 mg/100 g food[1]	*C. iubilans* *Hexamita*	Not 100% effective; may only reduce infestation
Fenbendazole	25–50 mg/kg in food for 3–5 days, repeat in 14–21 days[2] 2 mg/l prolonged immersion q 7 days × 3 treatments[2]	Intestinal nematodes	Biotest with novel species; change 50% water between each treatment
Formalin (37% formaldehyde)	0.125–0.25 ml/l bath q 24 hours × 2–3 days for up to 60 minutes[2] 0.015–0.025 ml/l (15–25 ppm) prolonged immersion, every 2–3 days × 6 days[2] Change 50% water on nontreatment days	Protozoan parasites, crustacean ectoparasites	Carcinogenic; depletes oxygen, additional aeration required; some fish are very sensitive; not for use in stressed fish; do not use if white precipitate forms; contraindicated at >27°C
Freshwater	Used as a dip up to 5 minutes[1,2]	Marine protozoan ectoparasites and some monogenean infestations	Not effective against all protozoans; a common quarantine procedure for marine fish, daily up to 5 days
Levamisole	1–2 mg/l bath up to 24 hours[1,2] 1.8 g/lb of food fed orally once weekly × 3 weeks[1] 50 mg/l × 2 hours[1]	Intestinal nematodes Monogeneans	—

(Continued)

Table 8.1 *Continued*

Antiparasitic agent	Dosage	Parasite treated	Comments
Lufenuron (Program®, Novartis Animal Health, East Hanover, NJ)	0.1–0.2 mg/L prolonged immersion[2]	Crustacean ectoparasites	Chitin inhibitor; may affect nontarget invertebrates
Mebendazole	1 mg/l prolonged immersion[1,2]	Monogeneans	—
Metronidazole	7–15 mg/l q 24–48 hours × 5–10 days Prolonged immersion Change 50% water between treatments 25–50 mg/kg (0.25% in food fed at 1% body weight/day) for 3 days	Some protozoal flagellates, including *Hexamita* and *Spironucleus*	Not very water soluble One oral treatment may be as effective as three water treatments
Hydrogen peroxide 22%/peracetic acid 5.0% (Minn Finn Max™, Aqua Solver LLC, Escondido, CA)	12.5 ml/100 gallons	Protozoans Monogeneans	New OTC drug (2009). More data on effectiveness and safety is needed. May be used extensively by hobbyists
Potassium permanganate	2 mg/l prolonged immersion[1,2] 5–20 mg/l 1 hour bath 100 mg/l × 5–10 min bath[2]	External infections, ectoparasites (protozoan, monogenean)	Inactivated by organic compounds in water; caustic; toxic in high pH water; stains; can be toxic to some fish species; can cause blindness (powder); watch for signs of stress with use; safer products are available
Praziquantel	2–10 mg/l 2–4 hours bath or prolonged immersion, q 7 days × 4–6 weeks for dactylogyrids, q 7 days × 2–4 weeks for gyrodactylids[2] 50 mg/kg/day oral—one dose[2]	Monogenean Cestodes	Add aeration; powders are not very water soluble; can be expensive in large systems Higher dosage levels reported to cause toxicity in *Corydoras* sp.
Sodium chloride	3–6 g/l prolonged immersion 10–30 g/l dip (minutes until fish is stressed)	Protozoan parasites Protozoan parasites	Dip is often used in quarantine protocols
Toltrazuril (Baycox®, Bayer Animal Health, Shawnee, KS)	7–10 mg/kg orally q 24 hours × 5 days 30 mg/l × 60 min q 48h × 3 treatments[2]	Coccidiosis Myxozoans	Caution with some species
Trichlorfon (organophosphate)	0.25–0.5 mg/l prolonged immersion or 1 hour bath every 5 days for 3–4 weeks[2] 0.5–1.0 mg/l prolonged immersion or 1 hour bath every 5 days	Freshwater crustacean ectoparasites, monogeneans, leeches Marine crustacean ectoparasites and monogeneans	Toxic to some species (neurologic signs); potentially carcinogenic; treatment extended in cooler water temperatures; increase aeration during treatment; EPA restrictions exist

[1] Stoskopf (1993).
[2] Wildgoose and Lewbart (2001).
[3] Yanong (2004).

110

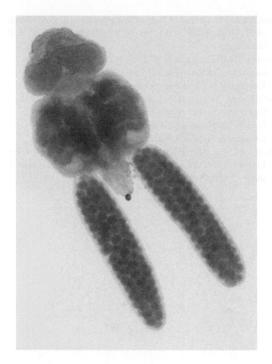

Fig. 8.7 A female *Ergasilus* sp. with two egg sacs, from a striped bass.

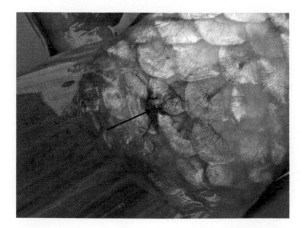

Fig. 8.8 Anchor worm attached to a koi, *Cyprinus carpio* (photo courtesy of Brian Palmeiro). Note the area of hemorrhage surrounding the posterior end of the protruding female parasite.

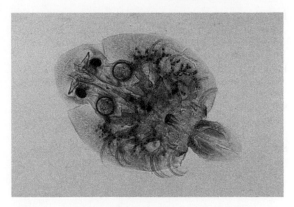

Fig. 8.9 *Argulus* sp., the "fish louse," from a koi, *Cyprinus carpio.*

husbandry practices is essential for an improved prognosis and recovery. Maintaining optimal water quality and hygiene of the tank or pond may reduce the severity of clinical signs in affected fish. Several parasites have life stages that can survive off the host, making environmental cleaning an essential component of treatment. Quarantine protocols should include screening new fish for parasites and treating if necessary during the quarantine period to reduce or eliminate the spread of parasites to other fish.

Treatment of the external parasites is fairly simple since most are susceptible to various waterborne chemotherapeutic compounds such as salt, formalin, or copper (Table 8.1). Care should be taken when administering these compounds as the fish is probably already in a compromised state of health and some of these compounds can be toxic to fish, invertebrates, and plants in the environment. Treatment of most of the internal parasites can be difficult to impossible. For the tissue- or coelomic-inhabiting stages, there are generally no effective treatments available. For most of these parasites, isolating and culling infected fish is probably the best method of control. For the adult parasites inhabiting the lumen of the gastrointestinal tract, some of the antiprotozoal and antiparasitical compounds have been shown to be efficacious.

References

Gratzek, J.B. (1993) Parasites associated with freshwater tropical fish. In *Fish Medicine* (Stoskopf, M.K., ed.), pp. 573–590. Philadelphia: W.B. Saunders.

Hoffman, G.L. (1999) *Parasites of North American Freshwater Fishes*, 2nd Edition. Ithaca, NY: Cornell University Press.

Khoo, L., Dennis, P.M., and Lewbart, G.A. (2006) Rickettsia-like organisms in the blue-eyed plecostomus, *Panaque suttoni* (Eigenmann & Eigenmann). *Journal of Fish Diseases* **18** (2): 157–164.

Lom, J. and Dyková, I. (1992) *Protozoan Parasites of Fishes*. Amsterdam, the Netherlands: Elsevier Science Publishers B.V.

Smith, S.A. (2006). Parasites of fish. In *Veterinary Clinical Parasitology, 7th Edition* (Zajac, A., ed.), pp. 265–279. Ames, IA: Blackwell Publishing.

Smith, S.A. and Noga, E.J. (1992) General parasitology of fish. In *Clinical Fish Medicine* (Stoskopf, M.K., ed.), pp. 131–148. Philadelphia: W.B. Saunders.

Stoskopf, M. (1993). Chemotherapeutics. In *Fish Medicine* (Stoskopf, M. ed.), pp. 832–839. Philadelphia: W.B. Saunders.

Yanong, R.P.E., Curtis, E., Russo, R., et al. (2004) *Cryptobia iubilans* infection in juvenile discus. *Journal of the American Veterinary Medical Association* **224** (10): 1644–1650.

Wildgoose, W.H. and Lewbart, G.A. (2001). Chemotherapeutics. In *BSAVA Manual of Ornamental Fish Health*, 2nd edition (Wildgoose, W.H. ed.), pp. 237–258. Gloucester: BSAVA Publications.

Woo, P.T.K., ed. (2006) *Fish Diseases and Disorders, Volume 1: Protozoan and Metazoan Infections*. Oxfordshire: CABI Publishing.

Chapter 9
Viral Pathogens of Fish

Brian Palmeiro and E. Scott Weber III

Introduction

Viruses are important pathogens in aquatic veterinary medicine. Given the significant diversity and number of fish species, it is likely that the majority of viral pathogens in fish have not been recognized. The following chapter will provide a basic understanding for the recognition, diagnosis, and treatment of viral disease in fish.

Clinical signs

Clinical signs for localized and systemic viral infections are nonspecific and can be seen with many types of infectious diseases and/or environmental problems. These clinical signs may include exophthalmia, petechiation, injected fins, increased respiratory rate, anorexia, overall darkening of the body, excess mucus production, clamped fins, lethargy, disorientation, spinal deformities, abnormal swimming patterns, increased prevalence of secondary bacterial, fungal, and parasitic infections, and varying morbidity and mortality (Noga, 1996; Roberts, 2001; Woo and Bruno, 2003; Ferguson et al., 2006).

Diagnosis of viral disease in fish

Virus isolation and identification

Virus isolation and identification can be difficult in aquatic animals. Since fish are poikilothermic, many of the assays, culture techniques, and diagnostic tools developed for mammals do not work or need modification for use in fish viral disease diagnosis. The key for success in virus isolation and identification is obtaining and preserving tissue samples appropriately and finding a suitable lab that specializes in diagnosing fish viral pathogens.

Tissue culture is the gold standard for isolation of fish viruses. In order to culture viruses, appropriate cell lines are needed. Although 120 cell lines have been developed from fish, they mainly represent economically important freshwater species; many viruses are species specific, and with 53,000 species and subspecies of fish, available cell lines can be a limiting factor for isolating live virus. Virus isolation typically takes between 2 and 3 weeks. Once a virus has been isolated, the cells or supernatant from the cells can be used for other molecular testing and microscopy for identification. Given the limitations of virus isolation, other molecular diagnostic assays or tests are used often for more rapid virus identification. Viral inclusion bodies may be visualized via light microscopy, whereas electron microscopy is required for viral particle identification. Molecular testing is designed either to detect antigenic components of the virus or antibodies to the virus. Some antigen/antibody approaches include enzyme-linked immunosorbent assay (ELISA) testing, serum neutralization, fluorescent antibody testing, immunofluorescent antibody testing, and immunostaining. In addition, there are other types of nucleic acid approaches to help detect virus in fish tissues, such as polymerase chain reaction (PCR), hybridization (*in situ* hybridization and dot blots), and sequencing.

Viral treatment

Although several viral diseases can cause catastrophic, economically significant losses, there are currently no successful commercially available therapeutics to treat viral infections in fish.

Avoidance and prevention are vital for successful control of viral disease in fish. Preventing a viral outbreak requires excellent husbandry practices such as quarantine, disinfection, and sanitation in conjunction with the appropriate diagnostic testing for potential pathogens. See the chapter on biosecurity for more details on pathogen control.

The most promising tool for preventing viral diseases in fish is the prospects of vaccine development. To date, there are few vaccines for fish to protect against viral disease, and the few available are inactivated virus or recombinant proteins. Development of vaccines using live-attenuated virus or DNA is ongoing for several fish pathogens, including koi herpesvirus (KHV) and infectious pancreatic necrosis (IPN).

Quarantine

The purpose of quarantine is to prevent the introduction of parasitic and infectious diseases into a retail/wholesale facility, farm, or an established collection. During quarantine, newly acquired animals are isolated from the established collection in such a manner as to prohibit physical contact, prevent disease transmission, and avoid aerosol and drainage contamination. See the biosecurity chapter for more details on quarantine systems.

With many fish viruses, maintaining a specific temperature range is vital, especially when screening fish for certain pathogens, as many viruses have a specific range when they optimally can infect the animals. When these viruses infect fish above or below these temperature ranges, latent or chronic infections may result, with the potential creation of asymptomatic carriers.

Virus taxonomy

Table 9.1 lists some of the virus families that have been identified in fish, with some disease examples and susceptible species.

Herpesviridae

Herpesviruses are double-stranded DNA viruses. There are three Cyprinid herpesviruses that are important pathogens of ornamental fish: carp pox (Cyprinid herpesvirus 1 [CyHV-1]), herpes viral hematopoietic necrosis (HVHN; Cyprinid herpesvirus 2 [CyHV-2]) and KHV (Cyprinid herpesvirus 3 [CyHV-3]). Other important viral diseases in the herpesvirus family include channel catfish virus (CCV) and pleco herpesvirus.

CyHV-1

Carp pox is caused by CyHV-1. In koi, it causes epidermal hyperplasia and results in papillomatous white to gray plaques on the fins and skin that are often described as "candle wax" in appearance. Although uncommon, CyHV-1 is reported to cause mortality in fry. Carp pox is typically seen in cooler water temperatures during the winter and spring, usually when the water temperature is colder than 15°C (59°F). Lesions usually regress as the water temperature is warmed to greater than 20°C (68°F). After lesion regression, the viral genome has been found in spinal nerves, cranial nerve ganglia, and subcutaneous tissue (Petty and Fraser, 2005). Treatment is typically not required, and an increase in water temperature typically results in spontaneous resolution. Lesions tend to recur in future seasons. Malignant transformation to squamous cell carcinoma has been anecdotally reported.

CyHV-2

CyHV-2, also referred to as HVHN or goldfish herpesvirus, has been associated with disease outbreaks and up to 50%–100% acute mortalities in goldfish. The disease is associated with necrosis of hematopoietic tissues and anemia with high mortality (Goodwin et al., 2006). CyHV-2 causes disease in all varieties of goldfish (*Carassius auratus*) when the water temperatures rises above 15°C (59°F) (Way, 2008). Clinical signs are similar to KHV and include lethargy, anorexia, and patchy pale areas of gill necrosis and skin lesions. The kidney and spleen are enlarged and the spleen often contains distinctive white nodules (Way, 2008). A quantitative sensitive and specific TaqMan® (Roche Molecular Systems, Inc., Pleasanton, CA) PCR test has been developed at the University of Arkansas, which can differentiate between active and carrier levels of

Table 9.1 Viral taxonomy in fish.

Herpesviridae	Cyprinid herpesvirus 1 (carp pox)	Koi
	Cyprinid herpesvirus 2 (herpes viral hematopoietic necrosis or goldfish herpesvirus)	Goldfish
	Cyprinid herpesvirus 3 (koi herpesvirus)	Koi
	Channel catfish virus	Channel catfish
	Pleco herpesvirus	Plecostomus
	Discus herpesvirus	Discus
Adenoviridae	—	—
Iridoviridae	Lymphocystis	Many species
	Megalocytivirus—systemic infection and can be transmitted from freshwater to marine species. Four viruses of this group have complete genomic sequence and are very homologous. Some are reportable for international export such as the Red sea bream iridovirus.	Many freshwater and marine species
	Skin and gill iridovirus	White sturgeon
	Epizootic hematopoietic necrosis virus	Many species
	Viral erythrocytic necrosis	Atlantic cod, Pacific herring
	European catfish virus	European catfish
	Ranaviruses—various systemic signs	Many Species
Poxviridae	Multiple species specific viruses	—
Retroviridae	—	"Lip fibromas" in angelfish
Birnaviridae	—	—
Reoviridae	—	—
Paramyxoviridae	—	—
Orthomyxoviridae	—	—
Rhabdoviridae	Spring viremia of carp	Multiple species
	Viral hemorrhagic septicemia	Multiple species
Caliciviridae	—	—
Nidovirales (order)	Coroniviridae	—
	Roniviridae	—
	Arteriviridae	—

infection (Goodwin et al., 2006). As with KHV, fish that survive infection may become carriers of the virus.

KHV

KHV is a double-stranded DNA herpesvirus (CyHV-3; carp interstitial nephritis and gill necrosis virus) that infects and causes massive mortality in koi and common carp (*Cyprinus carpio*). Approximately 80% nucleotide homology has been established between CyHV-1, CyHV-2, and KHV (Pokorova et al., 2005). KHV was first reported as a cause of massive fish mortality in Israel in 1998 and is now global in distribution (Hedrick et al., 1999). KHV is listed as a reportable disease by the World Organization for Animal Health (OIE) (Way, 2008). The respiratory system is predominantly affected, resulting in clinical signs such as piping (gasping at the water surface), elevated opercular rate, gathering near the surface or in well-aerated areas such as near waterfalls/filter input, excessive mucus from the gills, swollen gills, and mottled areas of gill necrosis/discoloration. The skin can also be affected with ulcerations, hemorrhages, sloughing of scales, and increased or decreased mucus production. Other common clinical signs include lethargy, anorexia, sunken eyes (enophthalmos) (Fig. 9.1), a notched appearance to the head dorsal to the nares (Fig. 9.2), erratic swimming, and "hanging" with a head down position in the water column.

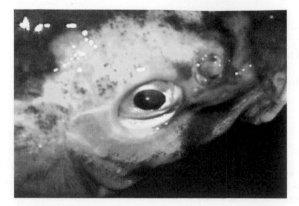

Fig. 9.1 Koi with koi herpesvirus showing enophthalmos (photo courtesy of Walt Oldenberg).

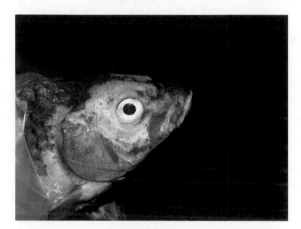

Fig. 9.2 Koi with koi herpesvirus with typical "notched" appearance to the skull in the area of the nares (photo courtesy of Walt Oldenberg).

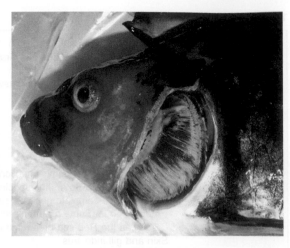

Fig. 9.3 Koi infected with koi herpesvirus with severe gill necrosis (photo courtesy of Dr. Helen Roberts).

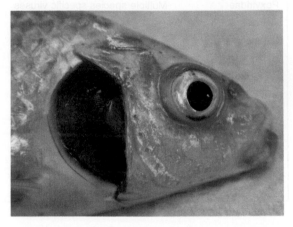

Fig. 9.4 Koi infected with koi herpesvirus with mild gill necrosis. Note the hyphema present in the right eye.

On postmortem examination, all fish have gill necrosis, which often presents as patchy regions of white discolorations. The necrosis can range from mild to severe. Figure 9.3 illustrates a KHV-infected koi with severe gill necrosis, whereas Figure 9.4 illustrates a koi with milder gill necrosis. Internal examination findings are nonspecific and include darkening or mottling of internal organs such as the spleen, kidney, or liver, and occasionally, fluid accumulation and adhesion formation (Hartman et al., 2004; Way, 2008). Wet mount examination of the gills will reveal gill necrosis with complete loss of normal lamellar architecture; secondary parasitic and bacterial infections are extremely common, both on the gills and skin.

Virulent virus is shed via the feces, urine, and skin and gill mucus (Way, 2008). The virus likely enters the fish through the gills, where it undergoes replication prior to disseminating through the bloodstream (by localizing in the white blood cells) to the kidney and other organs such as spleen, liver, and intestines (Pikarsky et al., 2004; Walster, 2008). The virus causes lysis of infected cells (Walster, 2008). Branchitis and interstitial nephritis are seen histologically as early as 2 days postinfection, but mortality does not typically occur until 6–8 days postinfection (Pikarsky et al., 2004; Walster, 2008).

Different strains that vary in virulence have been reported but are thought to arise from the same KHV ancestor (Aoki et al., 2007).

Water temperature contributes significantly to the course of the disease both directly by affecting viral replication and indirectly by augmenting the fish's immune response (Way, 2008). Natural or experimental infection between 16 and 28 °C (the permissive temperature range) results in *70%–100% mortality* over a course of 7–21 days (Gilad et al., 2003). Clinical disease is only seen when the water temperature is in this permissive zone (16–28 °C, 61–82 °F) (Walster, 2008). The virus has been shown to replicate in common carp at 13 °C and in cell culture at 4 °C, supporting the hypothesis that the virus can overwinter with the fish (Gilad et al., 2003, 2004); no growth occurs in cell culture at or above 30 °C (Gilad et al., 2003). Surviving fish, including those subjected to elevated water temperatures following infection, develop partial or complete resistance to reinfection (Gilad et al., 2003). A well-known characteristic of herpesviruses is their ability to persist in a latent state in their host, including those with both natural and vaccine-induced immunity; they can remain dormant and noninfectious for various periods of time but can become reactivated to result in clinical disease. Therefore, fish that survive KHV infection are considered lifelong carriers of the virus. It is currently unknown what percentage of surviving fish become carriers or where the latent phase of the virus resides in the fish. Common carp that recover from KHV infection can, in some cases, become persistently infected; these fish can shed the virus and infect naïve fish at water temperatures greater than 20 °C (St-Hilaire et al., 2005). In one study, the virus became reactivated and infected naïve fish up to 30 weeks after initial infection (St-Hilaire et al., 2005). Given that persistently infected fish are created, exposing fish to KHV at nonpermissive temperatures is not considered a safe method of disease prevention (St-Hilaire et al., 2005).

Diagnosis of KHV is based on clinical signs, combined with detection of the virus via virus isolation (on the KF-1 cell line) or DNA identification via PCR. In cases of acute infection, PCR is the most practical and rapid method of diagnosis. PCR is reported to be the most sensitive diagnostic tool available for the diagnosis of KHV (Haenen et al.,

2004). Gill, kidney, and spleen are the organs in which KHV is most abundant and should be submitted for virological testing (Way, 2008). Detection of KHV DNA via PCR is extremely difficult beyond 64 days after exposure (Gilad et al., 2004).

Currently, the most concerning aspect in the diagnosis of KHV is the ability to detect carrier fish. Detection of KHV antibodies is currently the only method of determining previous exposure to the virus if animals are not shedding active virus for detection of viral DNA via PCR (Way, 2008). A recent report describes use of an ELISA that detects antibodies in the serum of koi for periods of up to 1 year after previous exposure to the virus (Adkison et al., 2005). A quantitative KHV ELISA is now commercially available at the University of California Davis Veterinary Teaching Hospital and is the authors' test of choice for detecting carrier fish. False-negative serology results may occur early in the course of exposure as development of positive titers may take several weeks to develop.

There is no effective treatment for KHV. Depopulation and disinfection is recommended as fish that survive infection are considered carriers. In private collections, some owners may elect to treat their pet fish. The water temperature can be increased to greater than 29 °C (84 °F) to help reduce morbidity and mortality. Secondary bacterial and parasitic infections are extremely common and must be treated accordingly. Prolonged bath immersion with salt (0.1%–0.3%) can be used to decrease osmotic stresses associated with gill and skin disease. The owners must be thoroughly educated by the veterinarian that surviving fish are considered carriers and should not be mixed with naïve fish; when the owners refuse to depopulate and disinfect their systems, the authors recommend that surviving fish be maintained in a closed system, with no new fish introductions.

The virus can survive in pond water for at least 4 hours at temperatures of around 22 °C (Perelberg et al., 2003) and probably survives for much longer periods in droppings and pond mud (Dishon et al., 2005; Hutoran et al., 2005). Its ability to survive in water likely plays an important role in its rapid spread between fish (Walster, 2008). Common disinfectants that can be used on the system and equipment include chlorine (such as household bleach) at 200 mg/l and quaternary ammonium compounds

(Hartman et al., 2004). Other disinfectants that are reported to inactivate the virus include iodophores at 200 mg/l for 20 minutes, benzalkonium chloride at 60 mg/l for 20 minutes, and 30% ethyl alcohol for 20 minutes (OIE, 2006; Walster, 2008). Ponds and equipment can also be drained and dried, but the virus may survive in mud and pond sediment so complete drying for a minimum of 2 weeks is recommended; the authors commonly recommend combining drying with either chlorine bleach or quaternary ammonium compound disinfection.

KHV can be prevented by purchasing fish from reputable sources and quarantining all new fish for a minimum of 4–6 weeks at permissive temperatures. The authors recommend combining quarantine with ELISA serology to evaluate for the presence of carrier fish. Goldfish housed with infected koi have been shown to contain PCR detectable DNA identified as KHV, which may implicate other species as vectors in spreading KHV (El-Matbouli et al., 2007). No outbreaks of KHV in koi have been directly attributable to goldfish or other species to date. An antemortem test to screen for the presence of the KHV carrier state in goldfish is not currently available, and the duration of carriage in goldfish is unknown; therefore, caution should be taken when introducing goldfish into any existing koi population.

No KHV vaccines are currently approved for use in the United States or Europe. A live-attenuated vaccine is currently available for use in Israel. The virus was attenuated by 26 passages in cell culture followed by ultraviolet (UV) irradiation and selection by cloning (Walster, 2008). The vaccine is administered by intracoelomic injection or immersion and has been shown to protect fish from a KHV challenge that caused 95% mortality in non-vaccinated controls (Walster, 2008). The vaccine induces antibody against the virus, but the duration of the protection is unknown (Way, 2008). It is also unknown whether vaccinated fish may shed the virus, potentially exposing naïve fish. KHV is a notifiable disease by the OIE and is reportable in the United States and several other countries.

CCV

CCV is the most important viral disease of channel catfish; it is briefly discussed here as some koi and goldfish hobbyists also keep channel catfish. The mortality and speed at which signs develop are variable and directly related to the size of the fish, water temperature, and viral load to which the fish is exposed (Camus, 2004). During outbreaks, younger, more robust fish typically experience mortality first (Noga, 1996). Only young fry and fingerlings (<1 year) and small (<15 cm) fish show clinical signs (Noga, 1996; Camus, 2004). Mortalities are most rapid and severe during hot summer months in higher water temperatures, especially 25–30 °C (77–86 °F) (Noga, 1996; Camus, 2004). No mortality occurs in water that is <15 °C (59 °F).

The virus is transmitted horizontally in the feces and urine; vertical transmission is also reported (Noga, 1996; Camus, 2004). The virus can persist in a dormant form in fish that survive an outbreak, creating carrier fish; carrier fish such as broodstock can then shed the virus and infect young fish (Noga, 1996; Camus, 2004). Clinical signs include hanging in the water in a head-up position, disorientation (corkscrew spiral swimming), abdominal distension, swollen vent, exophthalmos, and hemorrhages of the fins and skin (Noga, 1996; Camus, 2004). Postmortem exam reveals yellowish to blood-tinged fluid in the coelomic cavity and punctuate hemorrhages of the viscera (Noga, 1996). The primary site of damage from CCV is the kidney (both excretory and hematopoietic), but the virus can affect all major organ systems (kidney, liver, spleen, gastrointestinal [GI] system, pancreas, muscle, central nervous system [CNS], gills) (Noga, 1996; Camus 2004). Definitive diagnosis of CCV requires identification of virus from target tissues. Serum neutralization of cell culture-isolated virus is the most widely used method for definitive diagnosis (Noga, 1996). There is no effective treatment for CCV. Treating secondary bacterial infections such as enteric septicemia and columnaris, decreasing water temperature, and a reduction of environmental stressors can decrease morbidity and mortality (Camus, 2004).

Pleco herpesvirus

A herpesvirus has been reported in blue-eyed plecos (*Panaque suttoni*). Affected fish are reported to have pale blotchy lesions on the skin that ulcerate; mortality occurs within days of appearance of skin lesions (Yanong, 1995). Herpesvirus-like particles were observed by electron microscopic examination of the skin lesions (Yanong, 1995). Similar lesions have also been reported in the common pleco (Petty and Fraser, 2005).

Discus herpesvirus

A herpeslike virus has been reported to cause high levels of mortality associated with skin ulceration and necrosis in discus (E.S. Weber and T. Waltzek, pers. comm.); further research on the classification of this virus is under way.

Iridoviridae

Iridoviruses are DNA viruses found in many poikilotherms, including invertebrates, amphibians, and fish (Daszak et al., 1999, 2003; Chinchar, 2002; Delhon et al., 2006). The family Iridoviridae has three genera found in fish that include the ranaviruses, lymphocystiviruses, and the megalocytiviruses (Chinchar et al., 2005). The genus *Megalocytivirus* is the group most frequently identified, causing systemic infections in both marine and freshwater fish. Several of the species of ornamental freshwater fish have included the dwarf gourami (*Colisa lalia*), chromide cichlids (*Etroplus maculates*), freshwater angelfish (*Pterophyllum scalare*), and the African lampeye (*Aplocheilichthys normani*) (Armstrong and Ferguson, 1989; Anderson et al., 1993; Rodger et al., 1997; Paperna et al., 2001; Sudthongkong et al., 2002). The mortality caused by iridovirus can reach 100% as observed in imported Banggai cardinal fish (*Pterapogon kauderni*) (Weber et al., 2009). Iridovirus infections have shown little species specificity for marine and freshwater hosts, and occur in diverse geographic areas, causing major impact on aquaculture for both the food and ornamental fish trades (Whittington and Chong, 2007). This lack of specificity may account for the genetic similarity of all the megalocytiviruses identified so far in fish, which share >93% DNA and amino acid sequence (Chinchar et al., 2005; Song et al., 2008). Another unique feature of iridoviruses are that the virus is very stable in the aquatic environment, and they can infect animals of the same and different species readily via waterborne transmission as shown in experimental studies between dwarf gouramis and Murray cod (*Maccullochella peelii peelii*), with cultured mandarin fish (*Siniperca chuatsi*), between red sea bream (*Pagus major*) and grouper (*Epinephelus malabaricus*), and in juvenile white sturgeon (*Acipenser transmontanus*) and sturgeon cell lines (Watson et al., 1998; He et al., 2000, 2002; Sano et al., 2002; Go and Whittington, 2006). Examples of iridovirus infections exhibiting systemic infection and greater than 50% mortality include outbreaks in ornamental fish such as orange chromide cichlids, in aquaculture for food fish such as red sea bream, and in wild populations of turbot (*Psetta maximus*) in the South China Sea (Inouye et al., 1992; Oh et al., 2006; Song et al., 2008).

Clinical signs associated with *Megalocytivirus* include lethargy, severe anemia, and branchial hemorrhages (Armstrong and Ferguson, 1989; Gibson-Kueh et al., 2003). On gross necropsy, the spleen is often enlarged, and on histopathology, virions can be found in multiple organs such as spleen, kidney, intestine, eye, pancreas, liver, heart, gill, and brain (Smail and Munro, 2001; Gibson-Kueh et al., 2003). Due to the large host range and multiple industries at risk to *Megalocytivirus* infection, this group of viruses may prove to be the most important infection of cultured fish and pose the greatest risk to endangered wild fish populations for ornamental and food fisheries and aquaculture.

Lymphocystis

The most common and well-researched viral disease of pet fish is lymphocystis (Weissenberg, 1965). Common species of fish affected include freshwater glass fish, freshwater cichlids, marine angelfish, and clown fish. Catfish and cyprinids are not susceptible (Petty and Fraser, 2005). Lymphocystis is transmitted when infected skin cells rupture and release viral particles into the water. Facilities with dense fish populations and excessive handling (such as retail and wholesale operations) are at higher risk for transmission and clinical disease (Petty and Fraser, 2005). The incubation period in experimental infections ranged from 5 to 12 days at 20–25 °C and was shorter with increasing temperature (Petty and Fraser, 2005).

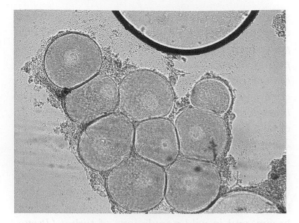

Fig. 9.5 Typical hypertrophied dermal fibroblasts on a wet mount exam of the skin from a fish with lymphocystis. Dermal fibroblasts appear like a "cluster of grapes."

The virus infects dermal fibroblasts, causing them to swell up to 100,000 times their normal size, resulting in coalescing white to gray nodules, typically on the fins. Lymphocystis is the only viral disease that can be diagnosed on wet mounts/skin scrapings, revealing the classic swollen/hypertrophied dermal fibroblasts that appear like a "cluster of grapes" (see Fig. 9.5). Hypertrophied fibroblasts are also seen on histopathology. Specific treatment is typically not required; improvement in environmental conditions and removal of underlying stressors typically results in spontaneous resolution. In some cases, surgical removal may be required.

Rhabdoviridae

Spring viremia of carp (SVC)

Rhabdoviruses are single-stranded RNA viruses that can cause disease in fish. The most significant viral disease of ornamental fish in the Rhaboviridae family is the spring viremia of carp virus (SVCV), also known as *Rhabdovirus carpio*. SVCV primarily affects fish in the Cyprinidae family; reported affected species include common carp (*C. carpio*), koi carp (*C. carpio koi*), grass carp/white amur (*Ctenopharyngodon idella*), silver carp (*Hypophthalamicthys molitrix*), bighead carp (*Aristicthys nobilis*), crucian carp (*Carassius carassius*), goldfish (*C. auratus*), tench (*Tinca tinca*), orfe, (*Leuciscus idus*), and sheatfish/European catfish/wels (*Siluris glani*) (Iowa State web sites, 2007). Common carp is the most susceptible species and considered the natural host (Iowa State, 2007). Experimental infections have been reported in roach (*Rutilus rutilus*), zebra fish (*Danio rerio*), guppies (*Lebistes reticulates*), northern pike (*Esox lucius*), golden shiners (*Notemigonus crysoleucas*), and pumpkinseed (*Lepomis gibbosus*) (Iowa State, 2007). The disease is considered endemic in Europe. In 2002, SVCV was found in cultivated koi in North Carolina and in wild common carp in Wisconsin and Illinois. Outbreaks were also reported in cultivated koi in Washington and Missouri in 2004 and in wild fish in the Upper Mississippi River in 2007 (Iowa State, 2007).

Transmission of SVCV is primarily horizontal (fish to fish) via the urine and feces of infected and carrier fish. Vector transmission with the carp louse (*Argulus foliceus*) and leech (*Piscicola geometra*) has also been reported (Petty et al., 2008). Infectious virus can persist in 10 °C water for more than 4 weeks and in 4 °C mud for at least 6 weeks (Iowa State, 2007). The disease typically occurs in the spring, when the water temperature is between 10 and 15 °C (50 and 59 °F) (Iowa State, 2007). Disease is most often seen in yearling fish. Clinical signs include lethargy, loss of equilibrium, swimming at the surface or edge of ponds, darkening and hemorrhages of the skin, pale gills, exophthalmos, abdominal swelling, swelling of the vent, and trailing mucoid fecal casts (Iowa State, 2007; Petty et al., 2008). Postmortem examination may reveal swollen or pale gills, ascites, inflamed dilated intestines, and petechiation of the intestines, other viscera, and swim bladder. The presence of pinpoint hemorrhages in the swim bladder is considered an important indicator of this disease (Petty et al., 2008). Mortality rate is variable (10%–100%) but is particularly higher in younger fish (Iowa State, 2007). SVC is listed as a notifiable disease by the OIE and is reportable in the United States; therefore, prompt notification of the state veterinarian's office and appropriate United States Department of Agriculture (USDA)-Animal and Plant Health Inspection Service (APHIS) Veterinary Services officials is mandatory.

Diagnosis of SVCV can be accomplished by various methods. Direct methods including virus isolation and identification using fathead minnow, epithelioma papillosum of carp, and primary carp ovary cells cell lines (Petty et al., 2008). Indirect tests for SVC include ELISA, virus neutralization (VN) and immunofluorescence (IFA) of suspect tissue. VN is currently the confirmatory identification test for SVCV (Petty and Fraser, 2005). In the United States, diagnostic testing can only be performed in USDA-approved laboratories. The virus can only be isolated from infected fish if the water temperature is less that 20 °C (Petty and Fraser, 2005). There is no effective treatment for SVC, and depopulation and disinfection is mandatory in active outbreaks, given the contagious nature of the pathogen and the possibility of nonclinical carriers that may not exhibit symptoms.

In 2006, the USDA-APHIS declared an interim rule on the importation of SVC-susceptible species. The rule established regulations to restrict the importation into the United States of live fish, fertilized eggs, and gametes of fish species that are susceptible to SVC.

Viral hemorrhagic septicemia (VHS)

VHS is caused by a member of the genus *Novirhabdovirus* in the family Rhabdoviridae. Polyclonal and monoclonal antibody neutralization suggests a single serotype consisting of three subtypes (I, II, III); both marine and freshwater isolates have been documented (OIE, 2006). Based on sequence analysis, four genotypes that correlate most with geographic distribution have been identified; North American isolates belong to genotype IV (OIE, 2006). Viral hemorrhagic septicemia (VHS) has been isolated from at least 50 species of freshwater and marine fish from the Northern Hemisphere. Species susceptible to infection include members of the Salmoniformes (salmon and trout), Pleuronectiformes (flounders, soles, and other flatfishes), Gadiformes (cod), Esociformes (pike), Clupeiformes (herring and anchovy), Osmeriformes (smelt), Perciformes (perch and drum), Scorpaeniformes (rockfishes and sculpins), Anguilliformes (eels), Cyprinodontiformes (mummichog), and Gasterosteiformes (sticklebacks) (Iowa State, 2007). Many species of marine fish appear to be infected asymptomatically, suggesting that VHSV is possibly endemic in marine environments (Iowa State, 2007). Species currently known to be affected include rainbow trout, lake trout, steelhead trout, turbot, Japanese flounder, Pacific herring, Pacific hake, Atlantic salmon, Pacific salmon (chinook), grayling, whitefish (*Coregonus* spp.), halibut, sea bass, tube snout, Atlantic cod, black cod, pilchard, ratfish, muskellunge, freshwater drum, round goby, shiner perch, yellow perch, smallmouth bass, white bass, walleye, bluegill, crappie, gizzard shad, redhorse sucker, bluntnose sucker, and northern pike (Iowa State, 2007). Anecdotally, koi/common carp have been reported to be infected by VHSV; however, the infection has not been confirmed at the USDA's National Veterinary Services Laboratory (National Aquaculture Association, 2007). Initially, the virus was not reported in warmwater fishes, but recent outbreaks in the Great Lakes have reported disease in warmwater species such as perch and drum (Iowa State, 2007). VHSV has become an emerging disease in the Great Lakes region of the United States; outbreaks have been detected in Lake Ontario, Lake St. Clair, Lake Erie, and the St. Lawrence River, as well as Conesus Lake (APHIS, 2006). Due to its high mortality and severe economic consequences, VHS is classified as a reportable disease by the OIE.

The virus is transmitted horizontally predominantly via the urine and reproductive fluids (Noga, 1996, Iowa State, 2007). Survivors of infection may become carriers, periodically shedding the virus; the virus is not consistently detectable in carriers until they are sexually mature (Noga, 1996). The virus can also be transferred by mechanical carriers such as birds (OIE, 2006).

Clinical signs of infection include anorexia, lethargy, abnormal swimming behavior, darkening of the skin, pale gills, hemorrhages of the eyes, fins, gills, and skin, exophthalmos, and ascites. Noga (1996) describes three phases of VHS outbreaks. In the acute phase, there is high mortality; fish are dark and lethargic, with hemorrhages and erythema of the fins. In the chronic phase, there is moderate mortality, and fish are hyperpigmented (black) with anemia, exophthalmos, and abdominal distension. In the nervous phase, there is low mortality, and fish exhibit abnormal swimming behavior, darting through the water and spiraling (Noga, 1996). Clinical disease and mortality vary with host factors such as species and age, VHSV strain, and various environmental factors. Young fish appear to be more severely affected. Temperature is also very important in the course of infection. The optimal temperature for active infection is 9–12 °C (48–54 °F); most outbreaks occur when water temperatures are less than 15 °C (59 °F) (Iowa State, 2007). VHS has not been reported when water temperature is above 18 °C (64 °F) (Iowa State, 2007).

Diagnosis of VHS can be achieved via virus isolation; recommended cell lines include BF–2 (Bluegill fry) and RTG–2 (Rainbow trout gonad) cells (OIE, 2006). Virus identity is confirmed by VN, IFA, ELISA, or PCR. Serology by VN or ELISA may be effective in detecting carriers but has not yet been validated for routine diagnosis (Iowa State, 2007). Suspected or confirmed cases of VHS should be reported to the appropriate state and federal authorities.

On October 24, 2006, USDA-APHIS issued an emergency order prohibiting the importation of 37 species of live fish from two Canadian provinces into the United States and the interstate movement of the same species from the eight states bordering the Great Lakes. The eight states in the federal order are Illinois, Indiana, Michigan, Minnesota, New York, Ohio, Pennsylvania, and Wisconsin; New York, Pennsylvania, Michigan, and Ohio have experienced fish die offs due to VHS (APHIS, 2006).

Retroviridae

"Lip fibromas," also called odontogenic hamartomas, present as nodular lesions around the lips of angelfish and have been associated with retrovirus-like particles (Francis-Floyd et al., 1993). The tumors do not typically result in mortality unless they interfere with feeding. The treatment of choice is surgical removal; typically, the lesions do not recur.

References and further reading

Adkison, M.A., Gilad, O., and Hedrick, R.P. (2005) An enzyme linked immunosorbent assay (ELISA) for detection of antibodies to the koi herpesvirus in the serum of koi, *Cyprinus carpio*. *Fish Pathology* **40** (2): 53–62.

Anderson, I., Prior, H., Rodwell, B., et al. (1993) Iridovirus-like virions in imported dwarf gourami (*Colisa lalia*) with systemic amoebiasis. *Australian Veterinary Journal* **70**: 66–67.

Aoki, T., Hirono, I., Kurokawa, K., et al. (2007) Genome sequences of three koi herpes virus isolates representing the expanding distribution of an emerging disease threatening koi and common carp worldwide. *Journal of Virology* **81**: 5058–5065.

APHIS Factsheet: Questions and Answers about VHS Federal Order. (2006) www.aphis.usda.gov/publications/animal_health/content/printable_version/fs_vhs_q_and_a.pdf (accessed October 1, 2008).

Armstrong, R.D. and Ferguson, H.W. (1989) Systemic viral disease of the chromide cichlid *Etroplus maculates*. *Diseases of Aquatic Organisms* **7**: 155–157.

Camus, A. (2004) *Channel Catfish Virus Disease*. SRAC Publication No. 4702. www.aquanic.org/publicat/usda_rac/efs/srac/4702fs.pdf (accessed October 1, 2008).

Chinchar, V.G. (2002) Ranaviruses (family Iridoviridae): emerging cold-blooded killers. *Archives of Virology* **147**: 447–470.

Chinchar, V.G., Essbauer, S., He, J.G., et al. (2005) Iridoviridae. In *Virus Taxonomy: 8th Report of the International Committee on the Taxonomy of Viruses* (Fauquet, C.M., Mayo, M.A., Maniloff, J., et al., eds.), pp. 163–175. London: Elsevier.

Daszak, P., Berger, L., Cunningham, A.A., et al. (1999) Emerging infectious diseases and amphibian population declines. *Emerging and Infectious Diseases* **5**: 735–748.

Daszak, P., Cunningham, A.A., and Hyatt, A.D. (2003) Infectious disease and amphibian population declines. *Diversity & Distribution* **9**: 141–150.

Delhon, G., Tulman, E.R., Afonso, C.L., et al. (2006) Genome of invertebrate iridescent virus type 3 (mosquito iridescent virus). *Journal of Virology* **80**: 8439–8449.

Dishon, A., Perelberg, A., Bishara-Shieban, J., et al. (2005) Detection of carp interstitial nephritis and gill necrosis virus in fish droppings. *Applied and Environmental Microbiology* **71**: 7285–7291.

El-Matbouli, M., Saleh, M., and Soliman, H. (2007) Detection of cyprinid herpesvirus type 3 in goldfish cohabiting with CyHV-3 infected koi carp. *Veterinary Record* **161**: 792–793.

Ferguson, H., Bjerkas, E., and Evensen, O. (2006) *Systemic Pathology of Fish: A Text and Atlas of Normal Tissue Responses in Teleosts, and Their Responses in Disease*, 2nd Edition. Ames, IA: Scotian Press.

Francis-Floyd, R., Bolon, B., Fraser, W., et al. (1993) Lip fibromas associated with retrovirus-like particles in angel fish. *Journal of the American Veterinary Medical Association* **202**: 427–429.

Gibson-Kueh, S., Netto, P., Ngoh-Lim, G.H., et al. 2003. The pathology of systemic iridoviral disease in fish. *Journal of Comparative Pathology* **129**: 111–119.

Gilad, O., Yun, S., Andree, K.B., et al. (2002) Initial characteristics of koi herpesvirus and development of a polymerase chain reaction assay to detect the virus in koi, *Cyprinus carpio koi. Diseases of Aquatic Organisms* **48**: 101–108.

Gilad, O., Yun, S., Adkison, M.A., et al. (2003) Molecular comparison of isolates of an emerging fish pathogen, koi herpesvirus, and the effect of water temperature on mortality of experimentally infected koi. *Journal of General Virology* **84**: 2661–2668.

Gilad, O., Yun, S., Zagmutt-Vergara, F., et al. (2004) Concentrations of a herpes-like virus (KHV) in tissues of experimentally infected *Cyprinus carpio koi* as assessed by real-time TaqMan PCR. *Diseases of Aquatic Organisms* **60**: 179–187.

Go, J. and Whittington, R. (2006) Experimental transmission and virulence of megalocytivirus (family Iridoviridae) of dwarf gourami (*Colisa lalia*) from Asia in Murray cod (*Maccullochella peelii peelii*) in Australia. *Aquaculture* **258**: 140–149.

Goodwin, A.E., Merry, G.E., and Sadler, J. (2006) Detection of the herpesviral haematopoietic necrosis disease agent Cyprinid herpesvirus 2 in moribund and healthy goldfish: validation of a quantitative PCR diagnostic method. *Diseases of Aquatic Organisms* **69**: 137–143.

Haenen, O., Way, K., Bergmann, S., et al. (2004) The emergence of KHV and its significance to European aquaculture. *Bulletin of the European Association of Fish Pathologists* **24** (6): 293–307.

Hartman, K.H., Yanong, R.P.E., Petty, D., et al. (2004) *Koi Herpes Virus (KHV) Disease*. University of Florida IFAS Extension Publication VM-149/VM113. http://edis.ifas.ufl.edu/VM113 (accessed October 1, 2008).

He, J.G., Wang, S.P., Zeng, K., et al. (2000) Systemic disease cause by an iridovirus-like agent in cultured mandarin fish *Siniperca chuatsi* (Basilewski) in China. *Journal of Fish Diseases* **23**: 219–222.

He, J.G., Zeng, K., Weng, P., et al. (2002) Experimental transmission, pathogenicity and physical-chemical properties of infectious spleen and kidney necrosis virus (ISKNV). *Aquaculture* **204**: 11–24.

Hedrick, R.P., Marty, G., Nordhausen, R.W., et al. (1999) A herpesvirus associated with mass mortality of juvenile and adult koi *Cyprinus carpio. Fish Health Newsletter* **27**: 7.

Hutoran, M., Ronen, A., Perelberg, A., et al. (2005) Description of an as yet unclassified DNA virus from diseased *Cyprinus carpio* species. *Journal of Virology* **79**: 1983–1991.

Inouye, K., Yamano, K., Maeno, Y., et al. (1992) Iridovirus infection of cultured red sea bream, *Pagus major. Fish Pathology* **27**: 19–27.

Lynch, M.J. (1998) Preliminary Investigation of Gourami Iridovirus Infections. MS Thesis, University of Florida, Gainesville, FL.

National Aquaculture Association. (2007) *VHS Found in Koi, Rainbow Trout and Gizzard Shad.* www.wisconsinaquaculture.com/Forms/073007_VHS_Found_In_Koi.doc (accessed October 1, 2008).

Noga, E.J., ed. (1996) *Fish Disease: Diagnosis and Treatment*. St. Louis, MO: Mosby.

Oh, M-J., Kitamur, S-I., Kim, W-S., et al. (2006) Susceptibility of marine fish species to megalocytivirus, turbot iridovirus, isolated from turbot, *Psetta maximus* (L.). *Journal of Fish Diseases* **29**: 415–421.

Paperna, I., Vilenkin, M., and Alves de Matos, A.P. (2001). Iridovirus infections in farm-reared tropical ornamental fish. *Diseases of Aquatic Organisms* **48**: 17–25.

Perelberg, A., Smirnov, M., Hutoran, M., et al. (2003) Epidemiological description of a new viral disease afflicting cultured *Cyprinus carpio* in Israel. *Israeli Journal of Aquaculture-Bamid-geh* **55**: 5–12.

Petty, B.D. and Fraser, W.A. (2005) Viruses of pet fish. *Veterinary Clinics of North America: Exotic Animal Practice* **8**: 67–84.

Petty, B.D., Riggs, A.C., Klinger, R., et al. (2008) *Spring Viremia of Carp*. University of Florida IFAS Extension Publication VM-142/VM106. http://edis.ifas.ufl.edu/VM106 (accessed October 1, 2008).

Pikarsky, E., Ronen, A., Abramowitz, J., et al. (2004) Pathogenesis of acute viral disease induced in fish by carp interstitial nephritis and gill necrosis virus. *Journal of Virology* **78**: 9544–9551.

Pokorova, D., Vesely, T., Piackova, V., et al. (2005) Current knowledge on koi herpes virus: a review. *Veterinary Medicine–Czech* **50** (4): 139–147.

Roberts, R.J. (2001) *Fish Pathology*, 3rd Edition. Philadelphia: W.B. Saunders.

Rodger, H., Kobs, M., Macartney, A., et al. (1997) Systemic iridovirus infection in freshwater angelfish, *Pterophyllum scalare* (Lichtenstein). *Journal of Fish Diseases* **20**:69–72.

Sano, M., Minagawa, M., and Nakajima, K. (2002) Multiplication of red sea bream iridovirus (RSIV) in the experimentally infected grouper *Epinephelus malabaricus. Fish Pathology* **37**: 1–6.

St-Hilaire, S., Beevers, N., Way, K., et al. (2005) Reactivation of koi herpesvirus infections in common carp *Cyprinus carpio. Diseases of Aquatic Organisms* **67**: 15–23.

Schuh, J.C.L. and Shirley, I.G. (1990) Viral hematopoietic necrosis in an angelfish (*Pterophyllum scalare*). *Journal of Zoo and Wildlife Medicine* **21** (1): 95–98.

Smail, D.A. and Munro, A.L.S. (2001) The virology of teleosts. In *Fish Pathology*, 3rd Edition (Roberts, R., ed.), pp. 169–253. Edinburgh: W.B. Saunders.

Song, J-Y., Kitamura, S-I., Jung, S-J., et al. (2008) Genetic EU variation and geographic distribution of megalocytiviruses. *Journal of Microbiology* **46**: 29–33.

Spring Viremia of Carp; Import Restrictions on Certain Live Fish, Fertilized Eggs, and Gametes. http://tal.ifas.ufl.edu/PDFs/APHIS-2006-0107-0002[1].pdf (accessed October 1, 2008).

Spring Viremia of Carp. Iowa State University. www.cfsph.iastate.edu/Factsheets/pdfs/spring_viremia_of_carp.pdf (accessed October 1, 2008).

Sudthongkong, C., Miyata, M., and Miyazaki, T. (2002) Iridovirus disease in two ornamental tropical fishes: African lampeye and dwarf gourami. *Diseases of Aquatic Organisms* **48**: 163–173.

Viral Hemorrhagic Septicemia. Iowa State University. www.cfsph.iastate.edu/Factsheets/pdfs/viral_hemorrhagic_septicemia.pdf (accessed October 1, 2008).

Walster, C. (2008) Koi herpesvirus: the international perspective. Paper presented at the WAVMA Conference /29th World Veterinary Congress, Vancouver, Canada, July 27–31.

Watson, L.R., Groff, J.M., and Hedrick, R.P. (1998) Replication and pathogenesis of white sturgeon iridovirus (WSIV) in experimentally infected white sturgeon *Acipenser transmontanus* juveniles and sturgeon cell lines. *Diseases of Aquatic Organisms* **32**: 173–184.

Way, K. (2008) Koi herpesvirus and goldfish herpesvirus: an update of current knowledge and research at Cefas. *Fish Veterinary Journal* **10**: 62–73.

Weber, E.S. (2008) Personal communication, ••

Weber, E.S., Waltzek, T., Young, D.A., et al. (2009) Systemic iridovirus infection in the Banggai cardinalfish (*Pterapogon kauderni* Koumans 1933). *Journal of Veterinary Diagnostic Investigations* **21**(3): 306–320.

Weissenberg, R. (1965) Fifty years of research on the lymphocystis virus disease of fishes (1914–1964). *Annals of the New York Academy of Science* **126**: 362–374.

Whittington, R.J. and Chong, R. (2007) Global trade in ornamental fish from an Australian perspective: the case for revised import risk analysis and management strategies. *Preventive Veterinary Medicine* **81**: 92–116.

Woo, P.T.K. and Bruno, D. (2003) *Fish Diseases and Disorders, Volume 3: Viral, Bacterial and Fungal Infections.* Oxford: CABI Publishing.

World Organization for Animal Health (OIE). (2006) *Manual of Diagnostic Tests for Aquatic Animals.* Paris: OIE; General Information. www.oie.int/eng/normes/fmanual/A_00022.htm (accessed October 1, 2008).

Yanong, R.P.E. (1995). Possible herpesvirus-associated disease in the blue-eyed plecostomus, Panaque suttoni. Proceedings International Association of Aquatic Animal Medicine. Mystic, Connecticut, May 6.

Chapter 10
Bacterial Diseases of Fish

Brian Palmeiro

Introduction

Bacterial disease is extremely common in both ornamental and food fish and is most frequently associated with bacteria that are ubiquitous in the environment acting as opportunistic pathogens secondary to stress. Less commonly, bacterial disease is caused by primary or obligate pathogens. Most bacterial infections of fish are caused by Gram-negative organisms, including the genera *Aeromonas, Citrobacter, Edwardsiella, Flavobacterium, Pseudomonas*, and *Vibrio* (Noga, 1996; Barker, 2001; Palmeiro and Roberts, 2009). Bacterial disease in fish is complex and involves the interplay of various factors, including the environment, the host (immune system function, host susceptibility, etc.), and pathogen-specific factors such as virulence. Various forms of stress often result in immune system dysfunction and are key in the pathogenesis of bacterial disease in fish; poor environmental conditions are the most common stressor involved in the precipitation of bacterial disease. The following discussion will primarily focus on the diagnosis and treatment of bacterial disease in ornamental fish species, with some discussion of pertinent food fish pathogens. Major bacterial pathogens in fish can be divided into the following four major groups (Palmeiro and Roberts, 2009):

(1) Ulcer-forming/systemic, Gram-negative bacteria. This group includes bacteria in the genera *Aeromonas, Vibrio, Edwardsiella, Pseudomonas, Flavobacterium*, and others. This is the most common group of bacterial pathogens that affect fish.
(2) External, Gram-negative bacteria. This group of bacteria most commonly cause external infections. Some of these bacteria may also cause systemic infections. Included in this group are *Flavobacterium columnare, Flexibacter maritimus*, yellow pigmented bacteria (YPB), *Cytophaga* spp., and others.
(3) Systemic, Gram-positive, rapidly growing bacteria. These bacteria generally cause systemic infections and include *Streptococcus* spp. and related species.
(4) Slow-growing, acid-fast bacteria. These bacterial pathogens cause systemic, chronic, granulomatous disease. The most common pathogens in this group are *Mycobacterium* spp.

Clinical signs of bacterial disease may be peracute (mortality without gross evidence of disease), acute, or chronic and varies with the particular pathogen and various host-related factors. The below sections will discuss more specific bacterial diseases in fish, including clinical presentation, diagnosis, and treatment.

Ulcer-forming and systemic infections caused by Gram-negative bacteria

This is the most common group of bacterial pathogens that affect fish and includes bacteria in the genera *Aeromonas, Vibrio, Edwardsiella, Pseudomonas, Flavobacterium*, and others (Noga, 1996; Barker, 2001; Palmeiro and Roberts, 2009). Clinical signs of ulcer-forming and systemic infections caused by Gram-negative bacteria include the following: lethargy, anorexia, abnormal swimming patterns/spinning, hemorrhagic lesions on the skin, ulcerative skin lesions, abdominal

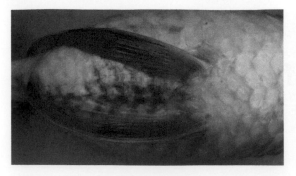

Fig. 10.1 Hemorrhages and erythema in a koi with septicemia due to *Aeromonas hydrophila*. This fish also has significant abdominal distension/ascites.

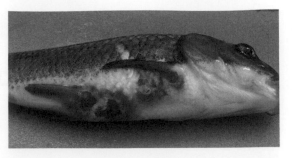

Fig. 10.2 A koi with ulcerative disease with typical cutaneous ulcers. Note the exposure of underlying musculature and peripheral annular rims of hemorrhage surrounding the ulcers.

distension/ascites, abnormal position in the water column, exophthalmia ("pop eye"), gill necrosis, and mortality (Noga, 1996; Barker, 2001; Palmeiro and Roberts, 2009). With gill involvement, respiratory signs such as increased opercular rate, piping (gasping for air at the water surface), and respiratory distress may be seen. Figure 10.1 illustrates the typical cutaneous hemorrhages of the skin and fins seen in a koi (*Cyprinus carpio*) with systemic bacterial disease due to *Aeromonas hydrophila*.

Motile aeromonad septicemia (MAS)

Motile aeromonads are the most common bacterial pathogens of fish and may result in a syndrome called MAS. MAS is most commonly caused by ubiquitous aquatic bacteria of the *A. hydrophila* complex, including *A. hydrophila*, *Aeromonas sobria*, and *Aeromonas caviae*. *A. hydrophila* is the most common isolate and is more commonly isolated from freshwater fish than from marine fish. MAS is almost always secondary to an underlying stressor. Common clinical signs include cutaneous hemorrhages and ulcers, visceral hemorrhages, edema, dropsy/ascites, and exophthalmia (Noga, 1996; Barker, 2001; Palmeiro and Roberts, 2009).

Ulcerative dermatitis (UD) in koi (*C. carpio*)

UD is a multifactorial syndrome seen in koi (*C. carpio*) and related cyprinids such as goldfish

(*Carassius auratus*) that results in ulcerative skin lesions. Clinical signs include raised/erythematous and missing scales, and ulcers that extend from the skin into the underlying musculature; in severe cases, bone may be exposed or penetration into the coelomic cavity may occur. Progression to septicemia can also occur resulting in clinical signs such as those seen with MAS (see above). Osmotic distress due to loss of epidermal integrity may result in fluid retention, exophthalmos, and dropsy. Figure 10.2 exhibits the typical ulcers in a koi with UD. Various bacterial pathogens have been isolated from these cases, including *Aeromonas salmonicida* and *A. hydrophila* (Barker, 2001; Hunt, 2006; Roberts and Palmeiro, 2009). *A. salmonicida* can be difficult to culture as it is fastidious and quickly overgrown by other rapidly growing bacteria such as motile aeromonads (Palmeiro and Roberts, 2009). In a recent abstract, *A. salmonicida* DNA was detected via polymerase chain reaction (PCR) in 77% of koi with ulcerative skin lesions (Goodwin and Merry, 2007). The author has isolated numerous pathogens from these cutaneous lesions via sterile swab and sterile tissue cultures, including *Aeromonas* spp., *Pseudomonas* spp., *Citrobacter* spp., *Chryseobacterium* spp., *Delfia* spp., and *Shewanella putrefaciens* (Palmeiro and Rankin, in press).

The author commonly divides causes of UD in koi into predisposing, primary, secondary, and perpetuating factors. Table 10.1 illustrates various predisposing, primary, secondary, and perpetuating causes of UD in koi.

Table 10.1 Predisposing, primary, secondary, and perpetuating causes of ulcerative dermatitis in koi.

Predisposing	Primary	Secondary	Perpetuating
Chemical stressors: poor water quality or other undesirable environmental conditions	Ectoparasites	Secondary bacterial invaders—motile aeromonads, *Pseudomonas*, *Flavobacterium*, *Citrobacter*, and so on	Fibrosis and scarring, granulation tissue, tissue weakening
Physical stressors: shipping, overcrowding, aggression, and so on	*Aeromonas hydrophila* complex	*Saprolegnia* Algae	Recruitment of inflammatory cells and enzymatic tissue degradation
Poor husbandry: filtration, tank/pond design, nutrition, and so on	*Aeromonas salmonicida*	Parasites that invade damaged epidermis—nematodes, flukes, *Trichodina*, *Ichthyobodo*, and so on	Osmotic stresses due to lack of epidermal integrity
—	Trauma	—	Septicemia
—	Koi herpesvirus	—	—

Genetic factors

In most cases, many of these factors interact together to result in clinical disease, which emphasizes the need for a thorough diagnostic evaluation in these cases. A detailed analysis of the environment for underlying stressors is critical in these cases as underlying environmental stressors such as poor water quality are commonly present. The author typically utilizes systemic antibiotics in the treatment of this condition. Prolonged bath immersion treatment with salt at 0.1%–0.3% is typically utilized to decrease osmotic stresses. In some cases, debridement of the ulcer and removal of necrotic tissue/scales may be necessary. Various topical treatments such as silver sulfadiazine can also be helpful. Further information on treatment can be found below under the section on treatment of systemic/ulcer Gram-negative infections.

A. salmonicida

A. salmonicida is a nonmotile species of *Aeromonas* that causes a chronic to subacute bacterial infection resulting in cutaneous ulcerations of the skin. There are three reported subspecies of *A. salmonicida*, including *A. salmonicida* subsp. *salmonicida*, subsp. *achromogenes* and *masoucida* (Noga, 1996). *A. salmonicida* subsp. *salmonicida* is usually associated with systemic infections and is the causative agent of furunculosis in salmonids (Noga, 1996). The atypical subspecies *achromogenes* is more commonly associated with ulcera-

tive skin lesions in nonsalmonid species such as goldfish, common carp, and eels. It is also the causative agent of carp erythrodermatitis and has been implicated as the causative agent of UD in koi (see above). *A. salmonicida* is considered an obligate pathogen of fish, but carrier fish can occur (Noga, 1996).

Pseudomonas spp.

Most *Pseudomonas*-associated septicemia cases in ornamental species are due to *Pseudomonas fluorescens* (Barker, 2001). Infections are more common in warmer water temperatures and are typically secondary to environmental stressors (Noga, 1996; Barker, 2001).

Edwardsiella spp.

Edwardsiella ictaluri is the causative agent of enteric septicemia of catfish (ESC), economically one of the most significant diseases of catfish in the United States (Noga, 1996). ESC is a seasonal disease, with outbreaks occurring with water temperatures between 24 and 28°C (75 and 82°F) (Noga, 1996). In the acute form (gastrointestinal septicemia), the ingested bacteria are absorbed through the intestines, causing a generalized infection with acute mortality. Affected fish hang their head up in the water column and have abnormal spiral swimming. In the chronic form, a typical "hole-in-the-head" lesion is created on the frontal bone of the skull.

Vibriosis

Bacteria of the genus *Vibrio* are ubiquitous in the marine and estuarine environment and are the most common causes of disease in marine fish. Species that have been shown to cause disease in fish include *Vibrio anguillarum* (most common), *Vibrio salmonicida*, *Vibrio ordalii*, *Vibrio alginolyticus*, *Vibrio parahaemolyticus*, *Vibrio vulnificus*, and *Vibrio damsela*; *V. anguillarum* and *V. ordalii* are the two most commonly identified from marine ornamentals (Barker, 2001). Clinically, vibriosis is very similar to MAS (see above) and results in hemorrhagic septicemia with cutaneous hemorrhages and ulcers (Barker, 2001). As with other bacterial infections, underlying environmental stressors are often present.

Diagnosis of Gram-negative, ulcer-forming/systemic infections

Diagnosis is based on history, clinical signs, and bacterial culture/sensitivity. Samples should be submitted to laboratories that are familiar with culturing aquatic pathogens. Most fish pathogens are best cultured at room temperature (22–25 °C), not 37 °C, which is the common protocol in mammalian microbiology laboratories. A nonselective agar such as blood agar is a good medium for the growth of most fish pathogens (Noga, 1996). In marine fish, a medium with high salt content may be needed. In some cases, selective specialized media can be used to enhance the growth and isolation of certain pathogens.

The organ of choice for bacterial culture (Fig. 10.3) in systemic infections is the posterior kidney (Noga, 1996; Barker, 2001; Palmeiro and Roberts, 2009). Dorsal and ventral approaches to the posterior kidney have been described (Noga, 1996). The author commonly utilizes the dorsal approach in small ornamental species and the ventral approach in larger species such as koi and goldfish. Other organs that may be cultured include the brain (especially when neurological signs are present), liver, spleen, and anterior kidney. Moribund fish showing clinical signs should be selected. Blood culture has been described as a nonlethal test in cases of systemic bacterial infections. A recent report described good correlation between blood

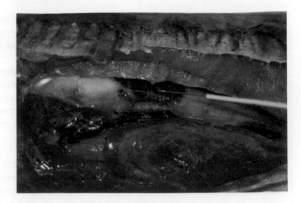

Fig. 10.3 Bacterial sampling from the posterior kidney.

culture results and posterior kidney tissue cultures in a small population of fish (Klinger et al., 2003). Blood cultures were obtained aseptically from the caudal vein; samples were incubated in brain heart infusion broth and then transferred to blood agar plates (Klinger et al., 2003). The author has also used blood culture as an antemortem survival procedure with good results; however, a larger-scale study comparing culture results from the blood and posterior kidney is needed. When culturing cutaneous ulcers, tissue cultures obtained aseptically are preferred to superficial swabs as secondary pathogens commonly invade ulcerative lesions. When culturing, samples should be obtained from the leading edge of the ulcerative lesion. *A. salmonicida* can be very difficult to culture as it is quickly overgrown by less fastidious secondary pathogens. Molecular techniques (such as PCR) can be utilized to illustrate the presence of *A. salmonicida* in ulcerative skin lesions (Goodwin and Merry, 2007).

Treatment of Gram-negative, ulcer-forming/systemic infections

Treatment of Gram-negative, ulcer-forming and systemic infections in fish should always involve a thorough analysis of the environment and improvement of any poor environment/husbandry-related problems or other related stressors. Without evaluation of the environment and removal of triggering stressors, treatment of bacterial disease in fish will be unsuccessful. The mainstay of treatment for Gram-negative,

Table 10.2 Dosage information for common antimicrobials in pet and ornamental fish.

Drug	Parenteral administration	Oral administration	Bath	Notes
Amikacin	5 mg/kg IM q 12 hours[1]	—	—	Not studied pharmacokinetically in pet fish Used commonly by koi hobbyists
Aztreonam	100 mg/kg IM, ICe q 48 hours[1]	—	—	Not studied pharmacokinetically in pet fish Used commonly by koi hobbyists
Ceftazidime	20 mg/kg IM q 72 hours[2]	—	—	Not studied pharmacokinetically in pet fish Used commonly by fish veterinarians
Enrofloxacin	5–10 mg/kg IM, ICe q 48–72 hours (koi)[3] 5 mg/kg IM q 48 hours (red pacu)[4]	5 mg/kg PO every 24–48 hours (red pacu)[4]	2.5 mg/l × 5 hours every 24–48 hours (red pacu)[4]	Only studied pharmacokinetically in koi[3] and pacu[4] but used commonly by fish veterinarians in many species
Florfenicol	Red pacu: 20–30 mg/kg IM q 24 hours[5] Koi: 25 mg/kg q 24–48 hours; shorter half-life in three-spot gourami may necessitate more frequent dosing[6]	50 mg/kg PO q 24 hours in koi; shorter half-life in gourami may necessitate q 12-hour dosing[6]	Minimal absorption as bath treatment in koi[6]	Studied pharmacokinetically in red pacu,[5] koi,[6] and three-spot gourami[4]
Kanamycin	—	300 mg/lb food per day × 10 days[7] 50 mg/kg/day in feed[1]	50–100 mg/l × 5 hours, repeat every 3 days for three treatments[1, 7]	Not studied pharmacokinetically in pet fish May cause renal damage
Oxolinic acid	—	150 mg/lb food per day for 10 days[7]	38 mg per 10 gallons for 24 hours, repeat as needed[7] 95 mg/gallon for 15 minutes, repeat twice daily for 3 days[7]	Not studied pharmacokinetically in pet fish May cause lethargy when used as bath treatment, inhibited by hard water

(Continued)

Table 10.2 *Continued*

Drug	Parenteral administration	Oral administration	Bath	Notes
Oxytetracycline	Red pacu: 7 mg/kg IM q 24 hours[8]	1.12 g/lb food per day for 10 days[7]	750–3780 mg per 10 gallons for 6–12 hours, repeat daily for 10 days (dose will depend on the hardness of water)[7] 50%–75% water changes between treatments	Studied pharmacokinetically in red pacu[8] Increased Ca and Mg inactivate, not useful in marine systems as bath treatment
Nitrofurazone	—	1.12 g/lb food per day for 10 days[7]	189–756 mg per 10 gallons for 1 hour, repeat daily for 10 days[7] 378 mg per 10 gallons for 6–12 hours, repeat daily for 10 days[7]	Not studied pharmacokinetically in pet fish Systemic absorption from bath treatment questionable, best reserved for external infections Carcinogenic Inactivated in bright light
Sulfadimethoxine/ormetoprim (Romet B®, Hoffman-LaRoche)	—	50 mg/kg per day for 5 days[1]	Not useful as bath treatment	Not studied pharmacokinetically in pet fish
Trimethoprim sulfa	—	30 mg/kg PO q 24 hours × 10–14 days[1]	20 mg/l × 5 hours q 24 hours × 5–7 days[1]	Not studied pharmacokinetically in pet fish

[1] Mashima and Lewbart (2000).
[2] Palmeiro and Roberts (2009).
[3] Lewbart et al. (2005a).
[4] Lewbart et al. (1997).
[5] Lewbart et al. (2005b).
[6] Yanong et al. (2005).
[7] Yanong (2006).
[8] Doi et al. (1998).
IM, intramuscular; ICe, intracoelomic.

systemic/ulcerative disease in fish is antimicrobials. Antimicrobials can be administered parenterally, orally, or as a bath treatment. Parenteral administration of antibiotics is the most effective method to achieve therapeutic blood levels that exceed the minimum inhibitory concentration for aquatic pathogens. Ideally, antimicrobials are selected based upon culture and antibiotic susceptibility tests (disk diffusion, automated broth microdilution techniques) as antimicrobial resistance is common in aquatic bacterial pathogens. Empirical first-choice antibiotics should be effective against Gram-negative bacteria. Few antimicrobials have been studied pharmacokinetically in ornamental fish. The antibiotics studied in ornamental fish include enrofloxacin, florfenicol, and oxytetracycline. Table 10.2 lists the common antimicrobials used in pet fish, including dosing information when applicable.

Injectable antibiotics are typically given as intramuscular (IM) or intracoelomic (ICe) injections. IM injections are most commonly given in the dorsal epaxial musculature. Owners of show fish should be notified that bruising and scale loss may occur after injection in this location. When treating show fish, the author has also utilized the pectoral musculature (on the ventral aspect of the fish at the base of the pectoral fin) as another potential site for IM injection. ICe injections can be given in the scaleless region at the base of the pelvic fin. Figure 10.4 illustrates an ICe injection in a koi.

Oral antibiotics are most commonly utilized when treating large numbers of fish and when injections are not practical. Antibiotics are either mixed with the feed or top-dressed on the feed using a binding agent such as canola oil. Gel-based diets (such as those by Mazuri®, Purina Mills, St. Louis, MO) offer the practitioner a convenient and palatable diet in which oral antibiotics can easily be mixed. Oral antibiotics can also be administered via oral gavage tube. Figure 10.5 illustrates the administration of oral medications to a koi with a red rubber catheter.

Administration of antibiotics in the water is commonplace in the aquarium industry, and numerous antibiotics are available over the counter to fish hobbyists. Problems associated with the use of bath antibiotics include limited absorption/insufficient dose, damage to the biofilter, and development of bacterial resistance (Palmeiro and Roberts, 2009). Pharmacokinetic data for bath antibiotics is lacking in ornamental fish; absorption is likely greater in marine fish due to increased water consumption. Bath antibiotics should be limited to cases of external infections (such as Columnaris disease and "fin rot") and in fish that are anorexic.

The food fish aquaculture veterinarian is limited to antibiotics approved for use in food species. Table 10.3 includes a list of approved antibiotics for use in food fish, including approved uses.

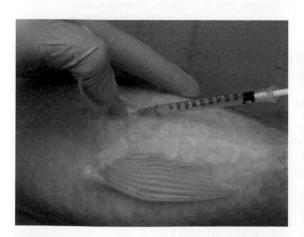

Fig. 10.4 Intracoelomic injection in a koi. The injection is administered in the scaleless region at the base of the pelvic fin.

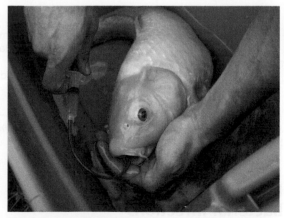

Fig. 10.5 Oral administration of medications in a koi using a red rubber catheter.

Table 10.3 Approved antibiotics for use in aquaculture.

Antibiotic	Species	Dosing/withdrawal time	Indication
Oxytetracycline dihydrate (Terramycin 200®, **Phibro Animal Health, Ridgefield Park, NJ**)	Salmonids	2.5–3.75 g per 100-lb fish per day for 10 days 21-day withdrawal time Water temperature not below 48.2 °F	Control of ulcer disease (*Hemophilus piscium*), furunculosis (*Aeromonas salmonicida*), bacterial hemorrhagic septicemia (*Aeromonas liquefaciens*), and *Pseudomonas* disease (*Pseudomonas* spp.)
Oxytetracycline dihydrate (Terramycin 200)	Freshwater-reared salmonids	3.75 g per 100-lb fish per day for 10 days 21-day withdrawal time	Control of mortality due to cold-water disease caused by *Flavobacterium psychrophilum*
Oxytetracycline dihydrate (Terramycin 200)	Freshwater-reared *Oncorhynchus mykiss*	3.75 g per 100-lb fish per day for 10 days 21-day withdrawal time	Control of mortality due to Columnaris disease (*Flavobacterium columnare*)
Oxytetracycline dihydrate (Terramycin 200)	Channel catfish	2.5–3.75 g per 100-lb fish per day for 10 days Water temperature not below 62 °F 21-day withdrawal time	Control of bacterial hemorrhagic septicemia (*A. liquefaciens*) and *Pseudomonas* disease (*Pseudomonas* spp.)
Sulfadimethoxine and ormethoprim (Romet®)	Channel catfish	50 mg/kg/day for 5 days 3-day withdrawal time	Control enteric septicemia (*Edwardsiella ictaluri*)
Sulfadimethoxine and ormethoprim (Romet)	Salmonids	50 mg/kg/day for 5 days 42-day withdrawal time	Control furunculosis (*A. salmonicida*)
Florfenicol (Aquaflor®, Schering-Plough Animal Health Corporation, Summit, NJ)	Channel catfish	10 mg florfenicol/kg fish/ day for 10 days 12-day withdrawal time	Control of mortality due to enteric septicaemia associated with *E. ictaluri* Control of mortality due to Columnaris disease associated with *F. columnare* (must use Aquaflor—CA1)
Florfenicol (Aquaflor)	Freshwater-reared salmonids	10 mg florfenicol/kg fish/ day for 10 days 15-day withdrawal time	Control of mortality due to furunculosis associated with *A. salmonicida* Control of mortality due to cold-water disease associated with *F. psychrophilum*

Sources: Food and Drug Administration, *Drugs Approved for Use in Aquaculture* (www.fda.gov/cvm/drugsapprovedaqua. htm); Gaunt (2006).

External Gram-negative bacterial infections

Bacterial diseases caused by Gram-negative bacteria that are typically more limited to the skin include Columnaris disease and fin rot. Columnaris disease is caused by *F. columnare* and results in cottony proliferative lesions on the skin and fins (Palmeiro and Roberts, 2009). Common locations for the lesions include perioral, periocu-

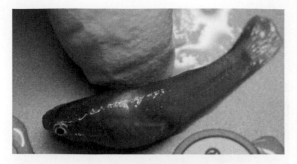

Fig. 10.6 Typical patchy white discolorations in the saddle region of a guppy with Columnaris disease.

lar, fins, dorsum, and tail regions. The synonym "cotton wool" disease describes the fluffy white cottonlike masses, patches, or plaques often seen with *F. columnare*. Given this clinical appearance, Columnaris disease is often misdiagnosed as fungal disease in aquarium fish; wet mount exam of affected area(s) can be used to differentiate between these two conditions. Columnaris disease is also commonly referred to as "saddleback disease" due to the typical discolorations that appear at the base of the dorsal fin resulting in a saddle appearance (see Fig. 10.6). *F. columnare* may also affect the gills, resulting in respiratory signs. A large number of other similar Gram-negative rods, including *Cytophaga* spp., *Flexibacter* spp., *Flavobacterium* spp., *Sporocytophaga* spp., and *Myxobacterium* spp., have been isolated from fish with similar lesions (Barker, 2001). All these Gram-negative bacteria form yellow to orange pigmented colonies and are occasionally collectively referred to as YPB (Barker, 2001). Columnaris-type infections caused by *F. maritimus* have been reported to cause a marine form of Columnaris disease with similar clinical signs to the freshwater counterpart (Noga, 1996; Barker, 2001).

Wet mount examination of the skin reveals characteristic long thin rods with gliding or flexing motion; "haystack" protrusions of rod-shaped bacteria may also be noted (Noga, 1996; Barker, 2001; Palmeiro and Roberts, 2009). Columnaris disease is common in live-bearers such as guppies, platies, mollies, and swordtails. Treatment of Columnaris disease can be achieved with antibiotic bath treatment with oxytetracycline (see Table 10.3 for dosing) repeated daily for

10 days. Other treatment options include potassium permanganate as a prolonged bath, copper sulfate, and diquat herbicide (Reward®, Syngenta Crop Protection Canada, Inc., Guelph, Ontario) dosed at 2–18 mg/l for 4-hour bath immersions (Palmeiro and Roberts, 2009). Treatment should be repeated daily for three to four treatments, with large water changes after each bath treatment. Systemic antimicrobials may be needed in more severe infections (see above). A recent study found that a single hydrogen peroxide (H_2O_2) treatment of 3.1 mg/l or more for 1 hour effectively eliminated external bacteria in the green swordtail *Xiphophorus helleri* (Russo et al., 2007).

Fin rot refers to a characteristic necrosis of the fins, resulting in an irregular notched to ragged appearance to the fins. Fin rot is almost always secondary to underlying stressors and poor husbandry. Several different species of bacteria can be isolated from these lesions in ornamental fish, including *F. columnare*, *F. maritimus*, and *Cytophaga* spp. (Barker, 2001). Treatment of this condition involves searching and removing underlying stressors and antimicrobials as for Columnaris disease.

Systemic, Gram-positive, rapidly growing bacteria

The most common bacteria in this group that cause disease in fish are *Streptococcus* spp.; other Gram-positive genera that are closely related to *Streptococcus* and cause disease in fish include *Lactococcus*, *Enterococcus*, and *Vagococcus*. Clinical signs are similar to those involving systemic Gram-negative infections such as skin discolorations, exophthalmos, ascites, skin ulcerations, and hemorrhages (Barker, 2001; Yanong and Francis-Floyd, 2006). Neurological signs are extremely common in fish with streptococcal infections, and abnormal swimming behavior such as spiralling or spinning is often reported (Yanong and Francis-Floyd, 2006). High mortality may also occur. Diagnosis is confirmed by culturing *Streptococcus* and related bacteria. As many cases invade the central nervous system (CNS), culturing the brain in suspected cases is critical. Antibiotics that may be effective against

Streptococcus and related species include erythromycin (1.5 g/lb of food fed for 10–14 days), amoxicillin/ampicillin, and florfenicol (Yanong and Francis-Floyd, 2006). Immunostimulants added to the feed, such as beta-glucans and nucleotides, have been shown to increase survival for *Streptococcus*-infected redtail black shark populations (Russo et al., 2006). *Streptococcus iniae* can cause disease in fish and in humans (see chapter on zoonotic diseases).

Slow-growing, acid-fast bacteria: mycobacteriosis

Mycobacteriosis in fish is caused by nontubercle-forming mycobacterium species that are ubiquitous in the aquatic environment. The two most common species associated with ornamental fish disease are *Mycobaterium marinum* and *Mycobaterium fortuitum* (Barker 2001; Decostere et al., 2004; Francis-Floyd and Yanong, 2006). *Mycobaterium chelonae* also causes disease in fish (typically cold-water salmonids) but is less commonly reported (Noga, 1996). Mycobacteriosis is zoonotic and can cause "fish tank granuloma" in people. A recent study in zebra fish illustrated that the primary route of infection is through the intestinal tract (Harriff et al., 2007). Fish can be infected by consuming contaminated feed, via cannibalism of infected fish and carcasses, or aquatic detritus (Noga, 1996; Decostere et al., 2004; Francis-Floyd and Yanong, 2006).

Mycobacterium spp. is ubiquitous in the aquatic environment; a recent report found 75% of water samples from decorative aquaria to be positive for *Mycobacterium* spp. (Beran et al., 2006). Environmental factors that favor growth of mycobacterium include low dissolved oxygen, low salinity, low pH, warmer water, and high organic loads (Francis-Floyd and Yanong, 2006).

Although mycobacteriosis has been reported in greater than 150 species of freshwater, brackish, and marine species, tropical aquarium fish are most commonly affected (Decostere et al., 2004). Members of the freshwater families Anabantidae (bettas and gouramis), Characidae (tetras and piranhas), and Cyprinidae (danios and barbs)

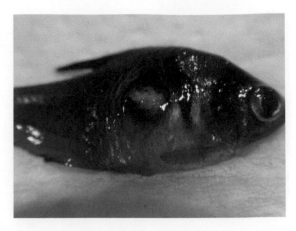

Fig. 10.7 Mycobacteriosis: ulcerative skin lesion in a serpae tetra (*Hyphessobrycon serpae*) with central caseous granulomatous exudate.

appear to be particularly susceptible (Decostere et al., 2004). In cultured finfish, striped bass (*Morone saxatilis*) are commonly affected.

In mycobacteriosis, clinical signs are usually nonspecific and can include ulcerative skin lesions, reduced appetite, emaciation, lethargy, exophthalmia ("pop eye"), swollen abdomen, anorexia, and fin/tail rot, and skeletal abnormalities (Barker, 2001; Palmeiro and Roberts, 2009). This disease is usually chronic, slowly progressive, and causes low to moderate mortalities. Mycobacteriosis is the most common chronic wasting disease of aquarium fish. Figure 10.7 illustrates a serpae tetra (*Hyphessobrycon serpae*) with chronic mycobacteriosis. On internal exam, granulomas will develop in the liver, kidney, spleen, heart, muscle, gill, and other tissues. Granulomas are typically pale gray to tan but are only visible to the naked eye in more advanced cases.

Diagnosis is based on clinical signs, the presence of granulomas, and the demonstration of acid-fast bacterial rods in tissues. Typical granulomas can be found on light microscopy of internal organ wet mounts (most commonly kidney, spleen, and liver). Granulomas can also be found in skin wet mounts, and less commonly, gill biopsies. Figure 10.8 illustrates the typical appearance of granulomas on light microscopy, with a dark brown center and surrounding capsule.

When granulomas are found, an acid-fast stain should be performed. Acid-fast stains can be per-

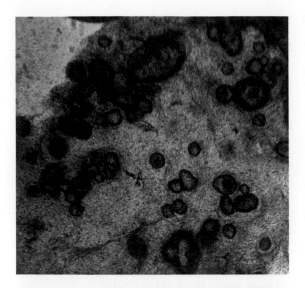

Fig. 10.8 Granulomas found on an internal wet mount exam of a fish with mycobacteriosis. Note the dark brown center with surrounding lighter capsule.

formed on cytological preparations or histopathological sections. A positive acid-fast stain reveals red to pink rod-shaped bacteria against a light green background. Culture of mycobacterium for definitive species identification can be lengthy and difficult but is best performed on mycobacterial selective media such as Lowenstein–Jensen agar. *M. marinum* is classified as a slow-growing mycobacterium, whereas *M. fortuitum* and *M. chelonae* are classified as rapidly growing (Decostere et al., 2004). Molecular diagnostics such as PCR are also useful in species identification.

There is no effective cure for mycobacteriosis in fish. In aquaculture, retail, and wholesale situations, depopulation and disinfection is often recommended. Treatment is often different in public aquaria/zoos and in private collections. Various antibiotics such as rifampin, erythromycin, streptomycin, kanamycin, doxycycline, and minocycline have been suggested as possible treatments, but a clinical cure is unlikely (Barker, 2001; Francis-Floyd and Yanong, 2006; Palmeiro and Roberts, 2009). Mycobacteria are resistant to many commonly used bactericidal agents at standard dosage rates, including chlorine bleach and quaternary ammonium compounds (Francis-Floyd and Yanong, 2006). As much as 10,000 ppm

chlorine has been reported necessary to kill mycobacteria (Francis-Floyd and Yanong, 2006). In a recent study comparing efficacy of common disinfectants against *M. marinum*, ethyl alcohol (50% and 70%), benzyl-4-chlorophenol/phenylphenol (Lysol®, Reckitt Benckiser, Slough, Berkshire, U.K.) (1%), and sodium chlorite (mixed as 1:5:1 or 1:18:1 [base:water:activator]) were the most effective disinfectants with elimination or reduction of *M. marinum* within 1 minute of contact (Marinous and Smith, 2005). Sodium hypochlorite (50,000 mg/l) was moderately effective but required a minimum contact time of 10 minutes to reduce bacterial counts (Marinous and Smith, 2005). Disinfectants that were ineffective after 60 minutes of contact time included ethyl alcohol (30%), *n*-alkyl dimethyl benzyl ammonium chloride (1:256), and potassium peroxymonosulfate–sodium chloride (1%) (Marinous and Smith, 2005).

References

Barker, G. (2001) Bacterial diseases. In *BSAVA Manual of Ornamental Fish*, 2nd Edition (Wildgoose, W.H., ed.), pp. 185–193. Gloucester: British Small Animal Veterinary Association.

Beran, V., Matlova, L., Dvorska, L., et al. (2006) Distribution of mycobacteria in clinically healthy ornamental fish and their aquarium environment. *Journal of Fish Diseases* **9**: 283–393.

Decostere, A., Hermans, K., and Haesebrouck, F. (2004) Piscine mycobacteriosis: a literature review covering the agent and the disease it causes in fish and humans. *Veterinary Microbiology* **99**: 159–166.

Doi, A.M., Stoskopf, M.K., and Lewbart, G.A. (1998) Pharmacokinetics of oxytetracycline in the red pacu following different routes of administration. *Journal of Veterinary Pharmacology and Therapeutics* **21**: 364–368.

Francis-Floyd, R. and Yanong, R.P. (2006) Mycobacteriosis in Fish. University of Florida IFAS extension publication # VM-96. http://edis.ifas.ufl.edu/VM055 (accessed October 1, 2008).

Gaunt, P.S. (2006) Veterinarians' role in the use of veterinary feed directive drugs in aquaculture. *Journal of the American Veterinary Medical Association* **229** (3): 362–364.

Goodwin, A. and Merry, G. (2007) Are all koi and goldfish ulcers caused by *Aeromonas salmonicida* Achromogenes? Paper presented at the Western Fish Disease Workshop, American Fisheries Society, Jackson Lake Lodge, WY, June 5, 2007.

Harriff, M.J., Bermudez, L.E., and Kent, M.L. (2007) Experimental exposure of zebrafish, *Danio rerio*, to *Mycobacterium marinum* and *Mycobacterium peregrinum* reveals the gastrointestinal tract as the primary route of infection: a potential model for environmental mycobacterial infection. *Journal of Fish Diseases* **30**: 587–600.

Hunt, C.J.G. (2006) Ulcerative skin disease in a group of koi carp (*Cyprinus carpio*). *Veterinary Clinics of North America Exotic Animal Practice* **9**: 723–728.

Klinger, R.E., Francis-Floyd, R., Riggs, A., et al. (2003) Use of blood culture as a nonlethal method for isolating bacteria from fish. *Journal of Zoo and Wildlife Medicine* **34** (2): 206–207.

Lewbart, G.A., Vaden, S., Deen, J., et al. (1997) Pharmacokinetics of enrofloxacin in the red pacu (*Colossoma brachypomum*) after intramuscular, oral and bath administration. *Journal of Veterinary Pharmacology and Therapeutics* **20**: 124–128.

Lewbart, G.A., Butkus, D., Papich, M., et al. (2005a) Evaluation of a method of intracoelomic catheterization in koi. *Journal of the American Veterinary Medical Association* **226**: 784–788.

Lewbart, G.A., Papich, M.G., and Whitt-Smith, D. (2005b) Pharmacokinetics of florfenicol in the red pacu (*Paractus brachypomus*) after single dose intramuscular administration. *Journal of Veterinary Pharmacology and Therapeutics* **28**: 317–319.

Marinous, M. and Smith, S. (2005) Efficacy of common disinfectants against *Mycobacterium marinum*. *Journal of Aquatic Animal Health* **17**: 284–288.

Mashima, T. and Lewbart, G.A. (2000) Pet fish formulary. *Veterinary Clinics of North America Exotic Animal Practice* **3** (1): 117–130.

Noga, E.J. (1996) *Fish Disease: Diagnosis and Treatment.* St. Louis, MO: Mosby.

Palmeiro, B. and Roberts, H. (2009) Bacterial disease in fish. In *Clinical Veterinary Advisor: Exotic Medicine* (Mayer, J., ed.), In press.

Palmeiro, B.S. and Rankin, S. (In press) *Culture & Susceptibility Characteristics of Ulcerative Dermatitis in Koi.*

Roberts, H. and Palmeiro, B. (2009) Ulcer disease in koi. In *Clinical Veterinary Advisor: Exotic Medicine* (Mayer, J., ed.), In press.

Russo, R., Yanong, R.P.E., and Mitchell, H. (2006). Dietary beta-glucans and nucleotides enhance resistance of red-tail black shark (*Epalzeorhynchos bicolor*, family Cyprinidae) to *Streptococcus iniae* infection. *Journal of the World Aquaculture Society* **37** (3): 298–306.

Russo, R., Curtis, E.W., and Yanong, R. (2007) Preliminary investigations of hydrogen peroxide treatment of selected ornamental fishes and efficacy against external bacteria and parasites in green swordtails. *Journal of Aquatic Animal Health* **19** (2): 121–127.

Yanong, R. (2006) *Use of Antibiotics in Ornamental Fish Aquaculture.* VM-84. Florida Cooperative Extension Service, UF-IFAS. http://edis.ifas.ufl.edu. (accessed October 1, 2008).

Yanong, R.P.E. and Francis-Floyd, R. (2006) *Streptococcal Infections in Fish.* University of Florida IFAS Extension Publication #57. http://edis.ifas.ufl.edu/FA057 (accessed October 1, 2008).

Yanong, R.P.E., Curtis, E.W., Simmons, R., et al. (2005) Pharmacokinetic studies of florfenicol in koi carp and threespot gourami *Trichogaster trichopterus* after oral and intramuscular treatment. *Journal of Aquatic Animal Health* **17**: 129–137.

Chapter 11

Fungal Diseases in Fish

Helen E. Roberts

Introduction

Fungal disease in fish is usually an opportunistic infection that results from acute or chronic exposure to stress, leading to a compromised immune system. There are a few fungal pathogens that can be a primary cause of disease, including *Aphanomyces* spp. and *Branchiomyces* spp. This chapter will discuss the predisposing factors associated with fungal disease, the clinical signs of fungal disease in fish, the diagnosis and identification of fungal elements, and the management and treatment strategies that may be employed.

Fungal diseases

Taxonomy and classification

The taxonomic classification of fungi is considered controversial, and can change depending on the method used for classification of the fungus, that is, genetic typing, method of reproduction, life cycle, hyphae morphology, and so on. (Khoo, 2000; Yanong, 2003). Fungi are heterotrophic and incapable of synthesizing nutrients without organic matter. Saprophytic fungi use dead organic matter for growth and reproduction. Parasitic fungi, in contrast, rely on living tissue.

Most freshwater fungal fish pathogens belong to the Oomycetes class. These fungi are found ubiquitously in the aquatic environment, with a worldwide distribution, and can affect virtually all freshwater fish species (Stoskopf, 1993; Khoo, 2000). Oomycetes, or water molds, reproduce primarily by asexual propagation of motile zoospores, and less commonly, by sexual reproduction via the production of oospores (Post,

1987; Noga, 1996; Khoo, 2000). Zoospores are the most common method of transmission of infection to fish and fish eggs. It is believed that zoospores are attracted and migrate to eggs and susceptible hosts via chemotaxis (Yanong, 2003; Grant, 2005). Encysted zoospores can survive in the environment for long periods of time (Grant, 2005).

Predisposing factors

Opportunistic fungal infections in fish generally occur once fish have been stressed or immunocompromised. The stress response in fish is similar to other vertebrates and causes cortisol and other chemical mediators to be released. These mediators cause a variety of physiological effects in the fish, including immune suppression and increased susceptibility to disease. Increased levels of cortisol can cause a reduction in the number of epidermal mucous cells (Khoo, 2000; Udomkusonsri and Noga, 2005). Healthy fish skin provides an effective means of defense against fungal disease under optimal conditions, including proper temperatures for the species involved. Intact skin with a healthy layer of mucus is unlikely to be colonized by zoospores. Fungal zoospores are trapped and removed as mucus is shed in healthy fish. Antifungal chemicals (proteins and naturally produced antibiotics) produced by the skin and found in the mucous layer serve to inhibit fungal growth (Udomkusonsri and Noga, 2005). Any activity (spawning, flashing due to parasitic infestations, and aggression) or process (netting and other handling methods, bacterial infections) that damages the skin or reduces the healing ability of damaged skin predisposes a fish to a secondary fungal infection.

Stressors most often implicated include poor water quality conditions, excessive chemotherapeutic use, spawning, parasitic, bacterial, and/or viral infections, and events that cause the loss of the protective mucous coat or affect epidermal integrity, such as handling, overcrowding, and traumatic injuries (Stoskopf, 1993; Noga, 1996; Khoo, 2000; Yanong, 2003; Grant, 2005; Udomkusonsri and Noga, 2005). Poor water quality conditions commonly specifically associated with opportunistic fungal infections include temperature changes (usually an acute drop), pH alterations, elevated ammonia and nitrite levels, and high levels of organic compounds. Dead or unfertilized eggs provide an excellent media for fungal growth.

In order to provide effective treatment and prevention of fungal infections, aquarists need to identify any potential predisposing factors and attempt to correct them. Without intervention or remediation of the contributing causes, infections are less likely to respond to treatment and are likely to worsen or recur.

Saprolegniasis

Saprolegniasis (also known as saprolegniosis, "winter kill syndrome," "winter fungus," "winter mortality," "fungus disease," or "sap") is a common term used to describe infections in fish caused by members in the genera *Saprolegnia*, *Achyla*, and *Dictyuchus* (Khoo, 2000; Yanong, 2003). Most species of freshwater fish are susceptible to saprolegniasis infections, and it is the most common fungal infection encountered in ornamental fish. Infections are commonly seen in cooler water temperatures in outdoor ponds and when temperatures decrease in indoor aquaria (heater failure, etc.). Fish transported in cooler weather may also break with saprolegniasis postshipping. Metabolic functions, including wound healing, are slower in cooler water. The delay in healing a small defect in the skin can lead to a secondary infection.

Clinical presentation

Fish infected with saprolegniasis will have fluffy, cottony lesions distributed in tufts that are

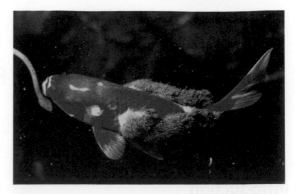

Fig. 11.1   A koi with saprolegniasis and secondary algal entrapment in the fungal mat creating a green appearance (photo courtesy of Ralph Woodruff).

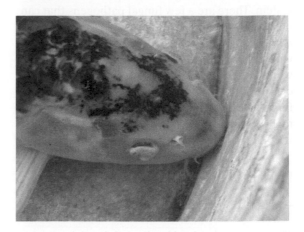

Fig. 11.2   A koi, housed in an outdoor pond, with fungal keratitis. This infection developed in February in upstate New York.

initially superficial and appear white, tan, or gray in color. Lesions that trap algal particles and suspended sediment can have a green, brown, or red appearance (Fig. 11.1). Lesions can appear anywhere but generally will be first noticed on the head, fins, and/or tail of the affected fish. Lesions can spread to include the skin, eyes, gills, and oral cavity (Fig. 11.2). Scales may appear elevated when the infection is located on a scaled surface of the body. Superficial infections can progress into the underlying dermis and musculature, sometimes very rapidly. Some strains of *Saprolegnia* may spread to infect internal organs, including the liver, spleen, kidney, nervous tissue, and the eyes

(Khoo, 2000; Grant, 2005). Extensive superficial infections and deep focal infections can cause loss of osmoregulation via necrosis and hemorrhage of the skin, leading to death in the severely affected fish. Mortality depends on the extent of the disease on the skin and gills (Noga, 1996) and on the location of the infection (Grant, 2005).

Unfertilized, nonviable, or damaged eggs are frequently infected by *Saprolegnia*, and the infection can eventually spread to viable eggs unless control measures are instituted (Khoo, 2000; Yanong, 2003; Pillay and Kutty, 2007). Prompt removal of the dead and unfertile eggs is recommended to reduce infections.

Diagnosis of saprolegniasis

A presumptive diagnosis can be made based on the clinical impression of the characteristic lesions and history. Many owners will assume that any white cottony growth is fungal disease, but lesions should be microscopically examined by a wet mount exam to differentiate from an *Epistylis* infestation or "Columnaris disease," caused by the bacteria *Flavobacterium columnare*. *Saprolegnia* appears as transparent, long, broad, branching nonseptate hyphae on wet mount cytology (Fig. 11.3). Lesions can be submitted for histopathology, special staining, and fungal culture for confirmation of the diagnosis. Before submitting

samples for culture, it is wise to contact the diagnostic laboratory to be sure they are comfortable with water mold culture and identification. Tissue samples should be taken from live, moribund, or euthanized fish (Khoo, 2000). Dead fish are frequently colonized by fungal elements postmortem regardless of the cause of death.

Treatment and management of saprolegniasis

Management of fungal disease in fish populations is a multiphase process involving the identification and elimination of key predisposing risk factors, good sanitation practices, maintenance of excellent water quality, and judicious use of chemotherapeutic agents for the treatment of the affected fish and eggs. Increasing the salinity of freshwater systems to reduce the osmotic gradient can be beneficial. An increased salinity may also have an effect on the fungal infection (Yanong, 2003). A potential therapeutic effect from the raised salinity levels may be the reason very few marine species experience water mold infections (Noga, 1996). There are few effective chemotherapeutic agents available to treat saprolegniasis. Once the infection is established in a population or shows severe extensive and deep lesions, prognosis is poor (Yanong, 2003). Table 11.1 lists the most common treatments used for the control and prevention of saprolegniasis and other fungal infections.

Branchiomycosis

Branchiomycosis, also known as "gill rot," is an acute infection primarily of the gills that can cause high mortalities and severe respiratory distress. *Branchiomyces sanguinis* and *B. denigrans* are the most commonly implicated species (Khoo, 2000; Holliman, 2001; Yanong, 2003) and infections can be found worldwide in several fish species, including koi, *Cyprinus carpio* (Holliman, 2001; Yanong, 2003). There is some controversy as to whether the two species are truly separate or variants of the same species (Khoo, 2000; Roberts, 2001; Yanong, 2003). *B. sanguinis* primarily occurs within the blood vessels of the gills, and *B. denigrans* can be found penetrating to the surface of the gill tissue.

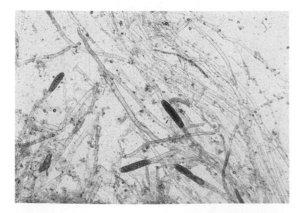

Fig. 11.3 Wet mount cytology of a skin scrape from a koi with cutaneous saprolegniasis showing long, broad, nonseptate hyphae (photo courtesy of Stephen A. Smith).

Table 11.1 Therapeutic agents used in the treatment of fungal diseases.

Drug	Dosage	Indications	Comments
Benzalkonium chloride	1–4 ml/l 1-hour dip/bath[1]	Branchiomycosis	—
Copper sulfate	Investigational: 10–50 ppm	Saprolegniasis infection in channel catfish eggs	Investigational stage*
	100 mg/l 24-hour bath or 10- to 30-minute dip[1]	Branchiomycosis	
Formalin	Eggs: 1–2 ml/l 15-minute bath 0.23 ml/l up to 60 minutes	Saprolegniasis in finfish eggs and finfish	Do not use if white precipitate has formed (paraformaldehyde is toxic to fish); precipitate forms when formalin is exposed to temperatures <4.4°C (40°F)† [1,3–5]
	Fish: 0.125–0.25 ml/l for 60 minutes 15 ml/l initial dip, then 25 ml/l immersion[1,2]		Do not use on eggs within 24 hours of hatching[2–4]
			Cannot be used with water temperatures >27°C (80°F), heavy algal blooms, and low dissolved oxygen;[3,5] toxicity enhanced with low water pH and reduced alkalinity[5]
			Do not use with potassium permanganate[5]
			Increase aeration with use;[2–5]
			Carcinogenic and potentially hazardous; shipping can be expensive; refer to material safety data sheet (MSDS)† [3]
Hydrogen peroxide	FDA approved use	Saprolegniasis in finfish eggs and finfish (investigational claim)	35% hydrogen peroxide Perox-Aid® (Western Chemical, Ferndale, WA); monitor for species sensitivity (has been shown to affect hatching success in some strains of rainbow trout eggs)†
	Eggs: 500–1000 mg/l for 15 minutes		
	Investigational label claim* ongoing for Finfish use: 50–100 mg/l for 30–60 minutes		Investigational claims can be evaluated at www.fws.gov/fisheries/aadap/summaryHistory11-669.htm (Aquatic Animal Drug Approval Program)*
	100–500 mg/l bath for 60 minutes[6]	Aphanomyces[6]	May not be effective

Malachite green	1–2 mg/l 30- to 60-minute bath treatment	Saprolegniasis	Carcinogenic, teratogenic, respiratory poison, and stains objects[4]
	0.1 mg/l prolonged immersion[2]	Saprolegniasis; branchiomycosis	Reported toxicity in eggs near hatching, small marine fish, young fry, some tetra, catfish, scaleless fish, loach species, and plants;[1-3] toxicity enhanced with warmer water temperatures and low pH[3-5,7]
	0.5 mg/l 60-minute bath[6]	Aphanomyces infection in fish and fish eggs	
	0.3 mg/l 24-hour bath[1]	Branchiomycosis	
	100 mg/l topical application[1]	Fungal skin lesions	Can be toxic when combined with formalin; use zinc-free solution;[1-3] remove from water with activated carbon;[2-4] rinse after topical application[7]
Sodium chloride	1–5 g/l prolonged immersion	Aid osmoregulatory function	Most sensitive species can tolerate at least 1 g/l prolonged immersion[3]
	Fish: 10–50 g/l for 1- to 2-minute bath	External fungal disease	
	10–20 mg/l 1-hour bath[6]	Aphanomyces	
Topical antifungal medications	Apply to affected area q 12–24 hours	Fungal skin lesions	Chlorhexidine ointment Pondone-iodine ointment, silver sulfadiazine cream

*www.fws.gov/fisheries/aadap/home.htm (Web site of the US Fish and Wildlife Service Aquatic Animal Drug Approval Program Partnership Program—lists status on drug approvals).

†www.wchemical.com (Western Chemical Inc. Web site with information and MSDS on hydrogen peroxide [35% Perox-Aid] and formalin [Parasite-S®]).

[1] Khoo (2000).
[2] Holliman (2001).
[3] Noga (1996).
[4] Carpenter (2001).
[5] Wildgoose and Lewbart (2001.)
[6] Yanong (2003).
[7] Stoskopf (1993).

Clinical presentation

Fish affected with branchiomycosis exhibit respiratory symptoms and a loss of equilibrium. Gills appear necrotic, eroded, and pale (Holliman, 2001). Mortalities can occur in as little as 48 hours (Roberts, 2001). Mortalities can be 50% or higher (Khoo, 2000; Roberts, 2001; Yanong, 2003).

Diagnosis of branchiomycosis

Gross evaluation of the gills in affected fish will show a patchy marbled appearance due to areas of ischemic necrosis and hemorrhage. Wet mount examination of the gill tissue will reveal hyperplasia, swelling, lamellar fusion, and fungal hyphae within the vessels of the gills or penetrating the necrotic gill tissue (Khoo, 2000; Roberts, 2001). Hyphae appear light brown, slightly refractile, branching, and nonseptate (Khoo, 2000; Holliman, 2001; Yanong, 2003). Special stains can be employed to identify the fungal elements. Various culture techniques can be used for positive identification.

Treatment and management of branchiomycosis

As with many fish diseases, elimination of predisposing factors will aid in the treatment and prevention of disease recurrence. Factors specifically associated with branchiomycosis include overcrowding, high levels of ammonia, algal blooms, high levels of organic material, warm water temperatures (20 °C/68 °F or higher), and poor hygienic practices (Roberts, 2001; Yanong, 2003). Husbandry practices that are used to control infection include prompt removal of infected and dead fish (Khoo, 2000; Holliman, 2001; Roberts, 2001), increasing pond water pH with quick lime (Khoo, 2000), and draining and liming ponds (Roberts, 2001). Although it is considered more effective to control the occurrence of branchiomycosis, specific chemotherapeutic protocols exist, including malachite green and formalin baths, copper sulfate and benzalkonium chloride dips, and oral administration of methylene blue (Khoo, 2000; Holliman, 2001). See Table 11.1 for dosage information.

Aphanomyces spp.

Aphanomyces invadans (also known as *A. invaderis* and *A. piscicida*) infections in fish are sometimes referred to as "atypical" water mold infections. The fungi are found in the eastern United States, Australia, Japan, South, and Southeast Asia (Khoo, 2000; Yanong, 2003), and infection has been reported in many freshwater and estuarine fish species, including several species of freshwater tropical fish (Khoo, 2000; Roberts, 2001; Yanong, 2003). *A. invadans* is considered a primary pathogen in fish and causes deep, ulcerative granulomatous lesions that can progress from the skin and underlying musculature to invasion of the body cavity (Yanong, 2003) or cranial vault (Roberts, 2001). Infections have been found in the spleen, kidney, gastrointestinal tract, liver, pancreas, and neurological tissue (Yanong, 2003). Disease syndromes associated with *Aphanomyces* infections include mycotic granulomatosis (Japan), red spot disease (Australia), epizootic ulcerative syndrome (Asia), and ulcerative mycosis (United States) (Khoo, 2000; Yanong, 2003; Sosa et al., 2007). Predisposing factors seen with outbreaks include reduced water temperatures (<25 °C/77 °F) and reduced salinity (due to freshwater flooding or heavy rainfall) in brackish systems (Yanong, 2003; Sosa et al., 2007).

Clinical presentation and diagnosis

Presentations can vary, but deep ulcerations of the skin are the most common clinical presentation seen with *Aphanomyces* infection in fish. The ulcers are gray or red, are frequently invaded by opportunistic fungi and bacteria, and are typically found on the sides of the body (Roberts, 2001). Affected individuals in a population may have lesions located in the same place (Roberts, 2001). Ulcerative lesions can progress to the underlying musculature and internal organs. Species susceptibility, extent of infection, and degree of mortality in a population varies. Goldfish can display hemorrhage, ascites, scale loss, and infection in the kidney and spleen (Yanong, 2003). Naïve populations will experience more severe outbreaks than previously exposed fish. Wet mount preparations of the lesions will show broad, nonseptate hyphae and inflammatory cells typically found in granulomatous diseases. Histopathology and culture can provide positive identification and a definitive diagnosis.

Treatment and management of Aphanomyces spp. infections

No specific treatment exists, but malachite green, hydrogen peroxide, and sodium chloride have all been used. See Table 11.1 for more details. Vaccine development against *Aphanomyces* spp. has been explored (Khoo, 2000).

References and further reading

Carpenter, J.W. (2001) Fish. In *Exotic Animal Formulary*, 2nd Edition (Carpenter, J.W., ed.), pp. 1–21. Philadelphia: W.B. Saunders.

Getchell, R. (2003) Pathogenic water molds infect fish. *Fish Farming News* **11**: 1–2.

Grant, A. (2005) Management of *Saprolegnia* on the farm—a veterinarian's view. *Fish Veterinary Journal* **8**: 81–92.

Holliman, A. (2001) Fungal diseases and harmful algae. In *BSAVA Manual of Ornamental Fish*, 2nd Edition (Wildgoose, W.H., ed.), pp 195–200. Gloucester: BSAVA Publications.

Khoo, L. (2000) Fungal diseases in fish. *Seminars in Avian and Exotic Pet Medicine* **9** (2): 102–111.

Noga, E.J. (1996) *Fish Disease: Diagnosis and Treatment*. St. Louis, MO: Mosby.

Pillay, T.V.R. and Kutty, M.N. (2005) *Aquaculture: Principles and Practices*, 5th Edition. Ames, IA: Blackwell Publishing.

Post, G. (1987) Mycotic diseases of fishes. In *Textbook of Fish Health*, Revised and Expanded Edition. Neptune City, NJ: TFH Publications.

Roberts, R.J. (2001) The mycology of teleosts. In *Fish Pathology* (Roberts, R.J., ed.), pp. 332–346. London: Harcourt Publishers.

Sosa, E.R., Landsberg, J.H., Stephenson, C.M., et al. (2007) *Aphanomyces invadans* and ulcerative mycosis in estuarine and freshwater fish in Florida. *Journal of Aquatic Animal Health* **19**: 14–26.

Stoskopf, M. (1993). Chemotherapeutics. In *Fish Medicine* (Stoskopf, M. ed.), pp. 832–839. Philadelphia: W.B. Saunders.

Udomkusonsri, P. and Noga, E.J. (2005) The acute ulceration response (AUR): a potentially widespread and serious cause of skin infection in fish. *Aquaculture* **246**: 63–77.

Wildgoose, W.H. and Lewbart, G.A. (2001) Therapeutics. In *BSAVA Manual of Ornamental Fish*, 2nd Edition (Wildgoose, W.H., ed.), pp. 195–200. Gloucester: BSAVA Publications.

Yanong, R.P.E. (2003) Fungal diseases of fish. *Veterinary Clinics of North America: Exotic Animal Practice* **6**: 377–400.

Chapter 12
Zoonotic Diseases of Fish

Stephen A. Smith

Introduction

As more clients bring fish into veterinary practices for diagnostic services, veterinary staff and other fish health professionals will increasingly come into contact with zoonotic diseases specific to aquatic animals that have historically been of little concern to practitioners dealing with the more common terrestrial species. These pathogens not only pose a potential threat to veterinarians and their staff but also to aquarium owners and aquaculturists working with finfish species. There is an extensive group of pathogens that are communicable to humans by consumption of aquatic species (Eastaugh and Shepard, 1989; Wolf and Smith, 2000); however, in contrast, there are only a few pathogens that might pose a risk to veterinary personnel that could be encountered during examination, handling, or treatment of fish. The complex interaction of the fish, the pathogen, and the aquatic environment increases the various routes of transmission possible. This is further complicated by the fact that many of the zoonotic pathogens do not cause disease in fish and reside as commensal organisms that normally cause little problem for aquatic species. Also, many of the clinical signs observed in fish have little relevance to the clinical signs exhibited in humans.

Fortunately, there are no parasitic, viral, or fungal zoonoses acquired from fish solely through the contact route, thus bacteria are the only pathogens of zoonotic potential acquired through handling of fish (Jahncke and Schwarz, 2002; Lowry and Smith, 2007) (see Table 12.1). There is a wide diversity of the bacterial species found in relation to fish that is largely attributable to the aquatic environment. Fish also live in a wide range of environmental conditions (i.e., freshwater, brackish, and marine) that can directly affect the species of bacteria that is associated with those fish species. For example, bacteria of the *Aeromonas* group are more commonly associated with freshwater fish species, while bacteria of the *Vibrio* group are generally associated with marine fish species. Although the majority of fish pathogens are Gram-negative, both Gram-positive and Gram-negative bacteria are represented in the potential zoonotic pathogens that are associated with fish. Most of the zoonotic bacterial infections are considered opportunistic infections in humans and are generally a result of trauma (e.g., cuts, abrasions, punctures) or associated with immunocompromised individuals.

Mycobacterial infections

Probably the best-known zoonotic infections acquired from fish are the aquatic *Mycobacterium* spp. infections. These Gram-positive, nonmotile, acid-fast rods are considered part of the nontubercular group of mycobacterial pathogens. Two major species of *Mycobacterium* that are commonly cultured from fish include *Mycobacterium marinum* and *Mycobacterium fortuitum*, but others such as *Mycobacterium chelonae*, *Mycobacterium ulcerans*, *Mycobacterium flavescens*, *Mycobacterium gordonae*, *Mycobacterium chesapaeki*, *Mycobacterium shottsii*, and *Mycobacterium pseudoshottsii* have been isolated from a wide range of freshwater, brackish, and marine species of fish as well (Nigrelli and Vogel, 1963; Falkinham, 1996; Smith, 1997; Chinabut, 1999; Decostere et al., 2004; Prearo et al., 2004; Kaattari

Table 12.1 Major zoonotic infections of fish.

Bacterial pathogen	Route of transmission	Clinical signs in finfish	Clinical signs in humans
Mycobacterium spp.	Contact with infected tissues, biofilms, or contaminated water	Lethargy, poor body condition, pigment changes, abdominal distention, exophthalmia, scale loss, skin ulcerations, and death	Granulomatous nodules to ulcerative skin lesions
Streptococcus iniae	Contact with infected tissues or contaminated water	Abdominal distention, hemorrhages of the skin, exophthalmia, and death	Cellulites, systemic arthritis, endocarditis, meningitis, and rarely, death
Aeromonas spp.	Contact with infected tissues	Ulcerative skin lesions, raised scales, abdominal distention, exophthalmia, and death	Localized edema and swelling at the site of infection
Vibrio spp.	Contact with infected tissues	Lethargy, skin ulcers, abdominal distention, exophthalmia, and death,	Edema, tissue swelling, and necrotizing fasciitis
Erysipelothrix rhusiopathiae	Contact with infected tissues or contaminated water	No apparent pathology	Localized to generalized skin infection, endocarditis, and death

et al., 2006). All of these aquatic *Mycobacterium* spp. can result in an acute to chronic disease in the fish and can present with no obvious clinical signs to a wide range of clinical signs. Generally, no clinical signs are apparent with the acute form of the disease, and often only a dead fish is found. Common clinical signs associated with the chronic form of the disease include lethargy, poor body condition, pigment changes, abdominal distention, exophthalmia, scale loss, and skin ulcers (Smith, 1997). To complicate management, many fish can be longtime carriers of the disease without any outward clinical signs of illness (Ross et al., 1962; Falkinham, 1996; Beran et al., 2006). Infected fish may also serve as reservoirs to spread the infection to other fish in the aquarium, tank, or pond. The most likely route of transmission between fish is, generally, orally through infected feces or tissues (Petrini, 2006; Harriff et al., 2007). Sloughed infected gill tissue or ulcerated skin lesions may also serve to allow dissemination of the *Mycobacterium* organism or infected material into the water (Smith, 1997). *Mycobacterium* infection in humans is often seen in individuals who handle or work with fish, leading to the name "fish handler's disease" or "fish tank granuloma." In humans, lesions generally appear on the extremities due to the organism's pref-

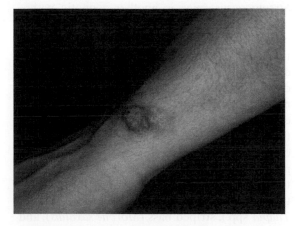

Fig. 12.1 Human "fish handler's disease" lesion on the arm (photo courtesy of Dr. Richmond Loh).

erence for lower temperatures (<30°C) and are either ulcerative lesions or raised granulomatous nodules (Huminer et al., 1986; Kiesch, 2000; Ho et al., 2006) (Figs. 12.1 and 12.2). However, a few cases of systemic mycobacteriosis have been rarely reported in humans and are typically seen in immunocompromised individuals, resulting in symptoms of respiratory disease (Lacaille et al., 1990; Tchornobay et al., 1992).

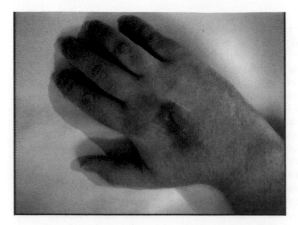

Fig. 12.2 Chronic infection of human mycobacteriosis on the hand (photo courtesy of Dr. Richard Lloyd).

Streptococcal infections

Streptococcus iniae is another zoonotic pathogen of fish that causes serious clinical disease in humans. This bacteria is a Gram-positive, nonmotile cocci that causes clinical signs of abdominal distention, petechial hemorrhage of the dermis, exophthalmia, and death in freshwater and marine species of fish (Perera et al., 1994; Eldar et al., 1995; Perl et al., 1999). Many species of tropical and ornamental fish can harbor the pathogen, but several species of food fish appear to be predisposed to infection, as well as being asymptomatic chronic carriers of *S. iniae*. These include tilapia (*Oreochromis* spp., *Sarotherodon* spp., and *Tilapia* spp.), striped bass (*Morone saxatilis*), and their hybrids (Kitao, 1993; Weinstein et al., 1997; Perl et al., 1999; Wolf and Smith, 1999). Clinical signs of infection of *S. iniae* in humans manifest as cellulites, systemic arthritis, endocarditis, meningitis, and occasionally, death (Weinstein et al., 1997). The majority of the human cases have occurred after handling live or dead fish and commonly involve a puncture wound or infection of an existing wound.

Aeromonad infections

Aeromonas spp. are Gram-negative, motile, facultative anaerobic rods that are ubiquitous in the freshwater aquatic and terrestrial environment. These bacteria frequently cause disease in ornamental, bait, and food fish. Clinical signs of *Aeromonas* infections in fish are seldom specific and include ulcerative lesions of the skin around the base of the fins and anus, raised scales, abdominal distension, and exophthalmia. Depending on the severity of infection, anemia, hepatomegaly, and ascites may also be observed. Aeromonad infections in fish are often secondary to stressors such as poor environmental conditions (suboptimal temperatures, elevated ammonia and nitrite levels), parasitism, and nutritional deficiencies. The primary route for transmission to a clinician or person handling fish is contact with infected or carrier fish mucus and tissues. Existing cuts and abrasions on hands, as well as direct trauma to the person from the fish, are possible routes of infection. *Aeromonas hydrophila, Aeromonas caviae, Aeromonas sobria*, and *Aeromonas schubertii* have all been implicated in human disease (Palumbo et al., 1989). In healthy individuals, the most common signs of an *Aeromonas* spp. infection includes localized swelling at the site of entry; however, in immunocompromised individuals, the bacterial disease can prove life threatening (Joseph et al., 1979; Moyer, 1987; Nemetz and Shotts, 1993; Tsai et al., 2006).

Vibrio spp. infections

Vibrio spp. are Gram-negative, facultative anaerobic rods that are commonly cultured from marine and brackish environments due to the bacteria's preference for higher salinities. However, despite being more prevalent in saltwater environments, *Vibrio* spp. can also be occasionally isolated from freshwater fish. These bacteria can be cultured from the skin and gastrointestinal tracks of fish that appear clinically normal. In stressed fish, these bacteria can cause disease, with clinical signs similar to those of other bacterial infections in fish (Bisharat et al., 1999). These clinical signs may include anorexia, lethargy, skin ulcers, exophthalmia, and erythema around the anus and base of fins. The species most commonly cultured from fish are *Vibrio vulnificus, Vibrio parahemolyticus*, and *Vibrio cholera*, with *V. vulnificus* being the most commonly fish-acquired species in human infections. In humans, the major route of exposure is through puncture wounds (Lehane and Rawlin, 2000; Oliver, 2005). Clinical manifestations in humans are edema, tissue swelling, and necrotizing fasciitis in the immediate area of the puncture wound or abrasion (Tang et al., 2006).

Erysipelothrix infections

Erysipelothrix rhusiopathiae is a Gram-positive organism that is ubiquitous in the soil, freshwater, and marine environments. Although no known pathology occurs in fish, the bacterium is often associated with the skin and mucus of the fish (Stenstrom et al., 1992). Human infections with *E. rhusiopathiae* are typically from contact or handling of contaminated animal tissues, subsequently infecting an existing wound or injury during animal handling (Gorby and Peacock, 1988; Rocha et al., 1989). In humans, the disease has three forms. One form is a localized skin infection usually associated with a wound or abrasion and is typically localized to the extremities, primarily the hands and fingers. The second form is a diffuse cutaneous progression of the localized infection to surrounding tissues. The third form is a systemic infection in which the heart and heart valves are affected, resulting in endocarditis.

Other zoonotic bacterial infections

There are sporadic reports of a number of other species of bacteria acquired from contact with fish as causing disease in humans, and these include bacteria of the genera *Edwarsiella*, *Escherichia*, *Salmonella*, and *Klebsiella* (Nemetz and Shotts, 1993; Gaulin et al., 2002; Senanayake et al., 2004). These are Gram-negative bacteria that are associated with freshwater fish species or freshwater aquatic environments. The greatest potential for infection to an individual is through a puncture wound while handling or examining fish, or by contamination of existing cuts and abrasions. Disease in fish with any of these potential pathogens produces nonspecific clinical signs that may include infection of the skin or systemic invasion. Infections with any of these bacteria in humans can remain localized at the point of entry or can become systemic, leading to severe cases of human illness (Jordon and Hadley, 1969; Vandepitte et al., 1983; Matsushima et al., 1996; Wilson et al., 1989).

Prevention of human infection and client recommendations

Veterinarians, veterinary staff members, and other fish health professionals working with finfish, whether ornamental, bait, or food fish, need to be aware of the possible zoonotic diseases that can be acquired from aquatic animals. Prevention is based on using standard safety and hygiene practices as would be used with mammalian patients. Avoiding contact with the fish and water is the single best way to prevent any chance of a zoonotic infection; however, to provide proper diagnostics and care to fish in home aquaria or aquaculture tanks, some contact will occur with the water, fish, or both. Basic hygiene and thorough hand washing after contact with fish or water containing fish is an excellent preventative protocol. Gloves should be worn at all times during handling and examination to protect the clinician from bacteria on the external surfaces of the fish. Using gloves to reduce contact with the fish or water, or to reduce potential injury from equipment, ornaments, coral, or being directly finned by fish, is a good way to prevent exposure to zoonotic pathogens. Gloves should be changed between fish from different tanks and between populations of fish to prevent the spread of potential pathogens. Areas with open sores, cuts, or scrapes should be prevented from coming into contact with aquarium water when cleaning or changing water. Also, whenever a brush, scrubber, sprayer, or other means of cleaning a tank can be used instead of the hands, it should be recommended. Clients should be cautioned that immunocompromised individuals may be at a higher risk for contracting a zoonotic infection and should limit contact with aquarium water and fish. Clients seeking advice regarding zoonotic diseases should also be advised to talk with their personal physician.

It is also important for veterinarians to inform clients of the health risks associated with handling and caring for aquatic animals. This is similar to the veterinarian's responsibilities when dealing with public health issues in pet animals and domesticated livestock. The most important information that a veterinarian can provide a client is reassurance that with proper precautions and proper hygiene, fish are safe to keep and maintain as pets or aquatic livestock.

Prevention in aquatic animals

Obviously, prevention is a much more effective and economical approach to avoiding zoonotic diseases than reacting to an existing infection. Thus, discussing basic biosecurity principles with the client with a home aquarium or ornamental pond or with the commercial producer with an aquaculture facility is paramount to reducing the introduction and spread of a pathogen in an aquatic animal population. There are several measures that can be recommended to clients to reduce the risk of introducing zoonotic pathogens into established populations.

(1) A quarantine area or tank separate from existing populations where new fish can be held is helpful in preventing not only zoonotic pathogens but also other disease agents (i.e., viral, bacterial, parasitic, and fungal) from entering a client's fish populations. The quarantine tank or area should be treated as a separate system with its own nets, feed, and tank-cleaning equipment to prevent contamination of existing fish. New fish should be held in quarantine for 30–45 days while observing behavior, feeding response, and development of any clinical signs. This length of time is generally long enough for most pathogens to present themselves as clinical disease in newly acquired fish. Unfortunately, chronic pathogens such as *Mycobacterium* spp. may not be detected during this time period.

(2) An "all-in-all-out" production cycle in facilities with large populations of fish is another method used to reduce the entrance and spread of some pathogens within a facility. A period of time between production cycles should be long enough to allow for the disinfection of tanks or systems for bacterial pathogens.

(3) And finally, a valid veterinary-client–patient relationship is also important for advising a client to have regularly scheduled appointments for fish examinations or site visits, and identifying problems contributing to the acquisition of an endemic or zoonotic pathogen in a fish population.

References

Beran, V., Matlova, L., Dvorska, L., et al. (2006) Distribution of mycobacteria in clinically healthy ornamental fish and their aquarium environment. *Journal of Fish Diseases* **29**: 383–393.

Bisharat, N., Agmon, V., Finkelstein, R., et al. (1999) Clinical epidemiological, and microbiological features of *Vibrio vulnificus* biogroup 3 causing outbreaks of wound infection and bacteriaemia in Israel. Israel *Vibrio* study group. *Lancet* **354**: 1421–1424.

Chinabut, S. (1999) Mycobacteriosis and nocardiosis. In *Fish Diseases and Disorders: Viral, Bacterial and Fungal Infections* (Woo, P.T.K. and Bruno, D.W., eds.), pp. 319–340. New York: CAB International.

Decostere, A., Hermans, K., and Haesebrouck, F. (2004) Piscine mycobacteriosis: a literature review covering the agents and the disease it causes in fish and humans. *Veterinary Microbiology* **99**: 159–166.

Eastaugh, J. and Shepard, S. (1989) Infectious and toxic syndromes for fish and shellfish consumption: a review. *Archives of Internal Medicine* **149**: 1735–1740.

Eldar, A., Bejerano, Y., Livoff, A., et al. (1995) Experimental streptococcal meningo-encephalitis in cultured fish. *Veterinary Microbiology* **43**: 33–40.

Falkinham, J.O. (1996) Epidemiology of infection by nontuberculous *Mycobacteria. Clinical Microbiology Review* **9**: 177–215.

Gaulin, C., Vincent, C., Alain, L., et al. (2002) Outbreak of *Salmonella paratyphi* B linked to aquariums in the province of Quebec, 2000. *Canada Communicable Disease Report* **28**: 89–93

Gorby, G. and Peacock, J. (1988) *Erysipelothrix rhusiopathiae* endocarditis: microbiologic, epidemiologic, and clinical features of an occupational disease. *Review of Infectious Diseases* **10**: 317–325.

Harriff, M.J., Bermudez, L.E., and Kent, M.L. (2007) Experimental exposure of zebrafish, *Danio rerio* (Hamilton), to *Mycobacterium marinum* and *Mycobacterium peregrinum* reveals the gastrointestinal tract as the primary route of infection: a potential model for environmental mycobacterial infection. *Journal of Fish Diseases* **30**: 587–600.

Ho, M.H., Ho, C.K., and Chong, L.Y. (2006) Atypical mycobacterial cutaneous infections in Hong Kong: 10-year retrospective study. *Hong Kong Medical Journal* **12**: 21–26.

Huminer, D., Pitlik, S.D., Block, C., et al. (1986) Aquarium-borne *Mycobacterium marinum* skin infection. Report of a case and review of the literature. *Archives of Dermatology* **122**: 689–703.

Jahncke, M.L. and Schwarz, M.H. (2002) Public, animal and environmental aquaculture health issues in industrial countries. In *Public, Animal, and Environmental Aquaculture Health Issues* (Jahncke, M., Garrett, E.S., Reilly, A., et al., eds.), pp. 67–102. New York: John Wiley & Sons.

Jordon, G.W. and Hadley, W.K. (1969) Human infection with *Edwardsiella tarda*. *Annals of Internal Medicine* **70**: 283–288.

Joseph, S.W., Daily, O.P., Hunt, W.S., et al. (1979) *Aeromonas* primary wound infection of a diver in polluted waters. *Journal of Clinical Microbiology* **10**: 46–49.

Kaattari, I.M., Rhodes, M.W., Kaattari, S.L., et al. (2006) The evolving story of *Mycobacterium tuberculosis* clade members detected in fish. *Journal of Fish Diseases* **29**: 509–520.

Kiesch, N. (2000) Aquariums and mycobacteriosis. *Revue Médicale de Bruxelles* **21**: A255–A256.

Kitao, T. (1993) Streptococcal infections. In *Bacterial Diseases of Fish* (Inglis, V., Roberts, R.J., and Bromage, N.R., eds.), pp. 196–197. New York: Halsted Press, John Wiley & Sons.

Lacaille, F., Blanche, S., Bodemer, C., et al. (1990) Persistent *Mycobacterium marinum* infection in a child with probable visceral involvement. *Pediatric Infectious Disease* **9**: 58–60.

Lehane, L. and Rawlin, G.T. (2000). Topically acquired bacterial zoonoses from fish: a review. *Medical Journal of Australia* **173** (5): 256–259.

Lowry, T.L. and Smith, S.A. (2007) Aquatic zoonoses of food, bait, ornamental and tropical fish. *Journal of the American Veterinary Medical Association* **231**: 876–880.

Matsushima, S., Yajima, S., Taguchi, T., et al. (1996) A fulminating case of *Edwardsiella tarda* septicemia with necrotizing faciitis. *Kansenshagaku Zasshi* **70** (6): 631–636.

Moyer, N.P. (1987) Clinical significance of *Aeromonas* species isolated from patients with diarrhea. *Journal of Clinical Microbiology* **25**: 2044–2048.

Nemetz, T. and Shotts, E. (1993) Zoonotic diseases. In *Fish Medicine* (Stoskopf, M.K., ed.), pp. 214–220. Philadelphia: W.B. Saunders.

Nigrelli, R.F. and Vogel, H. (1963) Spontaneous tuberculosis in fishes and other cold-blooded vertebrates with special reference to *Mycobacterium fortuitum* Cruz from fish and human lesions. *Zoologica* **48**: 131–144.

Oliver, J.D. (2005) Wound infections caused by *Vibrio vulnificus* and other marine bacteria. *Epidemiology and Infection* **133** (3): 383–391.

Palumbo, S.A., Bencivengo, M.M., Del Corral, F., et al. (1989) Characterization of the *Aeromonas hydrophila* group isolated from retail foods of animal origin. *Journal of Clinical Microbiology* **27**: 854–859.

Perera, R., Johnson, S., and Collins, M. (1994) *Streptococcus iniae* associated with mortalitiy of *Tilapia nilotica* and *T. aurea* hybrids. *Journal of Aquatic Animal Health* **6**: 335–340.

Perl, A., Frelier, P.F., and Bercovier, H. (1999) Red drum *Sciaenops ocellatus* mortalities associated with *Streptococcus iniae* infections. *Diseases of Aquatic Organisms* **36**: 121–127.

Petrini, B. (2006) *Mycobacterium marinum*: ubiquitous agent of waterborne granulomatous skin infections. *European Journal of Clinical Microbiology and Infectious Disease* **25**: 609–613.

Prearo, M., Zanoni, R.G., Campo Dall'Orto, B., et al. (2004) Mycobacterioses: emerging pathologies in aquarium fish. *Veterinary Research Communications* **28**: 315–317.

Rocha, M.P., Fontoura, P.R., Azevedo, S.N., et al. (1989) *Erysipelothrix* endocarditis with previous cutaneous lesions: report of a case and review of the literature. *Revista do Instituto de Medicina Tropical de São Paulo* **31**: 286–289.

Ross, B.C., Johnson, P.D.R., Oppedisano, F., et al. (1962) Detection of *Mycobacterium ulcerans* in environmental samples during and outbreak of ulcerative disease. *Applied and Environmental Microbiology* **63**: 4135–4138.

Senanayake, S.N., Ferson, M.J., Botham, S.J., et al. (2004) A child with *Salmonella enterica* serotype Paratyphi B infection acquired from a fish tank. *Medical Journal of Australia* **180**: 250.

Smith, S.A. (1997) Mycobacterial infections in pet fish. *Seminars in Avian and Exotic Pet Medicine* **6**: 40–45.

Stenstrom, I.M., Norrung, V., Ternstrom, A., et al. (1992) Occurrence of different serotypes of *Erysipelothrix rhusiopathiae* in retail pork and fish. *Acta Veterinaria Scandinavica* **33**: 169–173.

Tang, W.M., Fung, K.K., Cheng, V.C., et al. (2006) Rapidly progressive necrotising fasciitis following a stonefish sting: a report of two cases. *Journal of Orthopedic Surgery* **14** (1): 67–70.

Tchornobay, A.M., Claudy, A.L., Perrot, J.L., et al. (1992) Fatal disseminated *Mycobacterium abscessus* from Japanese medaka. *Journal of Aquatic Animal Health* **9**: 234–238.

Tsai, M.S., Kuo, C.Y., Wang, M.C., et al. (2006) Clinical features and risk factors for mortality in *Aermonas* bacteremic adults with malignancies. *Journal of Microbiology, Immunology and Infection* **39** (2): 150–154.

Vandepitte, J., Lemmens, P., and Stwert, L. (1983) Human edwardsiellosis traced to ornamental fish. *Journal of Clinical Microbiology* **17**: 165–167.

Weinstein, M.R., Litt, M., Kertesz, D.A., et al. (1997) Invasive infections due to a fish pathogen, *Streptococcus iniae, S. iniae* study group. *New England Journal of Medicine* **337**: 589–594.

Wilson, J., Waterer, R., Wofford, J., et al. (1989) Serious infections with *Edwardsiella tarda*: a case report and review of the literature. *Archives of Internal Medicine* **149**: 208–210.

Wolf, J.C. and Smith, S.A. (1999) Comparative severity of experimentally-induced mycobacteriosis in striped bass *Morone saxatilis* and hybrid tilapia *Oreochromis* spp. *Diseases of Aquatic Organisms* **38**: 191–200.

Wolf, J.C. and Smith, S.A. (2000) Human pathogens in shellfish and finfish. In *Marine & Freshwater Products Handbook* (Martin, R.E., Carter, E.P., Flick, G.J., et al., eds.), pp. 697–716. Weimar, TX: Technomic Publishing.

Fish Medicine

Chapter 13

Transport and Hospitalization of the Fish Patient

Helen E. Roberts

Fish that are unhealthy benefit from being examined in their own environment. This reduces stress from the processes of handling, capture, and transportation methods. Unfortunately, this is not possible for all patients. Either due to lack of portable and available diagnostic equipment or distance from the clinician, many pet fish will need to seen at the veterinary clinic.

Once a practitioner begins to see pet fish patients, the clients will need specific instructions on transportation to the clinic, and the hospital will need to devise ways to hold fish patients that need extensive treatments or surgical procedures. This chapter will discuss options for transport and hospitalization, from a simple plastic bag to more complex setups.

Stress

Capture, netting, handling, confinement, and transport are all stressful events to fish. Poor water quality that commonly occurs during transport adds even more stress to the fish. The stresses associated with these situations are often unavoidable but should be approached with understanding, and effort should be made to minimize these stressors. See Chapter 3 for an in-depth discussion of stress.

Initially, the stress response is beneficial but leads to further problems when the response becomes chronic. Acute stress alone has been shown to cause skin ulceration without any prior trauma or exposure to bacteria, viruses, parasites, or pathogenic fungal elements (Noga et al., 1998). When stressful events occur in the presence of pathogens, stressed fish have been shown to develop disease outbreaks in more than twice the number of nonstressed fish (Dror et al., 2006).

Capture of fish for transport

It is important that the fish owner take any measures that may reduce or mitigate the inherent stress associated with transporting their charges.

Recommendations include the following:

- Feeding a diet with an increased level of vitamin C for 10 days prior to the event. Studies have shown this to be beneficial in reducing the effects of stress and increasing resistance to disease (Lim et al., 2003; Fosså et al., 2007).
- Withholding food in small fish for 24 hours prior to handling and transport. Fasting for 48 hours is recommended for larger fish, goldfish, and koi (Lim et al., 2003; Fosså et al., 2007). Prolonged starvation will have the opposite effect; resistance to stress will be lowered.
- Removing obstacles that may interfere with capture nets such as decor, pump and filter intakes, and so on.
- Setting up a seine net in a pond to reduce the maneuvering room of the fish.
- Sedating fish. Very large fish can be sedated *in situ* by lowering the water level in the tank and adding a sedative, typically MS-222. Depending on the size of the tank, this is not inexpensive.
- Using netting with a fine mesh to reduce skin, fin, and tail damage.
- Being prepared to delay transport if the capture event becomes too stressful.

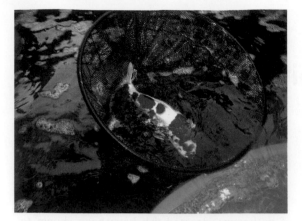

Fig. 13.1 To minimize handling stress and injury, without removing the fish from the water, a koi (*Cyprinus carpio*) is carefully moved from the net into a bowl.

- Adding 1%–3% (1–3 gm/L) sodium chloride to the transport water to minimize the osmotic gradient and reduce the energy expenditure. A higher level can adversely affect some fish species and the transport water quality (De Boeck et al., 2000; Fosså et al., 2007).

Capture methods should be discussed with the owner prior to capture. The image of a stressed, sick fish darting all over the tank or pond evading a net is one that is best avoided. Advance preparation can make a big difference on the health of the fish. Large fish, such as koi, need to be carefully supported when lifted out of the water. These fish often benefit from being guided into a suitable bowl once captured in a net (Fig. 13.1). Sock nets can also be used for capture of large fish, but care must be taken to prevent fins from becoming caught in the mesh. Again, large fish in these nets need to be properly supported when lifted.

Transportation

Many suitable containers exist to transport fish. The best choice depends on the length of time in transit, the size of the fish, and the amount of water that needs to be transported with the fish. Fish can be placed in plastic, polyethylene bags, with one-third of the volume filled with water and the remainder with air. Exhaled air should not be used due to its high carbon dioxide level (Francis-Floyd, 2004). Double bagging the fish adds an extra layer of security in case of a leak. For longer trips, oxygen can be used in place of room air. Insulated, Styrofoam coolers are ideal for placing plastic bags with fish inside to reduce thermal stress. Another method that can help prevent drastic temperature changes is to use layered newspapers or wrapped chemical heat or cooling packs around the bags. Extra padding, foam, or towels can also be placed around the bags to minimize movement. Keeping the fish in the dark can reduce some stress, so boxes, cartons, and coolers should have sturdy lids or be covered. Very large fish, such as koi, are prepared for transport the same way. Many hobbyists believe the box must be placed in the vehicle perpendicular to the road to prevent facial or head injury as a result of sudden stops.

Alternatively, a commercially available bag called Kordon® Breathing Bags™ (Kordon LLC, Hayward, CA) may be used. The company literature states that these bags contain a special plastic film that allows atmospheric oxygen to enter the bag and carbon dioxide to escape. The fish is added with water, but no air or oxygen is included in the packaging of the fish. While this author has not specifically seen any independent, peer-reviewed literature testing these bags, she has had clients travel many hours and long distances using these bags for their goldfish. Commercial 5-gallon minnow buckets with built-in aerators are also an effective method of fish transport for short distances (Fig. 13.2). While not always ideal, clients will sometimes devise their own methods of fish transportation, and despite "breaking the rules," some fish will show no adverse effects (Fig. 13.3).

Water additives during transport

In addition to anesthetic agents and sodium chloride as potential additives to transport water, several other options exist. Some of these have scientific merit, while others are questionable and are backed only by anecdotal information. Cation exchange resins, clinoptilolites, and zeolites are often added as unionized ammonia binding agents: examples of these are Ammo-Lock® and Ammo-Chips® (Aquarium Pharmaceuticals Inc., Mars

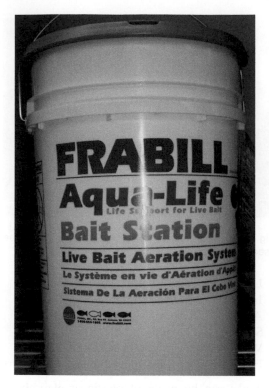

Fig. 13.2 A commercial minnow bucket with aerator can be a great transport container for short trips.

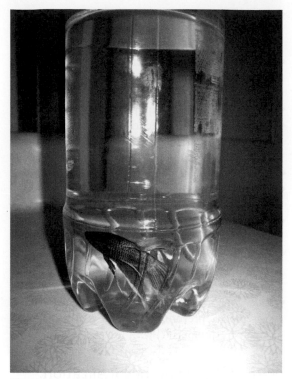

Fig. 13.3 Although not a recommended travel containment system, "Skye," a betta (*Betta splendens*), traveled by train from Chicago, IL, to Rochester, NY, in a one-liter water bottle with no adverse effects.

Fishcare, Chalfont, PA), AmQuel® (Kordon LLC), and Chloram-X™ (Aqua-Science Research Group Inc, North Kansas City, MO). Another popular additive includes synthetic "slime coat replacements": Stress Coat® (Aquarium Pharmaceuticals Inc., Mars Fishcare) and PolyAqua® or NovAqua® (Kordon LLC). Less commonly, antibiotics, proprietary vitamin mixes, and potassium permanganate are added. Investigation and inquiries should be made to the client if they are considering additives that may further stress the fish and cause potential damage.

Additional water

Depending on the size of the fish and the transport container, the client should be advised to bring several gallons (or more) of water from the tank or pond that can be used for recovery water (postanesthesia), water testing, and replacement water for the return trip. The water can also be used to acclimate the patient to a hospital tank if

needed. A minimum of 2 gallons is recommended for small fish, and much larger volumes will be needed for large fish, such as koi. Clients should not put anything, including fish, in the extra water.

Hospitalization

Hospitalizing fish patients can be more labor intensive and more involved than hospitalizing terrestrial animals. Luckily, in most situations, fish are dealt with on an outpatient basis. Occasionally, case management may require involved medical treatments or surgery, and hospitalization will be required.

Considerations include the following:

• Space and location requirement for the systems, including accessory equipment (e.g. pump, filter)

- The structural support required for the weight of the systems (water is heavy) and plumbing logistics for filling and drainage
- The maintenance of strict biosecurity measures to prevent pathogen exposure in hospitalized patients
- The use of separate equipment for each system
- Staff training in biosecurity practices, monitoring fish patients, monitoring water quality, and maintaining equipment
- Water quality measurement and maintenance
- Cleaning and disinfection of systems after hospitalization
- Using equipment that is disposable or can be easily disinfected
- Minimizing the stress of the patient while having reliable methods to observe the patient and administer treatments
- Lids, tops, or netting should be placed on all systems to prevent accidental deaths due to "escape attempts"

Water quality and hospitalization

The importance of excellent water quality in hospital systems cannot be overemphasized. Monitoring of important water quality parameters such as temperature, ammonia, nitrite, and pH should be done daily or, if needed, twice daily depending on the bioload of the system. Systems will need to be thoroughly cleaned and disinfected after each use, so providing a mature biological filter for each new setup can be difficult. In most cases, the hospitalization time is short and the nitrogenous wastes can be removed by water changes supplemented by efficient mechanical and chemical filtration methods. Alternatively, "seasoned" sponge filters can be maintained in a reserve system and moved as needed to hospital tanks. For small tanks with one or two small fish, this may be adequate.

When feasible, the client should provide the water for the hospital tank unless infectious disease is a concern.

Equipment suggestions

- Small tanks of various sizes with sturdy, close fitting lids

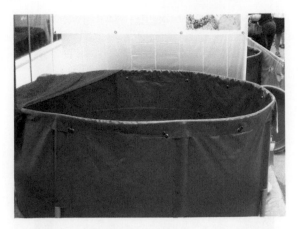

Fig. 13.4 A 300-gallon collapsible show tank can be used as a temporary hospital tank for large fish.

- Large tank, tub, or vat for larger fish
- Individual nets for each tank
- Airstones, air pumps, and airline tubing
- Submersible heaters and thermometers
- Water suction devices for water changes
- Filtration systems, including ultraviolet sterilizers

Tanks can be made of plastic or glass. Integrated systems with filtration systems, lighting, and hoods are convenient to set up and use for small fish (Eclipse® Systems by Marineland, United Pet Group, Spectrum Brands, Atlanta, GA). Heaters are added to complete the tank setup. Aquatic rack systems can be used when hospitalizing large numbers of fish. Each system should still have its own filtration system and equipment unless the fish are from a common source.

For large fish, Rubbermaid® stock tanks can make ideal temporary hospital tanks. Several sizes are available, from 50 to 300 gallons. Another option is the collapsible tanks used in koi shows. These can be easily assembled when needed (Fig. 13.4). The show tanks take up much less storage space than a stock tank when not in use.

Additional equipment and companion fish

It is important to remember that hospitalization in a new environment, treatments, and any handling will be stressful to fish patients. Hiding places should be used when possible. Polyvinyl chloride pipes of various diameters and plastic aquarium plants can provide hiding places and are easy to clean and disinfect for reuse.

Gravel or bottom substrate is not recommended for use in a hospital tank due to the likelihood of uneaten food and debris accumulating, leading to poor water quality conditions.

Social or schooling fish, such as koi or goldfish, may benefit from having a conspecific or tank mate from the home location during hospitalization. This practice may help reduce stress unless the healthy fish is also at risk for developing disease. The author uses this practice most often when keeping a fish for a short period postoperatively.

References and further reading

Butcher, R.L. (2001) General Approach. In *BSAVA Manual of Ornamental Fish*, 2nd Edition (Wildgoose, W.H., ed.), pp. 63–68. Gloucester: BSAVA.

De Boeck, G., Vlaeminck, A, Van Der Linden, A., et al. (2000) Salt stress and resistance to hypoxic challenges in the common carp (*Cyprinus carpio* L.). *Journal of Fish Biology* **57**: 761–776.

Dror, M., Sinyakov, M.S., Okun, E., et al. (2006) Experimental handling stress as infection facilitating factor for goldfish ulcerative disease. *Veterinary Immunology and Immunopathology* **109**: 279–287.

European Union. (2005) European Union Council Regulation No. 1/2005 of December 22, 2004. *Official Journal of the European Union*

Fagundes, M. and Urbinati, E.C. (2008) Stress in pintado (*Pseudoplatystoma corruscans*) during farming procedures. *Aquaculture* **276**: 112–119.

Fosså, S.A., Bassleer, G.M.O., Lim, L.C., et al. (2007) *International Transport of Live Fish in the Ornamental Aquatic Industry*. Maarsen, The Netherlands: Ornamental Fish International.

Francis-Floyd, R. (2004) Pet fish care and husbandry. *Veterinary Clinics of North America Exotic Animal Practice* **7**: 397–419.

Lim, L.C., Dhert, P., and Sorgeloos, P. (2003) Recent developments and improvements in ornamental fish packaging systems for air transport. *Aquaculture Research* **34**: 923–935.

Noga, E.J., Botts, S., Yang, M.-S., et al. (1998) Acute stress causes skin ulceration in striped bass and hybrid bass (Morone). *Veterinary Pathology* **35** (2): 102–107.

Stoskopf, M.K. (1993) Hospitalization. In *Fish Medicine* (Stoskopf, M.K., ed.), pp. 98–112. Philadelphia: W.B. Saunders.

Chapter 14

History

Helen E. Roberts

Introduction

Information gathered by a comprehensive history and a thorough physical exam can determine what course of action to take when evaluating the cause or causes of problems in sick fish. In addition, the history and physical exam can sometimes lead to a presumptive diagnosis. There are many types of fish clients and it is important to try to gain an understanding of their needs, level of experience in fish keeping, and understanding of fish health. Broad categories include single-tank owners, multiple-tank owners, breeders, pond or koi hobbyists, retail shop owners, and wholesalers (Stoskopf, 1988). It becomes important to determine into what category your client falls because an effective history is tailored to meet the needs and expertise of the type of client involved, in addition to the specific problem presented.

Many clients will initially seek the services of a fish veterinarian by telephone. By the time they seek the services of a fish health professional, most fish owners have been searching for assistance from many sources. Their fish may have been subjected to several unsuccessful therapeutic trials without the benefit of a diagnosis, making the initial problem or problems much worse. These owners can be frantic. Phone consultations can be very time consuming and in the end leave both the fish owner and the fish health professional frustrated. In the interest of limiting time spent on the phone, it is important to quickly determine the nature of the problem, how and if you can help, does the client want your assistance, and will the client be bringing the fish in or do you need to schedule a site visit (Stoskopf, 1988). In this author's experience, it is also important to find out quickly if the fish owner is seeking extensive "free advice" or is willing to allow for examinations and diagnostic testing. Requests for free help are not unique to a fish practice and a well-trained receptionist will be able to screen these calls. Sometimes the problem can be quickly solved by the recommendation of a few simple management changes. For clients who need *extensive* phone time and believe they cannot come in for an examination or live too far for a site visit, the author offers the option of a paid phone consultation with the consultation fee credited toward an examination. While this may seem to be a controversial practice, it does work to limit frustration on both ends and is time efficient.

Once a client has made an appointment, history forms can be emailed or mailed in advance of an office call or site visit.

Basic history

A basic history for fish problems should include details on the environment, that is, tank(s) or pond(s); the population that includes the affected fish; husbandry and management practices; the presenting problem; and information on previous attempts to correct the problem. As stated previously, it is critical to gauge the client's level of knowledge when asking questions. A question may need to be phrased a few different ways before understanding is reached.

Environmental assessment

Practitioners do not generally question owners on the specifics of the dog's bed or the cat's water bowl. In fish health assessment however, details

Table 14.1   Environmental history questions.

Tank: general questions	Comments
Volume of affected system (gallons or liters)	—
Depth (ponds)	—
How long has the tank been established?	Can offer clue to diagnosis (i.e., "new tank syndrome")
Bottom substrate, layer thickness, and substrate size	Sand, none used, gravel, river rock, etc.
Any shutoff periods for the equipment?	That is, pumps off at night
Ornaments/decor	Plastic, copper, spitter fountains (ponds), etc.
Tanks covered?	Yes/no
Location	Ponds—shaded/sunny
	Tanks—quiet/noisy, proximity to window, etc.
Filtration/life-support systems	—
Aeration?	—
Heater(s)? Wattage?	—
Temperature monitoring?	—
Ultraviolet (UV) sterilizer? Wattage? Age of bulb?	Flow rate through UV sterilizer should be questioned
Type of filter(s) and media	Canister, internal, external, wet/dry, etc.
Pump(s), type and volume	—
Gallons per hour of pump(s) (assesses water turnover)	Can be also asked in liters per hour
Lighting type/photoperiod	Natural, artificial, etc.
Other equipment	Ozonator, protein skimmers, CO_2 systems, refugia, chiller, reverse osmosis/deionization unit
Maintenance	
Water change schedule	—
Volume each change	—
Water treatments used with changes	Dechlorinating agents, proprietary blends, etc.
Equipment cleaning and maintenance	That is, change all filters at once or stagger? Vigorous cleaning?
Water quality	
Source of water	Tap, well, aged water, dechlorinated tap water, others
Pipe material (source water delivery)	Copper, lead, galvanized metal, polyvinyl chloride, plastic, others
Testing performed?	Yes/no
Test frequency and testing methods	Dry tab, electronic meters, liquid/drop, pet store testing, and so on
What parameters checked?	Ammonia, temperature, pH, dissolved oxygen, nitrite, nitrate, alkalinity, salinity, specific gravity, etc.
Last results	
Log of test results?	—
Water appearance	Clear, cloudy, colored, etc.
Quarantine system ("Q-tank")	Should be evaluated using the above parameters

on the aquatic environment, life-support equipment, and the variety of the tank or pond population can be critical. Many problems in pet fish are due to chronic stress. Poor water quality is the most common cause of stress in fish. A fish practitioner must question the owner extensively on the environment in which the fish live. If an onsite visit is not possible, clients can be instructed to send or bring in clear digital and video images of the environment and life-support equipment. Table 14.1 gives a detailed list of general questions on the aquatic environment, maintenance practices, life-support systems, and water quality. For a better understanding of the common types of equipment found in aquaria and ponds, please refer to Chapter 5 in this book.

Table 14.2 Fish patient history.

Fish population	Comments
Number of fish	Overcrowding? (Both size and numbers)
Species of fish	Some species are not compatible
Recent additions? (Species and number)	Failure to quarantine?

Nutrition	Comments
Food type, brand of food	Commercial food (flakes, pellets, frozen, etc.), live food, etc.
Live food source	If applicable
Age of food	It is not uncommon for owners to have old food on hand
Frequency and amount of feeding	Overfeeding is very common
Storage of food	In a cool, dry, pest free place?

Clinically affected fish	Comments
Number/species of affected fish	—
Description of problem	—
Behavior changes?	Abnormal swimming, flashing, listlessness, etc.
Duration of problem(s)	—
Previous treatments?	Treatments may have had impact on water quality,
Name of drug/dosage/duration of treatment	worsened condition, or led to deaths
Result of treatment	—
Deaths?	—

Patient history

Taking a specific history of the fish patient involves questions similar to those asked in histories of terrestrial species, with a few exceptions. Most owners do not have a problem recognizing the significance of behavioral changes such as anorexia, lethargy, and neurological disease in terrestrial species such as dogs and cats, but may fail to notice the significance of the same abnormalities in their fish. The questions should always be geared toward the owner's level of expertise and understanding. For example, a question on the presence of "flashing" may not yield the correct answer if the owner does not understand the term. Table 14.2 offers examples of questions that pertain to fish health.

References and further reading

Butcher, R.L. (2001) General approach. In *BSAVA Manual of Ornamental Fish*, 2nd Edition (Wildgoose, W., ed.), pp. 63–67. Gloucester: BSAVA Publications.

Noga, E.J. (1996) Fish disease diagnosis form. In *Fish Disease: Diagnosis and Treatment, Appendix I* (Noga, E.J., ed.), pp. 327–328. St. Louis, MO: Mosby.

Stoskopf, M.K. (1988) Taking the history. *The Veterinary Clinics of North America: Small Animal Practice* **18** (2): 283–291.

Stoskopf, M.K. (1993) Clinical examination and procedures. In *Fish Medicine* (Stoskopf, M.K., ed.), pp. 62–78. Philadelphia: W.B. Saunders.

Chapter 15
Physical Examination of Fish

Helen E. Roberts

A comprehensive physical examination of the fish patient includes an environmental examination, including evaluation of water quality and assessment of life-support systems, indirect visual examination of the patient(s), and a direct "hands-on" examination.

Environmental examination

Water quality evaluation is recommended for all sick fish, regardless of the presenting problem. Many owners will admit to having the water tested elsewhere and report the parameters were "all normal." It is important to get specific, numerical values for each parameter. In general, it is best to repeat the water quality tests and include parameters that may not have been evaluated, such as dissolved oxygen, alkalinity, salinity, and nitrates. (See Chapter 4 for a complete description of water quality, and Chapter 14, Table 14.1, for the environmental assessment history questionnaire.)

Whenever possible, an on-site evaluation of the environment is recommended. Life-support systems must be checked to ensure that they are adequate in size, to evaluate their condition (clean, filthy, damaged, etc.), and to find out what maintenance procedures are being performed. Many owners, particularly those with pond fish, are heavily influenced by current trends and fads in filtration systems and other equipment that may be inadequate, undersized, and ineffective for their facility. Aquaria should each have their own filtration systems and not be connected via a common filter system. Separation, although more expensive, can reduce the spread of infectious disease and limit the amount of medical treatment required. Fish owners may not be aware of

any deficiencies or may attribute known deficiencies to poor health in their fish. If a site visit is not possible, the client should be encouraged to bring good-quality images of the aquaria or pond, including photos and a diagram of the life-support systems and ancillary equipment such as ultraviolet filtration units, ozone generators, and so on.

Indirect examination

An initial evaluation and observation of the patient should ideally be performed with the fish in its own environment or, failing that, in the transport container. Details of the fish's position in the water column, orientation and swimming behavior, and reaction to external stimuli should be noted, in addition to the location of lesions. Other abnormal behaviors such as clamping of the fins and opercular rates should be recorded. Table 15.1 lists abnormal behaviors that may be seen on indirect physical exam of the fish patient. Body condition scoring and any asymmetry are also noted on the initial exam. Very thin fish might be experiencing malnutrition, anorexia, a wasting disease such as mycobacteriosis, or severe parasitism. Fish that appear to have coelomic distension or bloating should be further evaluated for the possibility of a coelomic mass, gas and air accumulation, a foreign body, generalized edema or "dropsy," obesity, and ascites (Weber and Innis, 2007). Polycystic kidney disease in goldfish may also present as coelomic distension (see Fig. 15.1). As with other pet species, obesity is also not an uncommon problem in pet fish. This information should be compared with the appearance and behavior of clinically normal fish in the same environment.

Table 15.1 Abnormal behaviors observed during physical examination of fish.

Behavior	Description	Comment/associated problem(s)
Bottom sitting	Fish, typically found in middle to top of water column, "sitting" on bottom, not resting	Differentiate from normal behavior; lethargy/depression.[1] May be seen in obese fish (HR, personal observation)
Circling	Purposeful movement in one direction[1,2]	Unilateral blindness/eye disorder;[1] unilateral fin damage[1]
Clamped fins	Fins held close to body wall	Systemic disease; lethargy; parasitism; poor water quality; depression; multiple causes
Coughing	Rapid opercular flaring	Occasional coughing is normal;[1] gill irritation; gill parasitism; other causes of gill disease
Curling	Body flexed laterally into a "C" shape	Can be associated with systemic disease, lethargy, and spinal disease; poor prognosis
Abnormal coloration	Darker or lighter color than normal healthy, fish coloration	Stress; secondary to drug use; systemic disease (sepsis); poor water quality; parasitism; differentiate from normal color or reproductive color changes[1]
Drifting	Movement without purpose in the water currents	Systemic disease; lethargy; poor prognosis
Feces: mucoid, bloody, long, with air bubbles, stringlike, pale[3]	Analogous to diarrhea in terrestrial animals	Gastrointestinal disorders; internal parasitism; high-fiber diet
Flared opercula	Opercula held open to expose gills	Severe hypoxia, usually agonal
Flashing	Rubbing on bottom of tank or pond and exposing the ventral aspect (a "flash" of pale color of the ventrum)	Parasitism; poor water quality
Gasping	Yawning-like behavior or rapid opening and closing of mouth	Hypoxia; gill disorders; relative hypoxia (anemia, nitrite poisoning); poor water quality
Hurdling[1]	Apparent "falling" in water column followed by rapid forward/vertical movement[1]	Neurological disease;[1] poor water quality–ammonia toxicity[1]
Jumping	Attempting to jump out of tank or pond ("suicide attempt")	Startled fish;[1] poor water quality (low oxygen, low pH)[1]
Listing	Leaning to one side	Buoyancy disorders
Pale coloration	Light version of normal is coloration	Systemic disease; stress
Petechiae/ecchymosis	Small red to purple spots on body surface, from pinpoint to larger focal areas (usually <0.3cm)	Sepsis; parasitism; systemic disease; trauma; sunburn (dorsal lesions)
Piping	Gulping of air at water surface	See "Gasping"; do not confuse with normal bubble nest building seen in fish such as Bettas
Postural abnormalities: head up, tail down	—	Systemic disease; parasitism; buoyancy disorders; water quality; "tail walking" has been associated with Pleistophora infection in neon tetras;[1] stress
Red streaks on tail/fin	Congestion of blood within capillaries	Septicemia; poor water quality; stress; trauma; fin/tail infections (fin and/or tail "rot")
Rubbing	Pruritis	See "Flashing"
"Shimmies"	Entire body moves back and forth	Systemic disease; poor water quality; neurological disease

Notes:
[1] Francis-Floyd (1988).
[2] Campbell (2005).
[3] Wildgoose (2001a).

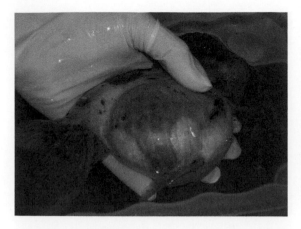

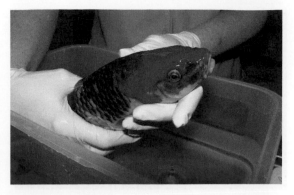

Fig. 15.2 A sedated koi is examined over a water-filled container in case of an accidental fall.

Fig. 15.1 A goldfish with coelomic distension due to polycystic kidney disease.

A camera is a valuable tool for documenting lesions and the overall general appearance of the fish. Digital images of lesions and abnormal behavior or posture can be retained for future reference and can also be included with any samples submitted for histological examination.

Direct physical examination

Direct physical examination of the fish may require some degree of sedation or anesthesia to facilitate the examination, reduce handling stress to the patient(s), and minimize further injury. It may be possible to examine debilitated, weak, or very small fish without sedation. Tricaine methanesulfonate, MS-222, is the only US Food and Drug Administration-approved anesthetic for finfish. (See Chapter 16 for further information on anesthesia in fish.) The use of rinsed, unpowdered latex or vinyl gloves is recommended when examining fish. The gloves offer some protection against zoonotic diseases and protect the delicate mucous layer of the fish. Some species of fish, catfish for example, have very sharp spines on their fins. Caution should be taken to prevent a painful injury to the practitioner and the client. Venomous, "electric," and toxic fish should only be handled by experienced personnel (Weber and Innis, 2007), and emergency treatment should be on hand in the event of envenomation. As a

matter of personal preference, the author does not handle venomous fish, reptiles, or amphibians.

It is very important to have a good grasp of the fish or to perform the examination over a container of water (see Fig. 15.2). Fish can be very slippery, and it is not uncommon to accidentally "drop" the fish. Owners do not take kindly to this and appreciate all steps taken to protect their pet from further injury. If the examination takes more than 1 or 2 minutes, the fish should periodically be placed in water or irrigated with water to prevent desiccation of the external surfaces. Chamois cloths, natural or synthetic, help maintain skin integrity and can be used to handle or transport the patient during examination and for diagnostic procedures such as radiographs (Weber and Innis, 2007).

A systematic, thorough method of examination should be used on all fish patients. The author prefers the "head to tail" method. Oral examination can be accomplished with an otoscope and cone in small fish, but larger fish need a high-quality flashlight to visualize the full depths of their oral cavity (Fig. 15.3). Gravel, stones, and tank decor are common foreign body objects that may be seen lodged in the oral cavity. Chronic obstruction of the oral cavity or pharynx may result in discoloration or an ulcer on the ventral aspect of the pharyngeal region. A penlight or flashlight should also be used to evaluate the eyes. The eyes should be checked for abnormalities such as parasites, air or gas bubbles, hyphema, hypopyon, corneal edema, exophthalmos, endophthalmos,

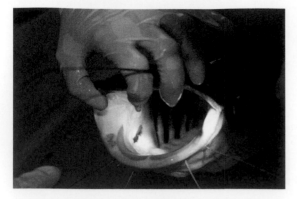

Fig. 15.3 A sedated tiger shovelnose catfish, *Pseudo-platystoma* sp., with a visible oral linear erosion made more apparent by the use of a flashlight.

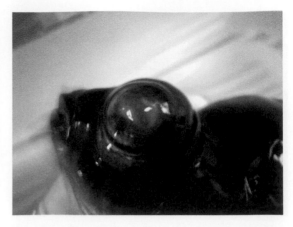

Fig. 15.5 Fluorescein uptake on the cornea of a goldfish with hyphema.

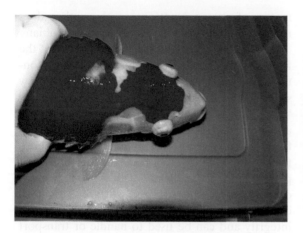

Fig. 15.4 Koi with bilateral exophthalmos (photo courtesy of Walt Oldenburg).

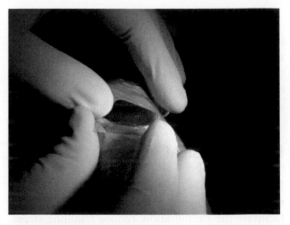

Fig. 15.6 The gills of a goldfish are lifted up and examined before taking a biopsy.

and cataracts (Weber and Innis, 2007; see Fig. 15.4 for an example of exophthalmos). Fish with prominent eyes or pendulous eyes (bubble-eyed goldfish) frequently experience traumatic injuries. Fluorescein dye can be used in fish to visualize corneal injury (Fig. 15.5).

The gills are best visualized by lifting the operculum, either gently with a thumb (Fig. 15.6) or sterile cotton swab. Grossly, the gills should appear dark red with no mottling, masses, or ragged edges. Pale gills can be indicative of anemia, and patchy areas of focal necrosis are sometimes seen in koi herpesvirus infections.

The fins and tail are examined for ragged edges suggestive of "fin rot," splitting, red streaking, hyperemia, and parasites (Fig. 15.7). Any lesions

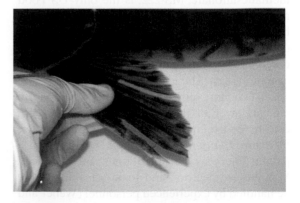

Fig. 15.7 The split left pectoral fin of a tiger shovelnose catfish.

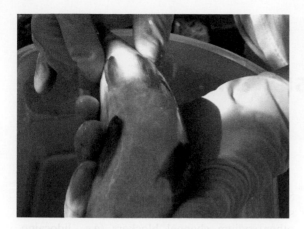

Fig. 15.8 Checking the sex of an anesthetized koi by applying gentle pressure to the caudal, ventral aspect of the coelomic cavity.

on the skin, such as ulcers, edema, lacerations, discoloration, and missing scales, should be noted. It is important to check the ventral aspect for lesions that may not have been initially visible to the owner or on indirect examination.

The coelomic cavity can be palpated gently for evidence of fluid accumulation, masses, and foreign bodies. *Gentle* expression of the area

cranial to the vent in adequately sized fish can cause the release of eggs or milt (Fig. 15.8), enabling sex identification in some species (e.g., koi and goldfish).

Following a complete examination, nonlethal diagnostic procedures can be performed while the fish is still sedated or anesthetized. (See Chapter 17 for a complete discussion of diagnostic procedures.)

References and further reading

Campbell, T.W. (2005) Performing a basic examination in fish. *Veterinary Medicine* **100** (12): 844–855.

Francis-Floyd, R. (1988) Tropical fish practice: behavioral diagnosis. *Veterinary Clinics of North America: Small Animal Practice* **18** (2): 305–316.

Weber, E.S. and Innis, C. (2007) Piscine patients: basic diagnostics. *Compendium on Continuing Education for the Practicing Veterinarian* **29** (5): 276–288.

Wildgoose, W.H. (2001a) Skin disease. In *BSAVA Manual of Ornamental Fish*, 2nd Edition (Wildgoose, W.H., ed.), pp. 109–122. Gloucester: BSAVA.

Wildgoose, W.H. (2001b) Internal disorders. In *BSAVA Manual of Ornamental Fish*, 2nd Edition (Wildgoose, W.H., ed.), pp. 123–134. Gloucester: BSAVA.

Chapter 16
Anesthesia, Analgesia, and Euthanasia
Helen E. Roberts

Introduction

The practice of fish examination, medical diagnosis, and treatment will, in most cases, require sedation or anesthesia of the patient to get diagnostic samples. Sedation and light anesthesia are also helpful to reduce the inevitable stress of handling and transport. Patients that are relatively tame, fragile, moribund, or extremely debilitated may be examined without sedation or anesthesia.

Commonly used anesthetic agents

Currently, the only anesthetic approved for finfish in the United States, the United Kingdom, and the European Union is tricaine methanesulfonate. In Canada, metomidate (Aquacalm® or Tranquil®, Syndel, Victoria, BC, Canada), is also available. Clove oil is used frequently by hobbyists and some retailers for sedation, anesthesia, and euthanasia. One anesthetic, Quin-Phos™, is currently being marketed as "the next generation anesthetic" by several online retailers for use in koi. This anesthetic is quinaldine and was described as a new anesthetic for ornamental fish in 1975 (Blasiola, 1975). Table 16.1 lists the stages of anesthesia in fish.

Tricaine methanesulfonate (MS-222)

Tricaine methanesulfonate, also known as tricaine, TMS, MS-222, and "triple two," is currently available in two brands: Finquel® (Argent Chemical Laboratories, Redmond, WA) and Tricaine-S® (Western Chemical Inc., Ferndale, WA). MS-222 was discovered accidentally when Sandoz researchers were looking for cocaine substitutes (Ross and Ross, 2008). In fact, as with other sodium channel blockers (e.g., lidocaine and benzocaine), tricaine will test positive in a law enforcement narcotics field test (Nark II®, Sirchie Finger Print Laboratories, Youngsville, NC). It is recommended when transporting tricaine for a house call or field research to keep it in its original container to avoid potentially embarrassing situations. MS-222 is a white, crystalline powder that is mixed with the patients' own water. Sodium bicarbonate is used to buffer an otherwise acidic solution that can have harmful effects to the fish, including corneal and epidermal damage. The ratio varies, depending on the local water supply buffering capacity and pH, but in most cases, two parts sodium bicarbonate to one part MS-222 is effective. Callahan and Noga (2002) found that *unbuffered* tricaine caused reduced mobility, rapid detachment, and mortality of *Ichthyobodo necator*, a protozoan parasite. Anecdotally, some people incorrectly state that in fish sedated and anesthetized with buffered MS-222, reduced levels of or no parasites will be found.

Most fish can be sedated with a 50–100 ppm (mg/l) solution in 3–5 minutes. Some finfish species may require a higher dose. The initial concentration should be decreased for sick, stressed, or debilitated fish. Likewise, novel species should always be approached with care when anesthetizing for the first time. It is always better to start with a lower dose and increase if needed. The anesthetic powder and sodium bicarbonate should be weighed on a gram scale for accurate dosing. MS-222 at a concentration of 1 g/l can be directly applied to gills with a spray bottle or bulb syringe for faster induction of anesthesia in larger species, such as elasmobranchs.

Table 16.1 Stages of anesthesia in fish.

Stage	Plane	Description	Signs
I	1	Light sedation	Responsive to stimuli; reduced motion; decreased ventilation
	2	Deep sedation	Similar to stage I, plane 1: some analgesia; less responsive to stimuli
II	1	Light anesthesia	Partial loss of equilibrium; good analgesia
	2	Deeper anesthesia	Loss of muscle tone; total loss of equilibrium; greatly reduced ventilation
III		Surgical anesthesia	Similar to stage II, plane 1; total loss of response to stimuli
IV		Medullary collapse	Ventilation ceases; cardiac arrest; death

Cooler water and hard water will result in a longer induction time compared with sedation/anesthesia used in warm or soft water (Ross and Ross, 2008). Gravid fish, older fish, and fish with a high body fat percentage can experience prolonged recovery (Ross and Ross, 2008). Tricaine, like other anesthetics in fish, has been reported to cause increased hematocrit, swelling of erythrocytes, hypoxia, hypercapnia, hyperglycemia, and changes in blood electrolytes (Ross and Ross, 2008). A working stock solution of 10 g/l MS-222 can be prepared in advance. The solution can be stored up to 3 months and must be protected from light and excess heat (Harms, 2003; Ross and Ross, 2008). Gloves should always be worn when handling MS-222 to reduce the potential for mucous membrane irritation and idiosyncratic allergic reactions. Retinal toxicity has been reported as a potential sequelae to long-term exposure, so protective goggles should be recommended during handling of the powdered form (Bernstein et al., 1997).

Isoeugenol

Aqui-S® (Aqui-S New Zealand Ltd.), isoeugenol, is a compound that is licensed for use in New Zealand, Australia, Chile, Korea, and Costa Rica. It is not approved for use in the United Kingdom or the United States. Aqui-S is used most often for the humane harvesting and transport of fish. Advantages of isoeugenol include a reduced cost compared with tricaine, some stress reduction, and a zero-day withdrawal period for release or slaughter. Aqui-S has a longer recovery time compared with tricaine; up to twice the length has been reported (Ross and Ross, 2008). Dosages range from 6 to 17 mg/l (Ross, 2001).

Aqui-S was evaluated extensively for approval in the United States, but a National Toxicology Program (NTP) exposure study in male mice revealed evidence of carcinogenic activity. As a result, the Food and Drug Administration (FDA) rescinded the investigational studies of this drug for use in food fish. It is unclear at this time (March 2009) what this will mean for pet fish sector use.

Clove oil

Clove oil (a mixture of isoeugenol, eugenol, and methyleugenol) is often used by koi and goldfish hobbyists to sedate their own fish. Dispersion in water can be improved by initially mixing with warm water and shaking the solution prior to adding to an anesthesia container (Ross and Ross, 2008). Clove oil is not approved for use in fish, but it is widely available without a prescription so its use is common. Disadvantages of use include poor water solubility, rapid induction rate, prolonged recovery rate, and narrower margin of safety when compared with tricaine. In addition, clove oil has fewer analgesic properties than MS-222, and the concentration of active ingredient can vary between lots. Clove oil does seem to have a measurable benefit in reducing short-term stress compared with MS-222 (Ross and Ross, 2008). Doses used range from 2 to 5 ppm for sedation and from 25 to 120 ppm for anesthesia (Harms, 2003; Ross and Ross, 2008). Hobbyists typically use three to five drops of the over-the-counter (OTC) product per gallon (personal observation). Induction and recovery are prolonged in cooler water. Methyleugenol and isoeugenol, components of clove oil, have both been found to be carcinogenic in NTP studies.

Metomidate

Metomidate is a water-soluble, light-sensitive, nonbarbiturate hypnotic anesthetic (Ross, 2001; Harms, 2003). It has a rapid induction and recovery compared with MS-222. Metomidate hydrochloride is absorbed from the water via the gills into the bloodstream, where it produces its sedation or an anesthetic affect on the central nervous system. Conversely, sodium channel blocker anesthetics, such as tricaine, act first on peripheral nerves, and then secondarily on the central nervous system. Color changes and transient muscle twitches may be observed in many species with metomidate. Gouramis may be more sensitive to metomidate than other species (Harms, 2003), and dosages (3–4.5 mg/l) required for anesthesia in larval goldfish resulted in high mortalities (Ross and Ross, 2008). Metomidate does not cause an elevation in blood cortisol levels due to suppression of cortisol synthesis, but its use is not considered to be stress free in fish (Ross and Ross, 2008). Metomidate does not possess any analgesic properties. Doses range from 0.5 to 1 mg/l for sedation and from 1 to 10 mg/l for anesthesia (Ross 2001; J. Brackett, pers. comm.).

Quinaldine and quinaldine sulfate

Quinaldine (2-4 methylquinoline) is an inexpensive, oily yellow liquid that must be dissolved in acetone or ethanol and buffered with sodium bicarbonate prior to use (Ross, 2001; Ross and Ross, 2008). Corneal damage and skin irritation have been reported with its use (Ross and Ross, 2008). Quinaldine sulfate is a water-soluble powder but is more expensive compared with quinaldine and tricaine. Both are more potent in warm water and in water at higher pH levels, and less potent in soft water. Dosages reported for carp (koi) are 12–37 mg/l (ppm) and up to 200 mg/l for tropical fish (Ross, 2001). Veterinary practitioners may be asked about this "new" anesthetic due to the recent increased OTC sales through fish retailers for use in koi.

Benzocaine

Benzocaine is sometimes used for anesthetizing fish, although it is not currently approved for use. It is insoluble in water and must be prepared with acetone or ethanol prior to use. A stock solution of 100 g/l can be made in advance and, if protected from light exposure, may be kept up to a year (Ross and Ross, 2008). The margin of safety is reduced in higher water temperatures. The dose for most species is 25–50 mg/l (ppm) (Ross and Ross, 2008).

Analgesia

Analgesia is defined as relief from pain (Ross and Ross, 2008). There is much debate on whether fish perceive pain, but most fish health professionals agree it is better to administer analgesics than not. Several compounds have been used to provide analgesia in fish. These include ketoprofen, carprofen, morphine, butorphanol, flunixin meglumine, and buprenorphine. These compounds are often administered as a single injection preoperatively or postoperatively, but could also be used in treating traumatic injuries that do not require complicated surgical procedures. Exact dosing and pharmacokinetic studies have not been done on most analgesic compounds, and doses used are generally extrapolated from other species. There are no approved analgesics for use in fish, and these drugs should never be used in food fish. See Table 16.2 for a list of analgesics used in fish.

Preparation, equipment, and procedure

Supplies needed for examination, anesthesia, and diagnostic testing should be gathered in advance to minimize anesthesia time for the fish and to increase efficiency (Fig. 16.1). Most fish can be transferred to a container for anesthesia induction. The container should have a lid to prevent possible injury or escape during hyperactivity/excitement, which may be initially noted in the induction phase. In situations requiring sedation or anesthesia of large fish that cannot be easily removed from their original tank or pond, sedation and anesthesia must take place *in situ*. Two options are available: applying a very concentrated solution of anesthetic to the gills with a spray bottle or a similar delivery device

Table 16.2   Analgesics used in fish.

Drug	Dose	Indication	Precautions
Butorphanol	0.1–0.4 mg/kg IM	Surgery; traumatic injuries; cutaneous ulcers	May be ineffective in some species; long-term effects unknown
Carprofen	2–4 mg/kg IM q 3–5 days	Surgery; traumatic injuries; cutaneous ulcers; inflammatory lesions	*Unknown* side effects; possibility of gastrointestinal ulceration, poor clotting, and so on; informed consent must be obtained
Flunixin meglumine	0.25–0.5 mg/kg IM q 3–5 days	Same as that of carprofen	See carprofen
Ketoprofen	2 mg/kg IM	Same as that of carprofen	See carprofen
Meloxicam	0.1–0.2 mg/kg IM	Same as that of carprofen	See carprofen
Morphine	0.3 mg/kg IM	—	Used in research; not generally used in private fish practice

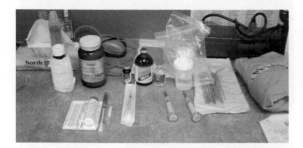

Fig. 16.1 Supplies gathered in advance preparation for diagnostic testing on an anesthetized fish: anesthetic, histopath vials, syringes, biopsy instrument kit, and clinical pathology supplies.

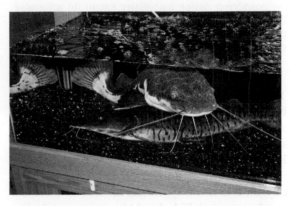

Fig. 16.2 These large fish will be anesthetized *in situ*. The tank volume has been lowered in preparation for the addition of the anesthetic mixture.

and extracting the sedated fish, or reducing the tank volume to a practical level and adding the anesthetic directly to the tank (Fig. 16.2). Other tank inhabitants, decor, and equipment must be considered. There can also be a significant cost factor with the amount of anesthetic, time, and labor involved.

If the fish will be anesthetized for a very short amount of time, no extra equipment will be needed beyond a container (Fig. 16.3) to hold the fish in anesthetic solution and a recovery container filled with fresh water (often the transport container). For surgical procedures, fish will need to remain anesthetized out of water. Lewbart and Harms (1999) describe a simple and effective way to build an anesthesia delivery system for use in fish. A fish anesthetic delivery system provides a method of positioning for surgery and constant delivery of a liquid anesthetic solution over the gills that can be recirculated (Figs. 16.4 and 16.5).

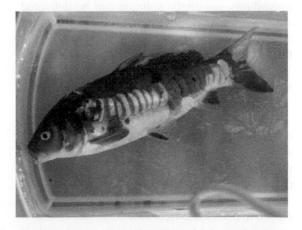

Fig. 16.3 A koi is anesthetized in a plastic container pondside for examination and treatment of multiple heron-induced skin defects.

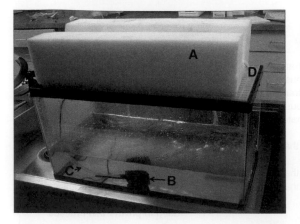

Fig. 16.4 Recirculating anesthesia delivery system: (a) positioning device (upholstery foam); (b) adjustable flow rate water pump; (c) tubing from pump to enter oral cavity and exit opercula of fish (bathing the gills); (d) return of anesthetic solution to container.

The concentration of anesthetic can be altered by adding fresh, conditioned water to dilute the anesthetic or by adding a volume of concentrated stock solution to increase the effect. The water in the anesthetic container should be aerated with air stones or diffusers to improve dissolved oxygen content. Oxygen gas can also be bubbled in when needed. Fish should be monitored during any anesthetic procedures for depth of anesthesia by evaluating the response to stimuli and gill movements or opercular rate. Anesthetic concentration should be adjusted accordingly. For short procedures, anesthetic solution can be delivered via a bulb syringe or a small syringe (Fig. 16.6). See Chapter 18 for a description of surgical preparation and monitoring.

If the patient stops ventilating, the gills should be lavaged via the oral cavity with fresh, conditioned, anesthetic-free water via a bulb syringe or oral syringe. Care should be taken not to damage the gills with excess water pressure. The fish can also be gently moved in the water in a forward direction (Ross, 2001). Once the fish has begun regular gill excursions, it can be monitored visually.

Recovery from anesthesia occurs when fish are placed in anesthetic-free water. The rate of recovery is influenced by water temperature, length of sedation or anesthesia, and the type of anesthetic used. Fish undergoing short, diagnostic proce-

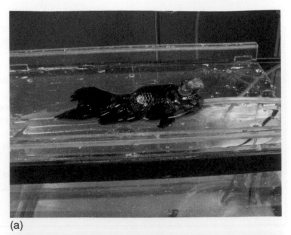

(a)

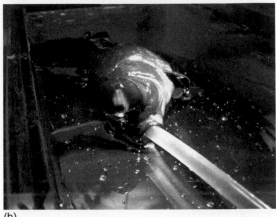

(b)

Fig. 16.5   a, b A goldfish on a recirculating anesthetic delivery device receiving anesthesia delivered via plastic tubing. The gills are bathed continuously with anesthetic solution during the surgical procedure.

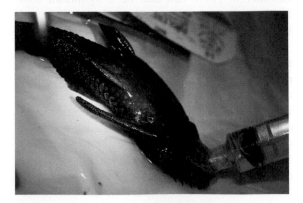

Fig. 16.6 A bristlenose plecostomus (*Ancistrus* sp.) receiving anesthetic delivered via a syringe through the oral cavity for a short-duration procedure.

dures generally recover within a few minutes and can be discharged with the owner.

Euthanasia

Euthanasia in fish should be relatively quick, humane, and with the written consent of the owner. Guidelines for euthanasia of fish have been published by both the American Veterinary Medical Association (AVMA, 2007) and the American Association of Zoo Veterinarians (2006). Methods used for euthanasia are divided into physical and chemical. Chemical method recommendations for veterinarians include injection of sodium pentobarbital 60–100 mg/kg intravenously or intracoelomically, immersion in or direct gill application of buffered tricaine >500 mg/l, and immersion in benzocaine >250 mg/l (AVMA, 2007). Fish should be left in solution until opercular movements have ceased for at least 30 minutes. Physical methods of euthanasia include decapitation followed by pithing or a sharp blow to the cranium (Ross and Ross, 2008). It is unlikely that pet fish owners will understand if these physical methods are used on their pets so chemical methods are recommended.

Owners will frequently call veterinary hospitals seeking advice on home methods of euthanasia. Although not recommended by the 2007 AVMA guidelines due to lack of adequate clinical trials, most fish practitioners recommend the use of concentrated clove oil (Ross, 2001). The author recommends clove oil at four to 10 times the anesthetic dose (20–50 drops per gallon) in a small container of warm water, observation of all gill movements ceasing for 30 minutes, followed by freezing (unless necropsy samples need to be obtained).

Acknowledgments

The author would like to thank the Town of Tonawanda Police Department Criminal Investigation Bureau for testing the MS-222 (Finquel and Tricaine-S) with the cocaine field test.

References and further reading

American Association of Zoo Veterinarians. (2006) *AAZV Guideline for Euthanasia of Nondomestic Animals.* Yulee, FL: American Association of Zoo Veterinarians.

American Veterinary Medical Association (AVMA). (2007) *Guidelines on Euthanasia.* www.avma.org/issues/animal_welfare/euthanasia.pdf.

Bernstein, P.S., Digre, K.B., and Creel, D.J. (1997) Retinal toxicity associated with occupational exposure to the fish anesthetic MS-222. *American Journal of Ophthalmology* **124** (6): 843–844.

Blasiola, G.C. (1975) Quinaldine sulphate, a new anaesthetic formulation for tropical marine fishes. *Journal of Fish Biology* **10** (2): 113–119.

Brackett, J. (2009) Personal communication, February.

Callahan, H.A. and Noga, E.J. (2002) Tricaine dramatically reduces the ability to diagnose protozoan ectoparasites (*Ichthyobodo necator*) infections. *Journal of Fish Diseases* **25**: 433–437.

Harms, C.A. (2003) Diagnostic procedures, anesthesia, and surgery. Paper presented at the Fish Health Management Seminar, North Carolina State College of Veterinary Medicine, Raleigh, NC, August 14–16,

Harms, C.A. (2005) Surgery in fish research: common procedures and postoperative care. *Lab Animal* **34** (1): 28–34.

Lewbart, G.A. and Harms, C.A. (1999) Building a fish anesthesia delivery system. *Exotic DVM* **1** (2): 25–28.

Ross, L.G. (2001) Restraint, anaesthesia and euthanasia. In *BSAVA Manual of Ornamental Fish*, 2nd Edition (Wildgoose, W., ed.), pp. 75–83. Gloucester: BSAVA Publications.

Ross, L.G. and Ross, B. (2008) *Anaesthetic and Sedative Techniques for Aquatic Animals*, 3rd Edition. Oxford: Blackwell Publishing.

Chapter 17

Nonlethal Diagnostic Techniques

Helen E. Roberts, E. Scott Weber III, and Stephen A. Smith

Introduction

Historically, several methods used to determine the cause of fish disease involve lethal sampling techniques. With the increase of pet fish owners seeking health care for their charges, animal welfare concerns, and research with endangered fish, the use and development of novel, nonlethal diagnostic techniques in fish health has grown in the past decade. Most of these techniques are simple, inexpensive, already performed to a similar degree in other species, and do not require additional expensive equipment beyond that which is already available in most veterinary hospitals (Smith, 2002). These techniques are best performed on anesthetized animals. Anesthesia makes the procedure easier to perform and less stressful for the fish (Smith, 2002; Weber and Innis, 2007). See Chapter 16 for a discussion on anesthesia. Gloves should be used when handling fish to protect the fish's skin and mucous layer and prevent the transmission of zoonotic diseases that may be present (Smith, 2002; Reavill, 2006; Weber and Innis, 2007).

Clinical diagnostic techniques should be considered only *part* of the investigation into fish disease. History, physical examination, and water quality evaluation tests are equally important in the minimum database (MDB) workup that should be employed in every fish health case.

Diagnostic cytology

Diagnostic cytology in fish starts with wet mount examinations of skin scrapes, gill biopsies or scrapes, fecal or cloacal wash fluid examination, and evaluation of aspirated fluid. The following section will give a detailed description on how to perform each

procedure. Materials should be gathered in advance to improve efficiency and ensure sample quality (Fig. 17.1). Samples need to be evaluated within a few minutes of collection in case the sample dries or parasites have become nonmotile or have died.

Skin scrape

A skin scrape of the mucous layer is one of several tests in the MDB and can easily be performed on an ambulatory visit, in addition to an office call at the clinic. If performing the test in the field or pond-side, be sure to protect the slides from heat exposure or drying will occur very rapidly. Equipment required includes the patient anesthetized in a container, a microscope, glass slides, coverslips, gloves, and a small amount of the patient's own water supply.

Procedure (see Fig. 17.2):

- Place a drop of water from the pond or tank on the slide.
- *Gently* scrape a *small* area of the skin with a coverslip or blade held at a 45-degree angle, moving in a cranial to caudal direction. Occasionally, a scale may be removed, but this is generally an indication of excessive pressure. Excessive trauma can also leave a defect in the skin, allowing for potential pathogen invasion. In small fish, sample very small areas to leave some remaining mucous covering.
- Sites preferred for sample collection include the following: the leading edge of lesions; under the mandible; and areas just caudal to the fins (Reavill, 2006). If no lesions are present, consider least hydrodynamic areas where parasites may be attached more effectively (Weber, 2009).
- Place the coverslip with the sample face down on the slide over the prepared water drop.

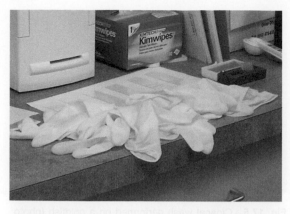

Fig. 17.1 Preparation of supplies: slides, gloves, and coverslips.

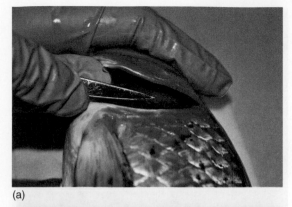

(a)

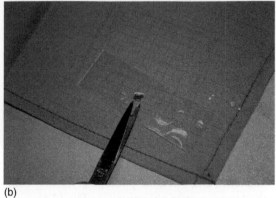

(b)

Fig. 17.3 (a) Gill biopsy sample taken from a koi (*Cyprinus carpio*). (b) Sample of gill tissue placed on a slide.

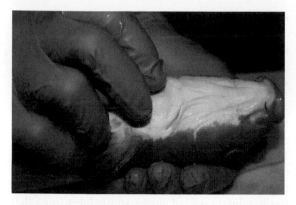

Fig. 17.2 A skin scrape being performed on an anesthetized koi (*Cyprinus carpio*).

- Evaluate starting with the lowest objective power first.
- Parasites can be identified by their size, shape, and characteristic movements.
- Fungal elements and bacteria can be identified further by drying and staining. Acid-fast stains can be used to identify possible mycobacterial pathogens.

Fin clip or fin biopsy

Fin biopsies are often recommended in an attempt to determine cause of disease. The procedure involves cutting a small piece of a fin and evaluating as a wet mount preparation for parasites, fungal elements, and bacterial disease. This technique should be reserved for fins severely affected by disease and as a premortem test as the finnage of most pet fish is prized by their owners. Fin

biopsy sites may never heal or appear normal after biopsying. This will dramatically affect the show career potential of some fish, such as koi.

Gill snip or gill biopsy

A gill biopsy involves taking a very small section of gill tissue and evaluating for morphological changes (such as hyperplasia, excessive mucus, and lamellar fusion), in addition to the search for parasites and bacterial and fungal disease elements. Equipment recommended is the same as for a skin scrape; with the addition of a small pair of scissors (iris tenotomy scissors or suture removal scissors work well). Bleeding may occur if the removed section is too large or if the fish is mature and/or gravid.

Procedure (see Fig. 17.3):

- Place a drop of water from the tank or pond on the slide.

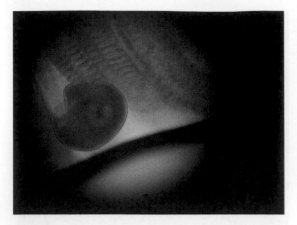

Fig. 17.4 *Ichthyophthirius multifilis* found on a gill snip.

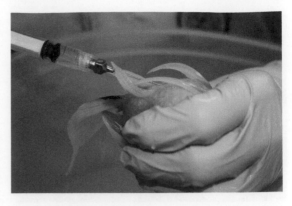

Fig. 17.5 Cloacal wash performed on a goldfish (photo courtesy of Marilynn Landsman-Podlewski).

- Gently lift the operculum with a gloved finger or thumb.
- With scissors, remove a very small piece of gill tissue and place on the slide in the water drop.
- Place a coverslip over the gill sample.
- Examine for gill pathology, parasites, fungal elements, and bacterial pathogens starting with the lowest power objective (see Fig. 17.4).

A gill scrape can be performed in lieu of a biopsy by using a coverslip and gently scraping a small section of the gill. This technique can result in more hemorrhage from the gill tissue.

Fecal exam and cloacal wash

An examination of the stool is performed as in other species. In most cases, a direct evaluation of a wet mount preparation will be sufficient. Most species of pet fish will not yield enough volume of stool to utilize flotation or centrifugation techniques. Fish will often defecate when anesthetized, making sample acquisition easy. It is important to examine *fresh* feces as colonization of feces in the environment by a multitude of organisms makes identification of pathogens somewhat confusing and inaccurate. A sample can sometimes be obtained by applying gentle pressure to the area just cranial to the vent in adequate-sized fish. The procedure requires the same equipment used in performing a skin scraping.

Procedure:

- Place a drop of tank or pond water on the glass slide.
- Place a fresh stool sample on the water drop and cover with a coverslip.
- Examine for parasite ova, larvae, and adult forms.

If fresh stool is not available, a cloacal wash can be performed to obtain a sample from the distal colon on an anesthetized fish (Weber, 2007) (Fig. 17.5): Supplies needed include a small tom-cat catheter, tear duct cannula, or red rubber feeding tube; glass slides; coverslips; a syringe prefilled with sterile saline; a pair of gloves; sterile lubricant jelly; and a container or tube to store the collected fluid.

Procedure:

- Sedate or anesthetize the fish.
- Place small fish in dorsal recumbency; large fish in lateral recumbency.
- Attach the syringe to the catheter/feeding tube/ cannula.
- Insert the lubricated cannula/catheter/feeding tube into the cranial opening (anus) in the vent.
- Gently instill a small amount of sterile saline.
- Gently aspirate some fluid.
- Place fluid in a container.
- Examine fluid immediately. Remaining fluid can be centrifuged or used to prepare dried slides for staining.

Masses, fluid aspirates, and impression smears

After samples have been obtained for bacteriological cultures, representative samples of cutaneous masses of fish can be obtained by standard aspiration techniques and by making impression smears. Slides made from aspirates or impression smears can be air-dried for staining. Fluid may accompany some cutaneous masses, ophthalmic lesions, swim bladder disorders, and coelomic cavity swelling. This fluid can also be evaluated using standard cytological techniques or submitted for bacterial culture and viral testing (if applicable).

Coelomic cavity tumors are often accompanied by a clear yellow or hemorrhagic fluid. Lymphocystis can be diagnosed by visualization of the characteristic hypertrophied cells seen on a wet mount sample taken from the raised mass. In goldfish and other fish, polycystic kidney disease results in multiple, fluid-filled cysts. These cysts can be aspirated. In most cases, the fluid will contain low protein levels and few, if any, cells (Reavill and Roberts, 2007). When the cysts rupture, the resulting fluid is usually hemorrhagic.

Hematology and clinical pathology

Serum or plasma biochemical tests and complete blood counts (CBCs) are valuable diagnostic tools in determining the cause of disease in many species. However, reference intervals, normal hematologic parameters, and diagnostic interpretation are not available for most pet fish species. Several reasons exist for this relative lack of data in fish. Published data exists for several significant food species but is not always applicable to pet fish. Environmental conditions such as water quality affect test results. Handling stressors, age, gender, photoperiod, and diet are other factors that can affect the results of a CBC and serum or plasma biochemistry (Clauss et al., 2008).

Venipuncture

A blood sample can be easily obtained in most fish. The most common site to obtain blood is the caudal vein using a ventral or lateral approach (Hrubec and Smith 2000; Southgate, 2001). Cardiac puncture has also been reported, although there is a higher risk of death using this technique. Fish blood clots very quickly so the needle and syringe

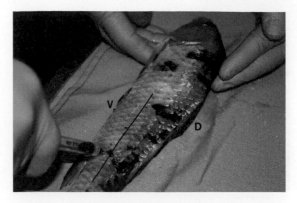

Fig. 17.6   Lateral venipuncture of a fish. D, dorsal aspect; V, ventral; solid line indicates the lateral line.

should be heparinized, although some serological tests may require unheparinized, whole blood. Lithium heparin tubes are recommended for use in most tests and with most fish species. Blood from stressed fish has been reported to clot even with the use of an anticoagulant (Hrubec and Smith, 2000). A blood volume collection of 0.5%–1.0% of the body weight can be safely taken from most fish. In most cases, 1 ml can be taken from 100-g fish and up to 3 ml in larger fish, such as koi (Groff and Zinkl, 1999). Most fish venipuncture can be done with a 1½-in. 21-gauge needle on a 3-ml syringe. A ½-in. 25-gauge needle on a tuberculin (1 ml) syringe is used for very small fish.

Procedure:

Lateral approach (see Fig. 17.6):

- Place the anesthetized fish in lateral recumbency.
- Identify the lateral line.
- With the bevel up, direct the needle under a scale just below and parallel to the lateral line.
- Advance the needle at a 45-degree angle, in a craniomedial direction toward the vertebrae until bone can be felt.
- Withdraw slightly, apply gentle negative pressure, and collect the blood sample.
- Apply digital pressure to the site as the needle is withdrawn to minimize bruising.

Ventral approach (see Fig. 17.7):

- Place the anesthetized fish in dorsal recumbency.
- Insert the needle between the anal fin and the tail.
- Advance the needle dorsally toward the spinal column applying gentle negative pressure.

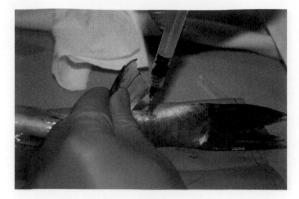

Fig. 17.7 Ventral venipuncture of a fish.

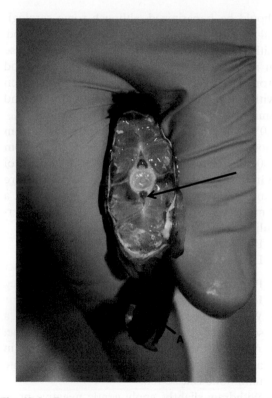

Fig. 17.8 Transverse section of a fish at the level of the caudal peduncle illustrating the caudal vein *in situ*, ventral to the vertebral column. Arrow points to vein. A, anal fin.

- Collect the sample and withdraw the needle, applying digital pressure to the site.

Figure 17.8 shows the location of the vein in relation to the vertebral column.

Interpretation of blood results

Interpretation of results in fish is difficult when compared with that in popular terrestrial species. Nucleated red blood cells and platelets prohibit the use of most analyzers used for mammalian blood counts. Manual evaluation by the hematocytometer–chamber method is the most common and easily performed in clinical practice (Groff and Zinkl, 1999). A few studies have been performed, and it is hoped that there will be many more in the future as the increase in pet fish medical care continues. In addition, two studies discussed below (Harrenstien et al., 2005; Palmeiro et al., 2007) evaluated the use of in-house blood analyzers for fish. The discussion on interpretation below highlights some references that have been published and is meant to serve as a guide.

CBC abnormalities

Packed cell volume (PCV, or hematocrit) results can vary within and between species depending on age, gender, activity level, diet, stocking density, and water quality (Clauss et al., 2008). Most hematocrits in fish range from 20% to 45% (Hrubec and Smith, 2000). Active species such as tuna have higher normal PCV levels, while young fish, elasmobranchs, and bottom dwellers have lower PCVs (Clauss et al., 2008). Male fish tend to have higher PCVs when compared with female fish of the same age and sex (Groff and Zinkl, 1999). Obligate air-breathers also have higher PCVs (Stoskopf, 1993c). Anemia is typically associated with a PCV less than 20 (except in some sharks where 20 or less is normal) (Clauss et al., 2008). Anemias in fish are classified in a similar manner to other species. Diseases and conditions that can contribute to or cause anemia include high ammonia and nitrite levels; hypoxia; heavy metal toxicities; poor acclimation to captivity; nutritional disorders, including starvation; increased stocking density; the use of chlorinated water; stress response; bacterial and viral diseases; inflammatory disease; and parasitism (Stoskopf, 1993a–c; Clauss et al., 2008).

An increased PCV (>45) is associated with dehydration (marine fish), hypoxia (marine and freshwater fish), stress, and anesthesia (MS-222 and benzocaine) (Clauss et al., 2008; Ross and Ross, 2008). The response to hypoxia can be very rapid, less than one hour (Stoskopf, 1993c). Elevated water temperature has been found to cause an elevated PCV in goldfish and koi (Stoskopf, 1993a; Groff and Zinkl, 1999).

White blood cell changes occur with many diseases and adverse environmental conditions. A stress leukogram in fish reveals a leukopenia with a lymphopenia and granulocytosis (Clauss et al., 2008). Elevated white blood cell counts can be found in freshwater fish held at higher water temperatures and those with sepsis (Stoskopf, 1993b; Groff and Zinkl, 1999). A decreased total count can be found during starvation (Stoskopf, 1993b). Increased lymphocyte counts can be found in normal juvenile fish, husbandry-related disorders, and any disease that stimulates the immune system (Clauss et al., 2008). Lymphopenia is associated with disorders that cause immune suppression, such as stress and bacterial sepsis (Stoskopf, 1993a; Clauss et al., 2008), and has also been found in ciliated protozoan infections (Stoskopf, 1993b). Inflammation from several causes, including external parasitism, is often accompanied by granulocytosis. Granulocytosis is also seen in sharks with bacterial septicemia, and neutrophilia can also occur in other species with septicemia (Clauss et al., 2008). Increases in the eosinophil count can occur with disorders causing inflammation, including parasitism.

Serum or plasma biochemical abnormalities

Muscle damage secondary to capture, anesthesia, and excess tissue trauma during sampling can increase creatine kinase (CK) levels similar to other species.

Palmeiro et al. (2007) determined alanine aminotransferase (ALT) to be the most liver-specific enzyme in koi in their study using a common in-house blood analyzer. Lowered blood glucose levels are seen as a subsequent response in hepatic disease and sepsis (Juopperi, 2003).

Blood glucose is found to be elevated during stress, anesthesia, and as an *initial response* in bacterial septicemia (Stoskopf, 1993a; Ross and Ross, 2008).

Serum calcium levels may be elevated in gravid females, although further reference interval studies that identify the sex of the fish are needed to substantiate this (Palmeiro et al., 2007).

Serum protein levels are found to be decreased in males and with bacterial septicemia, starvation, chronic stress, renal and hepatic diseases, during spawning, and failure to acclimate to captivity (Stoskopf, 1993b,c; Groff and Zinkl, 1999). Starvation is also accompanied by a decrease in blood urea nitrogen (BUN) (Stoskopf, 1993c). Serum protein levels can be increased in female cyprinids (koi and goldfish) and in cyprinids held at higher water temperatures (Groff and Zinkl, 1999). In one study (Harrenstien et al., 2005), rockfish with poor body condition had reduced total protein, albumin, glucose, cholesterol, and phosphorus values.

Elevated BUN, serum sodium, and chloride levels in marine fish can be indicative of gill disease (Stoskopf, 1993c; Harrenstien et al., 2005). BUN elevation, as well as *decreased* sodium and chloride, will be observed in freshwater fish with gill disease (Groff and Zinkl, 1999). Renal disease in marine fish can be accompanied by elevations in magnesium and sulfate levels and an elevation in creatinine (Stoskopf, 1993c).

Harrenstien et al. (2005) showed marine coldwater fish, rockfish (*Sebastes* sp.), with exophthalmia had decreased total protein, albumin, sodium, calcium, and chloride concentrations when compared with values taken from clinically normal fish. The study suggested this may have been a result of a chronic, low-level malnutrition secondary to the cause of exophthalmia.

Table 17.1 lists select hematology reference ranges for koi adapted from a study by Tripathi

Table 17.1 Hematology reference values for koi (*Cyprinus carpio*).

Packed cell volume	29.7–33.9
Hemoglobin	6.3–8.2
Red blood cell count × 10^6/μl	1.7–1.9
White blood cell count × 10^3/μl	19.8–37
Lymphocytes	74%–93%
	14.7–23.5 × 10^3/μl
Monocytes	0.5%–3.4%
	0.46–0.96 × 10^3/μl
Neutrophils	3%–14%
	1.6–3.9 × 10^3/μl
Basophils	3.5%–5.6%
	0.7–1.57 × 10^3/μl
Eosinophils	0%–1.0%

Table 17.2 Clinical chemistry reference ranges for koi (*Cyprinus carpio*)—(plasma).

ALP (U/l)	4–56
AST (U/l)	41–340
Alanine aminotranferase (U/l)	9–98
Creatine kinase (U/l)	1170–9716
Total protein (g/dl)	2–4.5
Glucose (mg/dl)	20–126
Blood urea nitrogen (mg/dl)	0.2–5
Creatinine (mg/dl)	0.07–0.09
Ca (mg/dl)	8.1–20
Na (mmol/l)	110–143
Cl (mEq/l)	123.6–127
K (mmol/l)	0.0–3.0
P (mg/dl)	3.8–12.6

et al. (2004) and results published by Groff and Zinkl (1999). Table 17.2 summarizes results from the benchtop analyzer study by Palmeiro et al. (2007) and results published by Groff and Zinkl (1999).

Diagnostic imaging

Fish represent the largest group of vertebrates, with over 53,000 species and subspecies recorded. One area that imaging can aid veterinarians is through systematically analyzing fish morphology to develop normal baselines for a variety of marine and freshwater species. Having high-quality normal baselines are vital for comparison when ill individuals present for examination. Once these baselines are established for a particular species, an evaluation of gross morphological abnormalities for a patient can be assessed. By correlating morphological abnormalities as compared with normal baseline images that are coupled with the presenting complaint and historical information for the patient, imaging can be used regularly to help assess fish health (Love and Lewbart, 1997).

Anatomical considerations

Before imaging any species of animal, one needs to be familiar with normal anatomical considerations. Some differences in the anatomy of fish for the musculoskeletal system, buoyancy regulation, digestion, and reproduction will be highlighted.

Musculoskeletal system

The fish musculoskeletal system is composed of muscle, bone, and/or cartilage. Major differences in the skeletal structure of fish include a lack of bone marrow and associated hematopoietic function and the complete absence of bone in certain groups such as the elasmobranchs. The skeletal system in fish can be divided into two parts: an axial region including the skull, vertebrae, and ribs; and an appendicular skeleton consisting of fins, pelvic and pectoral girdles. Some notable differences in the axial skeleton are the following. There is a great variability in skull bones from just over a dozen to over 300, depending on the species; most fish vertebrae do not interlock like terrestrial vertebrates but instead form a relatively incompressible spinal column; there are typically two cervical vertebrae that articulate with the skull; the trunk vertebrae are called dorsals and have ribs attached; the caudal vertebrae are flattened to articulate with the caudal fin rays; the spines located dorsally on the vertebrae are called neural arches and those located ventrally are called hemal arches for muscle attachment; and the ventral aspect of each vertebrae has fused transverse processes forming a hemal canal to protect the main blood vessels. The appendicular skeleton consists of the pectoral and pelvic girdles that are attached to a varying numbers of fin rays. Most often, the pectoral girdle may be fused to the skull, while the pelvic girdle is often free floating and may or may not have a midline fusion (Moyle and Cech, 2004; Bond, 2007).

Swim bladder

Buoyancy regulation in many species of fishes requires a specialized organ called the swim bladder (e.g., air bladder, gas bladder). Elasmobranchs lack a swim bladder and regulate buoyancy using oil (squalene) produced by their liver. Because the swim bladder is filled with gas, the organ can be regularly evaluated using imaging

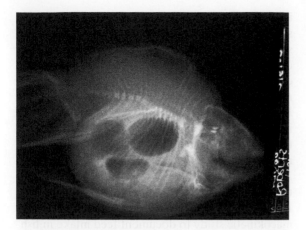

Fig. 17.9 Radiograph of a goldfish with diffuse enteritis, demonstrated by the gas pocket located in the ventral aspect of the body.

techniques (Fig. 17.9). The swim bladder is located in the coelom of the fish just ventral to the kidneys, running under the spinal column. In various fish species, it may be normal for the swim bladder to be absent (i.e., flounder), have one compartment (i.e., trout, angelfish), or have two compartments (i.e., carp, koi, cichlids). Swim bladders are characterized as physostomous, filled with air via a pneumatic duct that leads from the esophagus to the swim bladder, or as physoclistous, requiring a gas gland to diffuse gas across a complex of vessels called the rete mirabile (Moyle and Cech, 2004; Bond, 2007).

Digestive tract

The digestive tract is similar to that of other vertebrates. Fish may or may not have a stomach, and the stomach can have a variety of shapes. Pyloric cecae, if present, may be attached to the anterior portion of the intestine. This organ consists of several to multiple small blind-ended fingerlike projections to help with nutrient absorption. The length of the intestinal tract in fish varies depending on the dietary requirements of individual species, with carnivores generally having a fairly straight, short gastrointestinal (GI) tract and herbivores having elongated, coiled intestinal tracts. Many elasmobranchs have a specialized spiral colon to aid in nutrient absorption (Moyle and Cech, 2004; Bond, 2007).

Imaging techniques

Many types of imaging techniques used in veterinary medicine can be used for fish patients. These techniques include conventional radiography, xeroradiography, digital radiography, magnetic resonance imaging (MRI), ultrasonography, echocardiography, and computed tomography (CT). This chapter will focus on conventional and digital imaging methods but will include examples of many of these other techniques.

When imaging a species of fish for the first time, it is extremely helpful to have the clients bring a healthy conspecific of the same relative shape and size to provide a potential baseline comparison. As with other animals, multiple views are required for radiographs, as are appropriate markers. Most clinicians require a dorsal ventral and right lateral view for most fish species. Given the different body shapes, sizes, and anatomic configurations, this may be impractical for some species and may require moving the beam. Because of the great number of different species, keeping a record of technique is advised. Record the machine used, cassette type, mA, kilovolt peak (KVP), thickness used to calculate values (cm), the patient's morphometrics (total length [cm], widest girth [cm], weight [g]), and a digital picture of the patient. This information will help to create technique charts for other fish.

Diagnostic imaging of fish can be accomplished either in or out of water. If a fish is severely compromised or if the owners do not authorize the use of anesthesia, radiographic images can be taken in water with the animal lightly sedated or awake (Fig. 17.10). This is generally less stressful for the animal but has the limitations of positioning, movement, and the addition of water as a density. If sedation or anesthesia can be used, the best images can be taken with the animal out of water. All the preparations for the imaging should be done prior to taking the animal out of water to minimize the time for performing these diagnostics. When taking an anesthetized fish out of water, the patient will begin to undergo stress associated with hypoxia and also runs the risk of damage to the skin and mucus coat from handling. Bubble wrap or other nonabsorbent material can be used to support the animal, and latex gloves

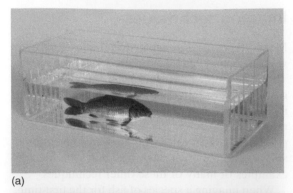

(a)

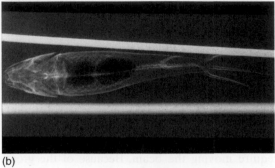

(b)

Fig. 17.10 Using a specialized aquarium (a) for taking dorsal ventral radiographs (b) of a fish patient (*Cyprinus carpio*) in water.

should be worn to minimize handling damage. Depending on the level of anesthesia, the patient will be immobile for several minutes, allowing time for performing radiographs and providing survey scans for helical CT.

Conventional and digital radiography

Conventional radiography is commonly used in fish medicine. The recent move toward digital radiography has greatly enhanced clinical efforts to include radiographs as an essential component included in the basic physical exam for fish patients. Digital radiology can both decrease time and help optimize contrast for fish. Radiographs help distinguish among several different densities in the fish patient, which includes: air, soft tissue/fluid, fat, bone, and metal/mineral. Morphological abnormalities identified via radiographs can be found in the skeletal system, swim bladder, GI tract, and reproductive system. In the skeletal system, bony and cartilaginous abnormalities include spinal scol-

iosis, kyphosis, and/or lordosis; fractures, compressions, and fusions of the appendicular and axial skeleton; osteochondroma; hypercalcification; and osteoporosis. Skeletal malformations are relatively common in fish and skeletal abnormalities can readily mimic coelomic masses (Bakal et al., 1998; Hansen and Yalew, 1988). Since the swim bladder is filled with gas, the size, anatomic location, wall thickness, and number of compartments can readily be assessed (Beregi et al., 1998; Britt et al., 2002). Masses and foreign bodies that are affecting the digestive tract can be visualized (Harms et al., 1995). Radiology has also been utilized in a pharmacokinetic study to document feed intake in fish with food containing X-ray-dense beads (Elema et al., 1994). Developing embryos and masses can also be identified in the reproductive tract (Weisse et al., 2002). Unfortunately, given the body composition and structure of certain fish patients, coelomic contrast in many patients is normally moderate at best and typically poor or absent. For extremely small patients, a dental or mammography unit can be used to increase detail.

Contrast radiography

To improve detail for conventional and digital radiography, contrast radiography can be used after survey radiographs have been performed to rule out stones or foreign bodies. Techniques used for contrast radiography have included using contrast material either orally and rectally in the GI tract, and also in the urogenital tract to visualize the ovaries or bladder. To perform contrast radiography, the animal should be anesthetized. Iodinated versus barium agents have been preferred to maintain water quality during the procedure. Barium agents can also cause hypoxia by coating the gill lamellae and can damage the fragile lamellae directly, decreasing oxygen diffusion across the gills. A dosage for nonionic agents is 5–10 ml/kg body weight, while the ionic agents dosing is 1–2 ml/kg body weight. If a barium agent must be used, water-soluble forms are preferred over oil- or fat-based forms. Barium sulfate has been successfully used at 5–10 ml/kg body weight for both gastrograms and enemas. Make sure that clean recovery water is readily available. Although adverse reactions have not reported in fish, animals should be monitored for several hours post-examination. If performing a gastrogram, some general knowledge regarding GI transit time may be available for more common species in fish physiology texts (Peres and Rigal, 1976; Gudmundsson et al., 1995; Heng et al., 2007). One should be prepared to radiograph the animal at various time intervals (1, 15, 30, 60, 120, 180, 240, 360, and 480 minutes). Due to various GI transit times in fish, radiographs may need to be repeated 24, 48, and 72 hours later to evaluate GI motility. If the animal is carnivorous and has a short GI tract, the entire GI tract can be filled with enough contrast to check the integrity of the tract simultaneously using a gastrogram and enema. Radiographic technique will vary from fish to fish and from machine to machine. Xeroradiography is a method of conventional radiography that uses paper instead of film, requiring higher radiation exposure, and has historically been used in human mammography. This technique has been useful for optimizing radiographic details in patients less than 500 g (Smith and Smith, 1994).

MRI

MRI has been used in fish patients (Fig. 17.11). It provides the best soft tissue contrast of all the imaging modalities discussed in this chapter. One of the greatest limitations of MRI in fish patients is the length of time necessary to complete the imaging study, often 20 minutes or longer. The fish has to remain anesthetized during this entire period, and an anesthetic delivery system that has no metal components has to be used. For large animals, this means a substantial amount of freshwater or saltwater in close proximity to the MRI unit. Based on magnetic principles, there also may be less resolution in marine solutions (paramagnetic ions) than in freshwater solutions. Because of these caveats and the expense of MRI studies, it is not frequently used for fish patients.

Ultrasonography

Ultrasound is regularly used in aquatic animal medicine. Some of the first reported studies using this modality were in salmon using diagnostic ultrasound examination and echocardiography (Fig. 17.12) (Sande and Poppe, 1995). Ultrasound can be done without anesthetizing the animals, although sedation reduces stress and allows for safer handling. The transducer needs to be protected by a waterproof seal. This can be done using a tight-fitting plastic cover over the transducer head, but waterproof probes are also available. The probe can be placed directly on the fish underwater, allowing water to act as the coupling agent. Ultrasound can be used for guided biopsies of specific organs, for centesis procedures, for evaluating the reproductive tract, for staging the size of oocytes and determining the gender of sexually mature fish, for echocardiography or to monitor the cardiac rate and flow during anesthesia, and for evaluating organs of the digestive system (Boyce,

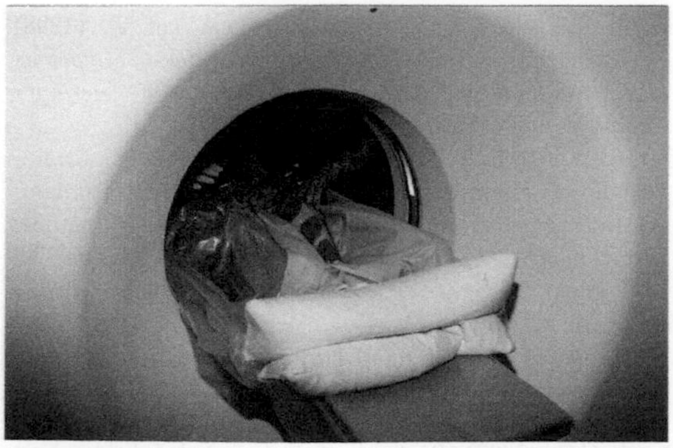

Fig. 17.11 A koi is prepared for a magnetic resonance imaging study.

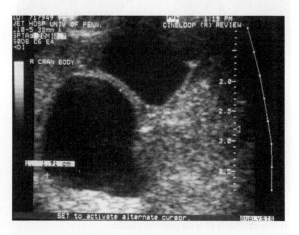

Fig. 17.12 Ultrasonographic image of a koi.

1985; Mattson, 1991; Blythe et al., 1994; Sande and Poppe, 1995; Gumpenberger, 2002).

CT

CT employs principles of conventional radiography diagnosis but by using cross-sectional or slice imaging, this technique can allow three-dimensional (3-D) viewing without reduction and superimposition of organs (Fig. 17.13). CT also can distinguish nearly a 40-fold difference in tissue densities as compared with the five densities indentified using traditional radiography. Through viewing different windows, CT offers improved spatial resolution, depth perception, and 3-D reconstruction of images. Some limitations of CT include poor contrast among soft tissues, distortion from metal objects, increased radiolucence of tissues when they are behind dense bone (beam hardening), and sometimes tissue margins can appear indistinct (volume averaging). Advances of CT scanning have led to the increasing use of helical or spiral CT, which scans patients in continuous motion rather than stopping the scan with

each consecutive slice. Although helical CT offers higher resolution and greater 3-D reconstruction, the greatest advantage for using this modality with fish patients is rapid imaging processing, dramatically decreasing the time for the patient. In some fish, this procedure has taken as little as 3 minutes for a survey and diagnostic scan using helical CT. As with conventional and digital radiography, IV iodinated contrast agents are extremely helpful when administered using the central vein in fish patients. Contrast has increased uptake in abnormally high vascular tissue such as the reproductive tract and areas of inflammation. There is also prolonged uptake of contrast agent in a variety of neoplasia caused by the decreased cellular integrity of tumor vessel wall. Some contrast can also penetrate the blood–brain-barrier to help identify brain abnormalities or anomalies.

Acknowledgments

E. Scott Weber III wishes to thank Dr. Tobias Schwarz, Senior Lecturer Diagnostic Imaging, Royal (Dick) School of Veterinary Studies, University of Edinburgh, whose excitement and enthusiasm for fish patients helped enhance diagnostic imaging for many of his fish patients.

References and further reading

Bakal, R.S., Love, N.E., Lewbart, G.A., et al. (1998) Imaging a spinal fracture in a Kohaku koi (*Cyprinus carpio*): techniques and case history report. *Veterinary Radiology & Ultrasound* **39**: 318–321.

Beregi, A., Molnar, K., Bekesi, L., et al. (1998) Radio-diagnostic method for studying swimbladder inflammation caused by *Anguillicola crassus* (Nematoda: Dracunculoidea). *Diseases of Aquatic Organisms* **34**: 155–160.

Blythe, B., Helfrich, L.A., Beal, W.E., et al. (1994) Determination of sex and maturational status of striped bass (*Morone saxatilis*) using ultrasonic imaging. *Aquaculture* **125**: 175–184.

Bond, C.E. (2007) *Biology of Fishes*, 3rd Edition. Fort Worth, TX: Saunders College Publishing.

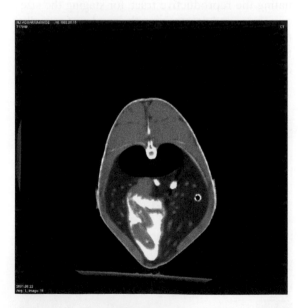

Fig. 17.13   A computed tomography image of a lipoma in the stomach of a largemouth bass.

Boyce, N.P. (1985) Ultrasound imaging used to detect cysts of *Henneguya salminicola* (Protozoa: Myxozoa) in the flesh of whole Pacific salmon. *Canadian Journal of Fisheries and Aquatic Sciences* **42**: 1312–1314.

Britt, T., Weisse, C., Weber, E.S., et al. (2002) Use of pneumocystoplasty for overinflation of the swim bladder in a goldfish. *Journal of the American Veterinary Medical Association* **221**: 690–693.

Clauss, T.M., Dove, A.D.M., and Arnold, J.E. (2008) Hematologic disorders of fish. *Veterinary Clinics of North America: Exotic Animal Practice* **11**: 445–462.

Elema, M.O., Hoff, K.A., and Kristensen, H.G. (1994) Multiple-dose pharmacokinetic study of flumequine in Atlantic salmon (*Salmo salar* L.). *Aquaculture* **128**: 1–11.

Groff, J.M. and Zinkl, J.G. (1999) Hematology and clinical chemistry of cyprinid fish. *Veterinary Clinics of North America: Exotic Animal Practice* **2** (5): 741–776.

Gudmundsson, O., Tryggvadottir, S.V., Petursdottir, T., et al. (1995) Measurements of feed intake and excretion in fish using radiography or chemical indicators. *Water Science and Technology* **31**: 131–136.

Guimaraes-Cruz, R.J., Santos, J.E., and Santos, G.B. (2005) Gonadal structure and gametogenesis of *Loricaria lentiginosa* Isbrücker (Pisces, Teleostei, Siluriformes). *Revista Brasileira De Zoologia* **22** (3): 556–564.

Gumpenberger, M. (2002) Ultrasound diagnosis— ultrasonographic detection of spinal malformation in a chub (*Leuciscus cephalus* L.). *Veterinary Radiology and Ultrasound* **43**: 584–585.

Hansen, H.J. and Yalew, Z.T. (1988) Morphologic features of perosomus ("short spine") in farmed salmon (*Salmo salar*): a preliminary report. *Veterinary Radiology* **29**: 52–53.

Harms, C.A., Bakal, R.S., Khoo, L.H., et al. (1995) Microsurgical excision of an abdominal mass in a gourami. *Journal of the American Veterinary Medical Association* **207**: 1215–1217.

Heng, H.G., Ong, T.W., and Hassan, M.D. (2007) Radiographic assessment of gastric emptying and gastrointestinal transit time in hybrid tilapia (*Oreochromis niloticus* × *O. mossambicus*). *Veterinary Radiology and Ultrasound* **48**: 132–134.

Harrenstien, L.A., Tornquist, S.J., Miller-Morgan, T.J., et al. (2005) Evaluation of a point-of-care blood analyzer and determination of reference ranges for blood parameters in rockfish. *Journal of the American Veterinary Medical Association* **226** (2): 255–265.

Hrubec, T.C. and Smith, S.A. (2000) Hematology of fish. In *Schalm's Veterinary Hematology*, 5th ed. (Feldman B.F., Zinkl, J.Q., and Jain N.C., eds.), pp. 1120–1125. Philadelphia: Lippincott Williams and Wilkins.

Juopperi, T. (2003) Fish clinical pathology. Paper presented at Fish Health Management Continuing Education Course, NC State College of Veterinary Medicine, Raleigh, NC, August 14–16.

Love, N.E. and Lewbart, G.A. (1997) Pet fish radiography: technique and case history reports. *Veterinary Radiology and Ultrasound* **38**: 24–29.

Mattson, N.S. (1991) A new method to determine sex and gonad size in live fishes by using ultrasonography. *Journal of Fish Biology* **39**: 673–677.

Meisner, A. and Burns, J. (1997) Viviparity in the halfbeak genera *Dermogenys* and *Nomorhamphus* (Teleostei: Hemiramphidae). *Journal of Morphology* **234**: 295–317.

Moyle, P.B. and Cech, J.J., Jr. (2004) *Fishes: An Introduction to Ichthyology*, 5th Edition. Englewood Cliffs, NJ: Prentice-Hall.

Palmeiro, B.S., Rosenthal, K.L., Lewbart, G.A., et al. (2007) Plasma biochemical reference intervals for koi. *Journal of the American Veterinary Association* **230** (5): 708–712.

Peres, G. and Rigal, A. (1976) Transit time in the digestive tract of fish. Critique of a radiographic method in trout (*Salmo gairdnerii*). *Bulletin de la Societe des Sciences Veterinaires et de Medecine Comparee de Lyon* **78**: 339–344.

Reavill, D.R. (2006) Common diagnostic and clinical techniques for fish. *Veterinary Clinics of North America: Exotic Animal Practice* **9**: 223–235.

Reavill, D.R. and Roberts, H.E. (2007) Diagnostic cytology of fish. *Veterinary Clinics of North America: Exotic Animal Practice* **10**: 207–234.

Ross, L.G. and Ross, B. (2008) *Anaesthetic and Sedative Techniques for Aquatic Animals*, 3rd Edition. Oxford: Blackwell Publishing.

Sande, R.D. and Poppe, T.T. (1995) Diagnostic ultrasound examination and echocardiography in Atlantic salmon (*Salmo salar*). *Veterinary Radiology and Ultrasound* **36**: 551–558.

Smith, S.A. (2002) Nonlethal diagnostic techniques used in the diagnosis of diseases of fish. *Journal of the American Veterinary Medical Association* **220** (8): 1203–1206.

Smith, S.A. and Smith, B.J. (1994) Xeroradiographic and radiographic anatomy of the channel catfish, *Ictalurus punctatus*. *Veterinary Radiology and Ultrasound* **35**: 384–389.

Stoskopf, M. (1993a) Clinical pathology of carp, goldfish, and koi. In *Fish Medicine* (Stoskopf, M., ed.), pp. 450–453. Philadelphia: W.B. Saunders.

Stoskopf, M. (1993b) Clinical pathology of freshwater tropical fishes. In *Fish Medicine* (Stoskopf, M., ed.), pp. 543–545. Philadelphia: W.B. Saunders.

Stoskopf, M. (1993c) Clinical pathology of marine tropical fishes. In *Fish Medicine* (Stoskopf, M., ed.), pp. 614–617. Philadelphia: W.B. Saunders.

Southgate, P.J. (2001) Laboratory techniques. In *BSAVA Manual of Ornamental Fish*, 2nd Edition (Wildgoose, W.H., ed.), pp. 91–101. Gloucester: British Small Animal Veterinary Association.

Tripathi, N.K., Latimer, K.S. and Burnley, V.V. (2004) Hematologic reference intervals for koi (*Cyprinus *carpio*), including blood cell morphology, cytochemistry, and ultrastructure. *Veterinary Clinical Pathology* **33** (2): 74–83.

Weber, E.S. and Innis, C. (2007) Piscine patients: basic diagnostics. *Compendium on Continuing Education for the Practicing Veterinarian* **29** (5): 276–288.

Weber, E.S. and Govett, P. (2009) Parasitology and necropsy of fish. *Education for the Practicing Veterinarian* **31** (2): Online E1–E7.

Weisse, C., Weber, E.S., Matzkin, Z., et al. (2002) Surgical removal of a seminoma from a black sea bass. *Journal of the American Veterinary Medical Association* **220** (2): 280–283.

Chapter 18

Surgery and Wound Management in Fish

Helen E. Roberts

Introduction

Surgical treatment and wound management of pet fish are essential practices of any companion aquatic animal practice. The most common indications for surgery include cutaneous ulcer disease management, exuberant tissue growth, cutaneous masses, ophthalmic diseases, exploration of the coelomic cavity and biopsy specimen sampling, elective gonadectomies, and coelomic mass removal. Simple procedures may be performed pond- or tankside, but more complex procedures are usually performed at the practitioner's clinic or hospital. Understanding the unique characteristics and healing of fish skin is essential to a successful outcome.

The skin of fish

Anatomy of the fish skin

Fish have developed unique strategies to deal with the adverse conditions present in an aquatic environment. The skin of fish serves as an impermeable barrier between the body and internal organs and the environment. The thickness of the skin varies between species, and with age, time of year, and anatomical location. The outermost layer of the skin is the cuticle. The cuticle, or mucous layer, consists of mucus secreted by goblet cells, cellular debris, and sloughed cells. Lysozymes, antibodies (immunoglobulin M-like [IgM-like]), and other substances present in the mucous layer provide antimicrobial properties that help inhibit pathogen growth. This layer is often referred to as the "slime layer" or "slime coat" by hobbyists.

The cuticle is the layer that is examined when performing a diagnostic skin scraping.

Below the cuticle is the avascular epidermis. In most species, it consists of nonkeratinized stratified squamous epithelial cells arranged in three layers—superficial, intermediate, and basal layers—similar to terrestrial animals. Epidermal cell mitosis and production occurs in all three layers, unlike in terrestrial animals, where it is confined to the basal cell layer. This can be an important factor in the healing of damaged skin. Lymphocytes in various numbers are also present in the epidermis and can increase in numbers during disease. Mucus-producing goblet cells, malpighian cells, and alarm cells are also present in this layer. The collagen filament-containing malpighian cells provide structure to the epidermis. The epidermis in fish is continuous; it extends over the fins and tail and also covers the scales. The epidermis and the cuticle provide a waterproof barrier for the fish.

The layer of the skin below the epidermis is the dermis. This consists of two layers: the superficial stratum spongiosum and the deeper stratum compactum. Pigment cells are located in the dermis. These consist of dark/black melanophores (with melanin granules), yellow and orange xanthophores (with rodopterin and carotenoid granules), white leucophores (with guanine), erythrophores (red pigments), and the light-reflecting iridophores (containing guanine and hypoxanthine) (Roberts and Ellis, 2001). Pigment cell tumors are not uncommon in several species of pet fish, including goldfish (*Carassius auratus*). For further information on neoplasia, see Chapter 20.

Scales emerge from shallow pockets in the dermis and are covered by a layer of epidermal tissue. They may overlap and provide additional structural integrity and protection to the fish. Scale loss is a significant injury to the fish, resulting in poor osmoregulation and allowing the entry of pathogens. Scales are made of collagen fibers and minerals, such as calcium phosphate and calcium carbonate forming hydroxyapatite crystals, organized in an organic matrix. Scales exist in four forms: ctenoid, cycloid, placoid, and ganoid. The dermis also contains mast cells that release substances in response to inflammation. These cells are located around scales and between melanophores. Finally, sensory tissue, neural tissue, fibroblasts, osteoblasts, and vascular tissue are also found in the dermis.

The deepest layer of the skin is the hypodermis or subcutis. This layer lies above the skeletal and muscular structures below the skin. Due to the loosely organized structure and large blood supply, this layer is very susceptible to bacterial invasion.

Skin's response to injury

When the skin is damaged, there is a very real risk of pathogens entering the body, with subsequent loss of osmoregulation. Depending on the depth and severity, cutaneous wounds in fish can have potentially fatal consequences. Because of this, fish have developed a rapid healing response to tissue injury. Fish healing is more efficient and more rapid compared with terrestrial animals. The effectiveness of wound healing is determined by the health status of the fish, concurrent diseases, water quality, and water temperature. Under ideal water conditions and in the absence of secondary infections or other pathogens, a small breach in the epidermis can be restored by epidermal cell migration within a few hours (Fontenot and Neiffer, 2004; Ferguson, 2006).

The initial response to injury is an inflammatory response, comparable with that in terrestrial animals. Inflammatory cells, such as macrophages, move into the site of injury and engulf debris. Epidermal cells migrate from the wound edges and begin to cover the surface within a few hours. The healing continues with the proliferation and organization of epithelial cells starts soon after reepithelialization. Fibroblast infiltration

and mucous cell development occur a few days after the initial trauma. In deep wounds, muscle tissue regeneration begins approximately a week after injury and is generally completed 2 weeks after the initial trauma if temperatures are in the species' optimal range. Scale formation will have been also completed by this time, depending on the depth of the injury. Very deep, severe injuries may show scars and no scale regrowth. Clients should always be informed of this possibility, especially if the patients are show fish.

Surgical patient evaluation

Koi and goldfish are relatively hardy fish and make good surgical candidates (Lewbart, 2001). Other species of pet fish may be more susceptible to the stress and trauma of surgery and anesthesia. As with any other pet species, care should be taken to thoroughly evaluate each patient prior to surgery to maximize survivability and surgical success.

A minimum database should be completed in all fish cases. In addition to an extensive verbal history (including questions on appetite, weight loss if applicable, behavior in the pond or tank, duration of presenting problem, and prior medical conditions and treatments) and a thorough physical examination of the patient, the clinician should also perform routine water chemistry testing and wet mount cytological exam for external parasites of the skin and gills. Flourescein dye can be applied to the skin and corneas to look for small ulcerative lesions and breaks in the epidermis that are not readily visible (Noga and Udomkusonsri, 2002). Other diagnostic techniques such as radiography and ultrasonography may help give further information prior to surgical exploration (see Chapter 17 on nonlethal diagnostic techniques).

Preoperative blood testing can be performed as in other species. In-house testing using the VetScan® (Abaxis Inc., Union City, CA) for plasma biochemical values has recently been explored by Palmeiro et al. (2007). Packed cell volume and total protein should also be evaluated preoperatively. Chapter 17 gives more information on abnormalities that may be found during blood tests. Septic, cachectic, anemic, or lethargic patients do not make good surgical candidates. Stabilization should be attempted whenever possible to reduce the risk of perioperative complications, including death.

The fish should remain off food for 24 hours prior to surgery to prevent possible water quality abnormalities (ammonia elevations, etc.) and particulate matter buildup in the water that may clog the gills (Murray, 2002).

Surgical principles are no different from that in other species: minimize surgical time whenever possible, use gentle tissue handling techniques, provide good hemostasis, and be familiar with the anatomy of the species. In the event the presenting species is a novel one, anatomy reference texts should be consulted if available. In addition, gentle handling of the patient is strongly advised to prevent the loss of the protective mucous layer of the skin that may predispose the fish to secondary infections (Murray, 2002).

Equipment

Instrumentation and suture selection

Most small animal practices have the necessary surgical instruments already in use (Fig. 18.1). Surgery on small fish species may require smaller instruments such as those used in ophthalmic surgeries or microsurgery. Self-retaining retractors

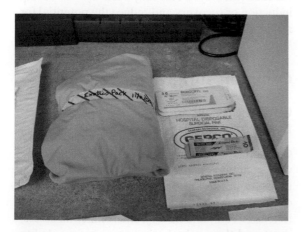

Fig. 18.1 An "exotic pack," clear plastic drape, and suture material gathered in preparation for surgery on a fish.

are very helpful in coelomic surgery to improve visualization and increase exposure (Wildgoose, 2000; Harms and Wildgoose, 2001; Lewbart, 2001; Harms, 2005). Visualization can be greatly enhanced through the use of head loupe magnification with mounted illumination (Harms and Wildgoose, 2001; Harms, 2005).

Absorbable suture material is not readily absorbed in most fish species. Monofilament suture is preferred over braided suture materials due to the potential for tissue reactions and bacterial infections that may occur due to wicking with braided sutures (Harms and Wildgoose, 2001; Harms, 2005). Monofilament sutures also exhibit less resistance passing through fish skin. A cutting needle works best on fish skin, which can be fairly tough (Harms and Wildgoose, 2001; Harms, 2005). A study by Hurty et al. (2002) evaluated the tissue and skin response to several suture materials in koi. The study found monofilament polyglyconate to cause the least reactions in koi, while organic suture materials such as silk, chromic cat gut caused the most severe reactions. The author uses polyglyconate (Maxon®, Covidien, Norwalk, CT), polydioxanone (PDS II®, Ethicon, Cincinnati, OH), poliglecaprone (Monocryl®, Ethicon), and nylon suture materials. Suture size is determined by the size of the patient and the procedure performed. Patterns of suture are generally a personal preference but should be chosen based on effectiveness, time involved, and ease of removal. Sutures are generally removed in 2–6 weeks, depending on appearance and healing of the incision. Healing can be enhanced by keeping fish in water temperatures at the upper limits of their preferred range (Harms and Wildgoose, 2001). Surgical glue, or tissue adhesive, has been shown to cause severe dermatitis in fish, increase the incidence of dehiscence (Harms and Wildgoose, 2001; Lewbart, 2001), and may inhibit healing time so it is not recommended for use in pet fish surgery.

Miscellaneous equipment

A surgery table used in fish surgeries may range from a plastic container lid used for very short procedures to an elaborate device placed on top of a liquid anesthesia delivery system (Fig. 18.2). Fish should be kept moist throughout any procedure

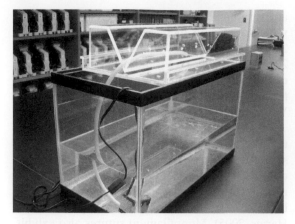

Fig. 18.2 A plexiglass trough for surgical positioning placed on top of a liquid anesthesia holding tank.

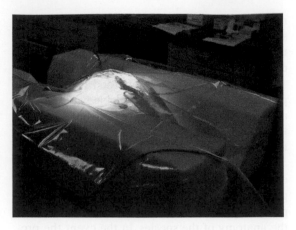

Fig. 18.4 A koi placed in readiness for surgery covered with sterile plastic drape.

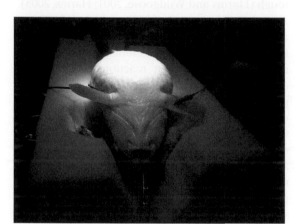

Fig. 18.3 A koi held in dorsal recumbency by a foam positioning device. Note the electrocardiogram (ECG) clips in place on the pectoral fins and the foam widely cut for gill excursions.

and not be subject to sliding on the surface they are placed on. Surgical assistants can gently irrigate the skin, taking care not to contaminate the incision site. Chamois towels or upholstery foam can be used to position fish and prevent movement due to the slippery conditions. Plexiglass troughs or upholstery foam cut into a V-shaped wedge help keep fish in ventral recumbency for exploratory coeliotomies (Figs. 18.2 and 18.3).

Clear plastic, sterile drapes improve visualization, minimize contamination, and help retain moisture (Lewbart, 2001; Harms, 2005) (Fig. 18.4). Sterile lubricating jelly can help keep the

drape attached to the skin, but small towel clamps can also be used. Bipolar cautery can be used successfully for hemostasis (Harms and Wildgoose, 2001; Lewbart, 2001; Harms, 2005), but care must be taken in small animals not to damage adjacent tissue. Small vessel bleeding is not usually a problem in fish surgery and can usually be controlled by direct pressure or temporary application of a hemostat. Monitoring devices such as pulse oximeters, electrocardiogram (ECG) monitors, and pulse Doppler probes can be used in fish surgery (Lewbart, 2001). Sterile ophthalmic lubricant is used to protect the eyes of the surgical patient. Moist towels can also be used to cover the lubricated eyes. This may calm the fish during induction or recovery and reduce the potential for retinal damage (Wildgoose, 2000).

Common surgical procedures

Cutaneous ulcers and traumatic injuries

Cutaneous wounds and ulcerative lesions are very common in pet fish. An understanding of the anatomy and response to diseases of the skin can better prepare the clinician in treating these lesions. A complete history, environmental assessment, and thorough physical exam are needed to enable effective management strategies to deal with all possible contributing factors resulting in these problems. Client education may help reduce the future recurrence of these wounds and ulcers.

Fish with traumatic injuries and ulcers should be examined thoroughly for potential causes and concurrent diseases. The entire body surface should be examined carefully, with particular attention to the ventral aspect of pond fish since lesions here are not always apparent when viewed in the pond. If a bacterial infection and/or septicemia are suspected, cultures should be taken prior to starting antimicrobial therapy. Cultures of ulcers should not be obtained from superficial tissue or mucus, the results of which will likely represent environmental contamination. The lesion should be rinsed with sterile saline (for marine species) or sterile water (for freshwater species) prior to sampling. Full-skin thickness biopsies can be helpful in evaluating the extent of an injury or disease in deeper structures such as the underlying musculature, dermis, and hypodermis (Fontenot and Neiffer, 2004).

All suspected traumatic wounds should be fully evaluated for depth and degree of damage (Fig. 18.5). Flushing is accomplished with dilute chlorhexidine, sterile saline, or a dilute povidone–iodine solution (Wildgoose, 2001; Fontenot and Neiffer, 2004). Ragged edges and further contamination can be removed by debriding, leaving a "clean" surface where healing can take place. Sterile cotton or gauze swabs can be used effectively in most cases. Wounds that can be closed or

partially closed should be sutured (Fig. 18.6). This will reduce the area of skin that is vulnerable to the osmotic changes in the tissues (influx of water in freshwater fish and efflux of water in saltwater fish) and exposure to pathogens. Most ulcers and superficial wounds in fish are left to heal by secondary intention. Fish skin is relatively inelastic and is tightly adhered to the underlying body tissues, making primary closure difficult in most cases. Deep wounds that cannot be sutured may benefit from the application of a topical medication or commercially available bioadhesive product containing 2-octyl cyanoacrylate (Colgate Orabase Soothe-N-Seal®, Colgate-Palmolive Company, New York, NY) or carmellose sodium (a mucoprotectant contained in Orahesive Powder, Convatec, Princeton, NJ) (Wildgoose, 2001; Fontenot and Neiffer, 2004; Harms, 2005). Some products require the area of application to be dry in order to adhere properly, and the manufacturer's directions should be followed. The use of an occlusive paste or gel on the wound may be beneficial in protecting the wound against osmotic pressures and allows faster healing, but it may also trap pathogens inside the wound. Many koi hobbyists advocate the use of a homemade paste that includes potassium permanganate, but this may be harmful to the operator and has the potential to cause blindness, respiratory irritation, and skin damage in humans. (Consult a Material Safety Data Sheet on potassium permanganate for all potential hazards; an example can be found at www.sciencelab. com/xMSDS-Potassium_permanganate-9927406.)

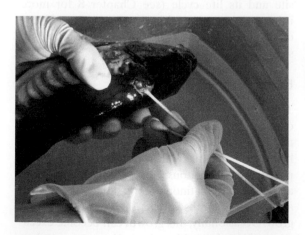

Fig. 18.5 The wounds of this koi, *Cyprinus carpio*, are carefully probed with sterile cotton swabs to evaluate the depth of the injury.

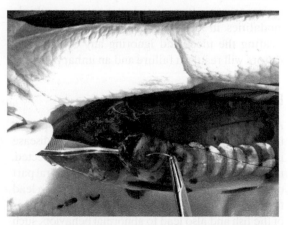

Fig. 18.6 Closure of a large skin defect with suture.

Impaired wound healing and pain in the patient makes this practice controversial and the practice may be of limited benefit.

Topical medications containing bacitracin, silver sulfadiazine, neomycin, polymixin B, mupirocin, povidone–iodine, and various other antibacterial products have been used in pet fish. There are few scientific reports of adverse effects with the use of these products, and most aquatic health professionals have found them to be relatively safe in ornamental fish. The "extra-label use" of these unapproved topical products is prohibited in food fish. The client should always be informed as to the relative lack of data available with the use of any unapproved products. Petroleum-based products may have an increased risk of causing toxicity in sensitive species. A novel tris-EDTA topical solution, Tricide® (Molecular Therapeutics LLC, Riverbend Laboratories, Athens, GA), has been used extensively by veterinarians and hobbyists in the treatment of ulcerative disease in fish (Ritchie et al., 2004). Tricide® can be used by adding an antibiotic or antifungal product, or can be used as a prepared solution containing neomycin, Tricide-Neo®(Molecular Therapeutics LLC). These solutions can be used in a spray bottle and applied to the wound directly instead of being used as a dip, which must be discarded after use. The solutions are not recommended as water additives due to the adverse effects on the biofilter. Systemic antimicrobial treatment is indicated in severe or extensive wounds and systemic bacterial infections.

It is very unusual to find just one abnormality contributing to a disease in pet fish. Treatment regimens are often aimed at applying multiple modalities in order to achieve success. Simply treating the ulcer and ignoring any contributing factors will result in failure and an unhappy client.

Environmental disorders

Abnormal water quality can be a significant contributor to the development of ulcers and disease in fish. In most cases, several fish will be affected, making environmental management an integral part of disease management. Poor water quality can lead to physical changes in the protective mucous layer of the fish and also lead to abnormal behaviors, such as jumping and flashing, which directly cause traumatic lesions. Water quality parameters associated with disease include abrupt changes in pH, excessively low or high pH, abrupt water temperature changes, and low dissolved oxygen. In addition, high levels of organic debris and detritus, water pollution, and overcrowding can contribute to disease.

Pond fish are also susceptible to injury from intense sunlight and ultraviolet radiation given the right conditions. Lesions are typically seen on the dorsal aspect of the fish and located in the pale or nonpigmented areas of the skin. Affected fish are usually found in shallow ponds with no shade. This type of injury is most often seen in warm climates and during the summer months. Conditions that bring fish to gasp and congregate at the water surface, such as diseases that affect the gills causing hypoxia or a relative hypoxia (e.g. nitrite poisoning) can increase the likelihood of sunburn developing.

Ectoparasites

External parasites can cause epithelial trauma through pruritic behavior in fish (flashing) and direct damage by their attachment and subsequent inflammatory response in the skin. A few parasites will not generally cause disease on their own but will compound the effects of other stressors. Effective parasite control will involve treating the entire population rather than just the presenting individual. Duration of therapy and method of application are determined by the identified parasite and its life cycle (see Chapter 8 for more information on parasitic diseases). The efficacy of treatment should be monitored with follow-up skin scrape examinations.

Exuberant wen growth

The wen is the head growth seen on some varieties of fancy goldfish (*C. auratus*) (and some mature male Cichlids). This group includes orandas, lionheads, and ranchus. The wen in goldfish is composed of myxomatous, fibrous connective tissue and has a gelatinous consistency. Beginning around 3–4 months of age, the wen will start to grow. Occasionally, this growth can become excessive and interfere with eating and movement when it covers the eyes (Fig. 18.7a). It can also become very heavy and cause some abnormal swimming

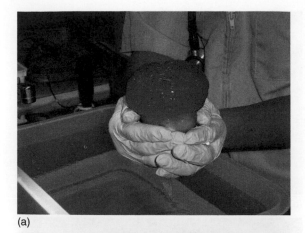

(a)

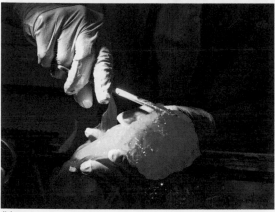

(b)

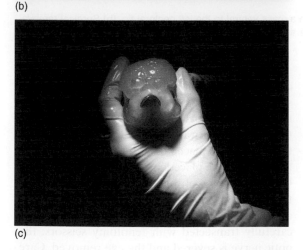

(c)

Fig. 18.7   (a) An oranda with excessive head growth (wen). (b) Surgical removal of excess wen growth in an oranda. (c) An oranda after excess wen removal.

and may resemble a buoyancy disorder. Owners find excessive growth to be distressing and often request a "haircut." After anesthetizing the fish, excess wen tissue can removed with small, sharp scissors such as tenotomy scissors (see Fig. 18.7b). Hemostasis is rarely a problem and can be accomplished by applying direct pressure with a sterile cotton swab. The eye should be protected when trimming close and avoid removing tissue too close to the base of the head. Trim carefully to achieve a balanced, symmetrical appearance (Fig. 18.7c). The wen will regrow over time and need trimming periodically. Preoperatively, the author gives a single injection of butorphanol and, if needed, an injection of ceftazidime.

Cutaneous masses

External masses are commonly reported to fish health practitioners by owners. These growths can occur anywhere on the body; they may interfere with movement or eating. Masses can result from inflammatory reactions, granulomas, neoplasia, or parasitic disease. In most cases, the skin cannot be closed over the remaining defect and must be left to heal by second intention. When closure can be used, suture material should be chosen based on fish size and are removed when the incision is healed (Fig. 18.8). For suspected neoplastic masses, margins must be wide and deep as they extend into the underlying musculature. Additional treatment includes the use of topical medications on the site of excision, analgesic injections, and antibiotic injections. Masses should be submitted to a diagnostic laboratory familiar with cutaneous fish pathology.

In the removal of external masses, use of carbon dioxide lasers may be beneficial due to improved hemostasis and reduction in surgical time and postoperative pain (Stetter, 2005). Debulking and removal of masses can also be accomplished through the use of liquid nitrogen cryosurgical units. A recent report evaluated the successful use of an over-the-counter wart removal system in cryotherapy following surgical debulking of a recurrent external mass (Harms et al., 2008).

Ophthalmic surgery

Ophthalmic problems that require surgery are not uncommon in pet fish. The most common

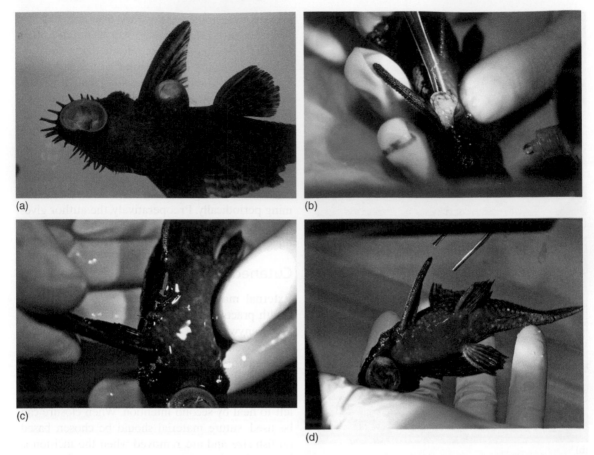

Fig. 18.8 (a) A bristlenose plecostomus (*Ancistrus* sp.) with a mass ventral to the left pectoral fin. (b) Surgical removal of the mass. (c) Sutures at the surgical site. (d) Surgical site at suture removal (1 month postoperative).

indications for ophthalmic surgery are trauma, neoplasia, inflammatory, and infectious diseases (Harms and Wildgoose, 2001). Goldfish are the most common pet fish species presented to the aquatic practitioner for ophthalmic disorders for several reasons, including the high frequency of neoplasia seen in goldfish (O'Hagan and Raidal, 2006) and traumatic injuries. Traumatic injuries are particularly common in fancy goldfish with protruding eyes (telescope eye/dragon eye, bubble eye, celestial eye) kept in outdoor ponds.

As with other presenting cases, a full workup including a detailed history, physical exam, water quality analysis, and diagnostic cytology is recommended. Flourescein dye application can be used to detect corneal lesions in fish as with terrestrial species. Medical treatment and water

quality management should be attempted prior to surgery in cases where immediate enucleation is not required. Enucleation of the fish eye is a relatively straightforward procedure. Once anesthetized, the fish is placed in lateral recumbency, with the affected eye placed upward (Wildgoose 2005). Gently cleansing of the eye can be achieved with the use of dilute povidone–iodine solution (Harms and Wildgoose, 2001). Attachments of the eye are carefully transected with tenotomy scissors; the optic nerve is severed and the eye removed. Care must be taken not to apply excess traction on the optic nerve to prevent secondary problems with the opposite eye. Hemostasis is not usually a problem. The author clamps the optic stalk for a few minutes or applies gentle pressure with a sterile cotton swab. Cautery can also be used

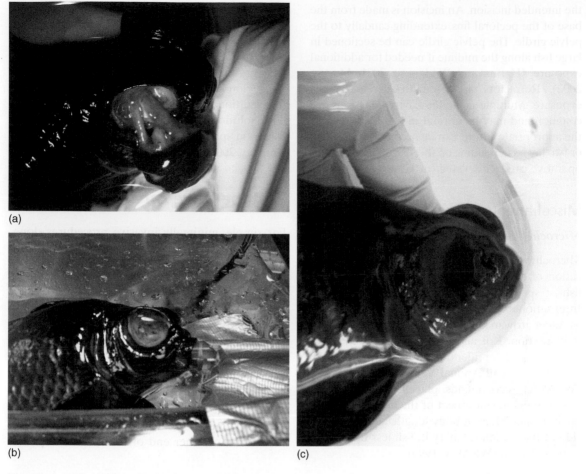

Fig. 18.9   (a) A goldfish with a severe traumatic injury to the eye. (b) Goldfish immediately postsurgical removal of the eye. (c) Goldfish enucleation 2 weeks after surgery.

(Harms and Wildgoose, 2001) with caution, especially in small patients. The eye should be submitted for histopathological examination in cases of suspected neoplasia, inflammatory, or infectious diseases. Figure 18.9 demonstrates an enucleation secondary to traumatic injury in a goldfish.

Other ophthalmic surgical procedures include cataract removal, management of deep or severe corneal injuries, and prosthesis placement following enucleation.

Coelomic cavity surgery

Intracoelomic surgery is performed for many reasons, including foreign body removal, mass removal, elective gonadectomies, exploration and organ biopsy, and buoyancy, gastrointestinal, and reproductive disorders. Preoperative evaluation, including radiography and ultrasonography, can be valuable in determining a presumptive diagnosis and prognosis prior to surgery.

For most coelomic surgeries, the patient is placed in dorsal recumbency and held in place with a positioning device (Fig. 18.3). The ventral midline is carefully cleaned to remove excess mucus and debris with sterile saline, dilute povidone–iodine, or dilute chlorhexidine (Harms and Wildgoose, 2001; Murray, 2002; Harms, 2005). Scales can be carefully removed individually in fish with prominent, large scales along the midline. A clear plastic drape is placed and held with a small amount of petroleum jelly at the margins of the intended incision. An incision is made from the base of the pectoral fins, extending caudally to the pelvic girdle. The pelvic girdle can be sectioned in large fish along the midline if needed for additional exposure (Harms and Wildgoose, 2001; Murray, 2002). Retractors are used to increase visual exposure. Multiple coelomic cavity adhesions are common and may be normal in koi. Closure, with the appropriate suture, can be accomplished in one or two layers depending on the size of the fish. Post-operative care is discussed further in this chapter.

Miscellaneous procedures

Microchip implantation

Microchips are placed in fish for unique identification of the individual fish. Legal, captive-bred fish of species protected by the Convention on International Trade in Endangered Species, such as Asian arowanas, can be identified by microchip implantation. Koi and other fish are sometimes microchipped for identification in case of theft. The World Small Animal Veterinary Association (WSAVA) recommends placement on the left side at the anterior aspect of the dorsal fin in fish greater than 30 cm in body length, and in the left side of the coelomic cavity in fish less than 30 cm in body length (WSAVA, 1999).

Intracoelomic catheterization

A method of temporary intracoelomic catheter placement using a butterfly catheter sutured in place has been described in koi (Lewbart et al., 2005). Treating a sick fish may involve multiple injections over a long period of time. Intracoelomic catheterization offers a method of delivery that can reduce handling stress and reduce injury to the fish and owner (Lewbart et al., 2005). In the study, the catheters were left in place for at least 7 days. Further studies are needed to determine if the catheter can be left for a longer period of time.

Laparoscopic surgery

Minimally invasive surgery with the use of laparoscopic techniques is becoming more popular in many segments of veterinary medicine, including pet fish medicine. Laparoscopic assisted surgery provides faster surgical time (depending on the surgeon's experience), less trauma and stress to the patient, less incision dehiscence, and faster recovery time (Boone et al., 2008). Insufflation of the coelomic cavity can be accomplished through the traditional use of gas or with the use of sterile fluid solutions. Several articles have been published on specific laparoscopic procedures in fish (Murray, 2002; Stetter, 2005; Boone et al., 2008).

Postoperative care

For simple, minimally invasive procedures done pondside or tankside, the fish can be monitored in a recovery container until it is upright and swimming normally before being placed back into its own environment or a hospital tank (Fig. 18.10). Hospital tanks or containers should be prepared in advance and contain water from the patient's home system whenever possible. Water quality should be monitored closely to prevent secondary stress. The water should be acclimated to the same temperature as the water used in the anesthetic solution. If it is at the cooler end of the species' optimal temperature range, a gradual increase over to the warmer end of the range can prove

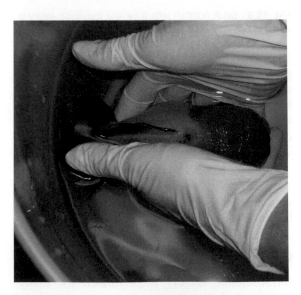

Fig. 18.10 This goldfish is being held and monitored in the water during recovery after a surgical procedure.

beneficial in healing and recovery from surgery (Harms and Wildgoose, 2001). Sodium chloride (1–3 g/l) can be added to reduce the osmotic gradient for freshwater patients. In most cases, a hospital tank should not have gravel or decorations, although a hiding place should be provided to reduce stress. A companion or "buddy" fish from the home environment can also help to reduce stress in social species such as koi or goldfish.

Depending on the indication for surgery and anticipated length of surgery, preoperative antibiotics and perioperative or postoperative analgesics may be used. The author gives 10 mg/kg enrofloxacin intramuscular (IM) (Baytril®, Bayer Health Care, Animal Health Division, Shawnee Mission, KS) or ceftazidime 20–30 mg/kg IM (Fortaz®, GlaxoSmithKline, Research Triangle Park, NC) when indicated. Butorphanol 0.1–0.4 mg/kg IM (Equanol®, Vedco, St. Joseph, MO) can be given just prior to recovery for postoperative analgesia (Lewbart et al., 1998; Harms and Wildgoose, 2001; Harms, 2005). Nonsteroidal anti-inflammatory drugs such as a single injection of ketoprofen 2 mg/kg IM (Ketofen®, Fort Dodge Animal Health, Fort Dodge, IA) have also been used (Harms 2005). The author has used carprofen 2–4 mg/kg IM (Rimadyl®, Pfizer Animal Health, New York, NY) as a single injection postoperatively without complications in multiple freshwater fish species. The owner should always be informed that the use of such medications is not approved by the Food and Drug Administration (FDA) and the possibility of adverse side effects is unknown.

Fish should be monitored postoperatively for the presence of secondary infections, return of appetite, and return to normal function and behavior.

Conclusion

As the availability of aquatic veterinarians and the information on ornamental pet fish health increases, surgery in these animals will become a more common part of exotic animal practice.

Acknowledgment

The author would like to thank her son, Jonathan, for taking pictures of multiple procedures and cases, including many of the photographs used in this section.

References and further reading

Boone, S.S., Hernandez-Divers, S.J., Radlinsky, M.G., et al. (2008) Comparison between coelioscopy and coeliotomy for liver biopsy in channel catfish. *Journal of the American Veterinary Medical Association* **233** (6): 960–967.

Dror, M., Sinyakov, M.S., Okun, E., et al. (2006) Experimental handling stress as infection facilitating factor for goldfish ulcerative disease. *Veterinary Immunology and Immunopathology* **109**: 279–287.

Fontenot, D.K. and Neiffer D.L. (2004). Wound management in teleost fish: biology of the healing process, evaluation, and treatment. *Veterinary Clinics of North America: Exotic Animal Practice* **7**: 57–86.

Ferguson, H.W. (2006) Skin. In *Systemic Pathology of Fish*, 2nd Edition (Ferguson, H.W., ed.), pp. 64–89. London: Scotian Press.

Harms, C.A. (2005) Surgery in fish research: common procedures and postoperative care. *Lab Animal* **34** (1): 28–34.

Harms, C.A. and Wildgoose, W.H. (2001) Surgery. In *BSAVA Manual of Ornamental Fish*, 2nd Edition (Wildgoose, W.H., ed.), pp. 259–266. Gloucester: BSAVA.

Harms, C.A., Christian, L.S., Burrus, O., et al. (2008) Cryotherapy for removal of a premaxillary mass from a chain pickerel using an over-the-counter wart remover. *Exotic DVM* **10** (2): 15–17.

Hunt, C.J.G. (2006) Ulcerative skin disease in a group of koi carp (*Cyprinus carpio*). *Veterinary Clinics of North America: Exotic Animal Practice* **9**: 723–728.

Hurty, C.A., Brazik, D.C., McHugh Law, J., et al. (2002) Evaluation of the tissue reactions in the skin and body wall of koi (*Cyprinus carpio*) to five suture materials. *Veterinary Record* **151**: 324–328.

Lewbart, G.A. (2001) Surgical techniques in the koi patient. *Exotic DVM* **3** (3): 43–47.

Lewbart, G.A., Spodnick, G., Barlow, N., et al. (1998) Surgical removal of an undifferentiated abdominal sarcoma from a koi carp (*Cyprinus carpio*). *Veterinary Record* **143**: 556–558.

Lewbart, G.A., Butkus, D.A., Papich, M.G., et al. (2005) Evaluation of a method of intracoelomic catheterization in koi. *Journal of the American Veterinary Medical Association* **226** (5): 784–788.

Murray, M.J. (2002) Fish surgery. *Seminars in Avian and Exotic Pet Medicine* **11** (4): 246–257.

Noga, E.J. and Udomkusonsri, P. (2002) Fluorescein: a rapid, sensitive, nonlethal method for detecting skin ulceration in fish. *Veterinary Pathology* **39**: 726–731.

Noga, E.J., Botts, S., Yang, M.S., et al. (1998) Acute stress causes skin ulceration in striped bass and hybrid bass (*Morone*). *Veterinary Pathology* **35** (2): 102–107.

O'Hagan, B.J. and Raidal, S.R. (2006) Surgical removal of retrobulbar hemangioma in a goldfish (*Carassius auratus*). *Veterinary Clinics of North America: Exotic Animal Practice* **9**: 729–733.

Palmeiro, B.S., Rosenthal, K.L., Lewbart, G.A., et al. (2007) Plasma biochemical reference intervals for koi. *Journal of the American Veterinary Medical Association* **230** (5): 708–712.

Ritchie, B.W., Wooley, R.E., and Kemp, D.T. (2004) Use of potentiated antibiotics in wound management. *Veterinary Clinics of North America: Exotic Animal Practice* **7**: 169–189.

Roberts, R.J. and Ellis, A.E. (2001) The anatomy and physiology of teleosts. In *Fish Pathology*, 3rd Edition (Roberts, R.J., ed.), pp. 12–54. London: Harcourt Publishers.

Stetter, M. (2005) Laparoscopic and laser techniques in fish. North American Veterinary Conference Proceedings, Orlando, FL, January 8–12.

Stoskopf, M.K. (1993) Fish histology. In *Fish Medicine* (Stoskopf, M.K., ed.), pp. 31–47. Philadelphia: W.B. Saunders.

Wildgoose, W.H. (2000) Fish surgery: an overview. *Fish Veterinary Journal* **5**: 22–36.

Wildgoose, W.H. (2001) Skin disease. In *BSAVA Manual of Ornamental Fish*, 2nd Edition (Wildgoose, W.H., ed.), pp. 109–122. Gloucester: BSAVA.

World Small Animal Veterinary Association (WSAVA). (1999) *Microchip Implantation Sites Update—October 1999*. WSAVA. www.wsava.org/site1099.htm (accessed January 2, 2009).

Chapter 19

Necropsy of Fish

Drury Reavill

Introduction

As many of the problems with fish health are related to water quality and other husbandry issues, a necropsy is only one part of a complete evaluation in order to determine the entire disease process. Many of the issues with water quality and husbandry practices may not result in direct identifiable pathology. However, the combination of these issues with the findings of a complete post mortem will help identify all the factors associated with morbidity and/or mortality.

History

A good postmortem examination of a fish requires a thorough history of the animal. This type of history is the same as that used in clinical cases. The owner should be questioned as to past and current husbandry practices, possible changes in the external environment, the numbers and types of other animals housed with the fish in question, and the clinical appearance before the fish either died or was euthanized. See Chapter 14 for information and the questions used in taking a thorough history.

Selection and handling

For best results, a complete fish necropsy should utilize a moribund or appropriately selected fish for humane euthanasia. A live fish gives the practitioner a chance to evaluate the fish's behavior for any possible neurological clinical signs and for color changes or other lesions on the external surface, which may not be evident after death. As with the

basic diagnostics in evaluating a clinical case, it is recommended that a gill biopsy, skin scrape, and fin exfoliative cytology be collected on this live specimen. Protozoal parasites, particularly protozoa that are poorly attached to the external surface of the fish, will be adversely affected by euthanasia and death of their host (Callahan and Noga, 2002). In a population of fish, several individuals should be evaluated. Choosing fish at various stages of the disease process will help identify the primary problem from the secondary complications.

The practitioner should be prepared to perform the complete postmortem examination. Although fresh dead fish (less than 6 hours and kept refrigerated) can provide some useful information, the rapid autolysis will result in difficulty interpreting any bacterial cultures and will degrade the quality of the histological samples (Noga, 1996). Fish decompose more quickly than mammals, precluding the shipping of the body to a laboratory for a necropsy. It is possible to freeze the fish; however, this also results in tissue degradation and possible misinterpretation of any lesions (Westenend, 2004).

Postmortem equipment

The equipment suggested for a complete postmortem includes a digital camera, microscope, glass slides, coverslips, scalpel blades and handles of various sizes, surgical-quality curved and straight scissors, tissue forceps and hemostats, rongeurs and bone-cutting shears, needle and syringe, sampling materials for microbiological pathogens, and sample containers with the fixative of choice. A reference book with a description of normal

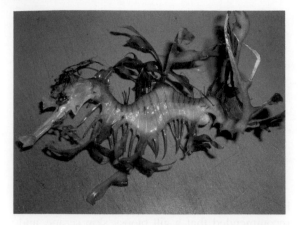

Fig. 19.1 A formalin-fixed leafy sea dragon (*Phycodurus eques*) submitted for examination. Note the unusual anatomy.

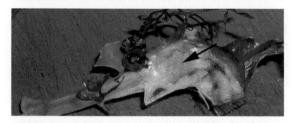

Fig. 19.2 The head of the dragon from Figure 19.1. The operculum has been removed and the arrow marks the location of the gills.

anatomical structures may prove helpful (Figs. 19.1 and 19.2).

Blood

Once examination of the live fish is completed, the fish can be anesthetized and then humanely euthanized for evaluation. Many anesthetic solutions can be used for euthanasia either by an overdose and/or by increasing the exposure period. Blood samples should be collected when the fish is anesthetized or immediately after death. The procedure and sites for collection are described in Chapter 17. It will be difficult to get a blood draw from external sites after death. Blood smears should be made immediately. Be aware that reference ranges may not exist for many fish, making interpretation complicated.

Radiographs

Radiographs are also very useful for a postmortem examination before you cut into the body cavity. As with mammals, two views are suggested (lateral and dorsoventral), especially to evaluate the swim bladder. Radiographs can help pinpoint lesions of the skeletal system that may not be evident on gross examination. See Chapter 17 for more information on diagnostic imaging.

Photographs

With many of the diverse fish forms and disease processes, it is not always obvious what structures represent actual lesions. Taking photographs as you perform the necropsy will help both the pathologist performing the histological examination and the practitioner when trying to correlate the histology findings with the gross pathology and clinical presentation. The first images should be for identification of the case; they should include the fish and any case identification. Before opening the fish, document any external lesions. Once the body has been opened, carefully evaluate and photograph the arrangement of the organs within the coelomic cavity. Extensive pathology such as tumors or severe inflammatory lesions of the coelom may obscure or distort organ systems. As samples are collected, label and photograph all abnormalities.

Cultures

Cultures can be collected for both bacterial and fungal isolates. Most fungal organisms will be evident grossly on the external surfaces, and these can be tentatively identified by cytology pending culture results. Determining the pathogenic bacteria involved with external lesions may be difficult. If cultures are collected after anesthesia or euthanasia, be aware that there may be alterations in culture growth, especially if high concentrations of tricaine methanesulfonate (MS-222) was used (Fedewa and Lindell, 2005). For superficial lesions, it may be prudent to collect the sample as early as possible before death. With frayed fins, cut off a section and put it directly on culture media. Samples from skin lesions can be prepped with a 1:10 chlorhexidine scrub, rinsed, and then cultured deep into the wound. After death, open lesions should be seared, and a piece of the tissue excised and inoculated onto media. Some fish pathogens may require extended incubations (3–6 weeks).

For cultures of internal organs, there are several approaches. A culture of the brain should be considered in a fish with neurological clinical signs. Using an alcohol prep, disinfect the dorsal surface of the head, on the midline and slightly caudal to the eyes. Cut into the brain with a sterile blade and collect the culture.

In cases of suspected systemic infections, a culture from the posterior kidney will generally identify the pathogen. To avoid contamination that can occur when the coelomic cavity is opened, cut off the dorsal fin, sear the fish at the site of the dorsal fin, cut perpendicular to spine with a sterilized pair of scissors, and break the spine, exposing the kidney. The posterior kidney will be sitting ventral to the spine. The kidney can also be approached after the lateral body wall has been removed to examine the internal organs. Coelomic cavity fluid and fluid accumulating around the heart are also good samples to consider. Bacterial isolates from the liver and spleen may also represent systemic pathogens.

For practices with a heavy case load, running cultures in-house can be considered. However, the setup, and in some cases the special media, may not be a sound investment if the case load is low. Consulting with an outside laboratory about their willingness to work with aquatic animal cultures before submitting samples is prudent.

Cytology

Impression smears are very helpful in both the biopsy and necropsy situations. Any additional information that can be obtained will be useful in refining the differential diagnosis list. In general, before the fish is dead, collect and examine cytology preparations of the gills, skin, and any lesions on the fins. These should be examined immediately while any protozoa are still moving to help with identification. The specific techniques are described in Chapter 17.

At postmortem, cytology samples from the organs, any fluids, and mass lesions should be collected and examined. Masses, gastrointestinal contents, swim bladder, and coelomic cavity or pericardial fluid can be aspirated with an appropriately sized needle and syringe and expelled onto a glass slide for direct or stained examination. Remember to make multiple slides, as several stains may be considered, including modified Wright's, Gram's, and acid-fast stains. Scraping the cut surface of firm masses may be necessary to obtain cells for examination. Impression smears are useful, especially in postmortem samples. There is an additional classic form of cytology preparation that is valuable for rapid diagnosis at postmortem examination of fish. This is the tissue squash method. Cut small samples of the liver, intestines, or kidney, place on a slide, and gently squash with a coverslip. These are examined as wet mount preparations or can be stained. Parasites, granulomas, and melanomacrophage centers (MMCs) are the most common findings with this method. MMCs are present in the liver, kidney, and spleen. Cytologically, they are nodular masses of brown to black cells that are large round to polyhedral. The cytoplasmic pigment, which ranges from brown to black, is within a foamy cytoplasm. The exact function of the MMCs is not completely determined, but they are suspected to be involved with antigen processing (Agius and Roberts, 2003) (Fig. 19.3).

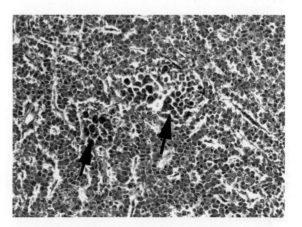

Fig. 19.3 Histology of melanomacrophage centers (shown by arrows) in the liver. H&E stain.

Toxicology

For toxicological evaluation, the first step to take is to identify the potential toxin. Most toxicities are due to deficiencies in the husbandry, and water conditions and may be identified during anamnesis (Roberts and Palmeiro, 2008). For toxins introduced into the system, a consultation with a toxicologist or the product manufacturer is suggested in order to collect the appropriate samples. Some toxins have target organs and specific requirements as to collection and storage. For some toxins, it may not be possible to collect appropriate samples, as either the animals may not have enough tissue for the tests currently available or these toxins may have already been degraded and can no longer can be measured. In general, collect sections of liver, kidney, fat, stomach contents, a section of the brain, and serum. These can be held frozen until more specific information is obtained. Generally, with toxic exposures in fish, there are multiple animals affected, and it is suggested that dead specimens that are not appropriate for histological evaluation be held frozen for further toxicological or other testing. There are some toxins, such as heavy or toxic metals (lead, copper, zinc, iron, cadmium, and arsenic), that can be evaluated from formalin-fixed tissues, if this clinical information of exposure comes after the samples have been collected and shipped to a pathologist (Anderson, 1996). Again, early communication is important in order to have the appropriate sample held and submitted for such analysis.

Parasitology

The most common parasitology procedure will be to evaluate for external protozoan or metazoan organisms on the moribund, but still living, fish. Again, it might be important to test before the fish is anesthetized or sedated, as this can affect the protozoal organisms, making them more difficult to identify (Callahan and Noga, 2002). Collection is in the same manner as that in antemortem diagnostics.

After the fish has been opened, if there are grossly identifiable parasites within the coelomic cavity, these should be collected. A direct smear and/or a wet mount can be performed on the gastrointestinal contents to evaluate for any parasites, both metazoan and protozoan. Having a relationship with a parasitologist and knowing how they would like the samples preserved is helpful when confronted with the plethora of parasites that can be found on fish. In general, nematodes should be preserved in 70% ethanol. Parasites in tissue sections can be processed for histology to be evaluated either by the pathologist or sent out for secondary consultation with a parasitologist.

Additional means for identification can include electron microscopy or polymerase chain reaction (PCR) techniques. Although specimens preserved in glutaraldehyde for electron microscopy and frozen sections for PCR are preferred, it is also possible to run these diagnostic procedures from the paraffin-embedded, formalin-fixed tissue. Tissues held wet in formalin may be too degraded for accurate results (Wacharapluesadee et al., 2006).

Virology

In general, tissue samples can be held frozen or in medium such as Hanks' balanced salt solution (HBSS) for virus isolation. For viral diseases or other etiologies that may have PCR diagnostics available, collect representative organ samples, such as gill, liver, or section of the kidney, and preserve those as directed by the laboratories that can run these particular diagnostics. It is helpful to periodically confirm the current diagnostic techniques for some of the more important pathogens such as koi herpesvirus and spring viremia of carp (a reportable disease) and post the protocols for sampling in the necropsy area (Miller et al. 2007).

General approach

Primarily, due to the rapid autolysis of dead fish, most, if not all, postmortems will be performed in-house. One of the most important factors to consider when performing a fish necropsy is to be consistent in your necropsy protocol from collection to handling. Whatever format you choose, do it the same way each time! If you get into a routine, you reduce the chance of missing lesions or forgetting to collect an important sample.

To ensure death, sever the vertebral column from the head once it is determined that the fish appears dead (no opercular movements). This will be the appropriate time to collect measurements that may be important later on. Measure the fish from snout to tail base and from snout to tip of tail and get a body weight.

Placing the fish in right lateral recumbency, the incision to open the body cavity for a most fish is along the midline of the ventrum from just in front of the cloacal or anal opening to the level of the gills at the point where the opercula are at their ventral aspect. From here, the incision is up along the operculum dorsally and then rounding out along the vertebral column caudally to curve down back to the original incision in front of the anus. The lateral body wall is then lifted gently from the underlying organs, attempting to prevent contamination of the organs and distortion of their arrangement. In this orientation, the spleen should be evident on the left side of the body, closely associated with the stomach.

Many of the small fish, particularly those coming from hobbyist aquariums, can be difficult to evaluate without some magnification (Fig. 19.4). The necropsy protocols will be similar as described for larger animals. The coelomic cavity is carefully opened along the midline, and bacterial cultures can be collected from the hematopoietic kidney. Once the coelomic cavity has been examined, the entire fish can be placed in buffered 10% formalin. In a disease outbreak with multiple fish involved, select representative fish for fixation in formalin and hold other fish frozen for other diagnostics.

After cultures have been collected, representative samples of the organs are harvested and preserved in 10% buffered formalin at 1 cm thickness to allow adequate fixation. The size of the tissue collected and preserved in formalin does matter. Formalin penetrates tissue at approximately 0.2 cm in 24 hours, so your tissue sections should be no thicker than 1 cm. Opening a tubular organ enhances formalin penetration. Formalin preservation is slower in very bloody, dense tissue such as a congested spleen or liver. As the tissues are collected for histological preservation, samples should also be collected for cytology. Aspirates of the gastrointestinal tract, cystic structures, or the swim bladder are suggested. Wet mounts or squash preparation are recommended from all identifiable organs (Fig. 19.5) It is important to also remember to collect sections of the gills,

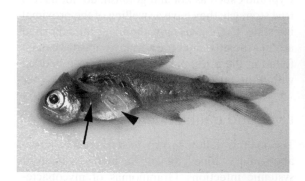

Fig. 19.4 Magnification is suggested for examination of small aquarium fish, such as this 3-cm-long black neon tetra (*Hyphessobrycon herbertaxelrodi*). The fish has significant loss of body condition, with muscle wasting and no coelomic cavity fat. The arrow head marks the swim bladder pulled away from the body and the arrow marks the liver.

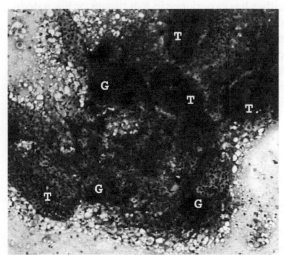

Fig. 19.5 Squash preparation of a kidney from a goldfish. Renal tubules and glomeruli are supported in a background of dense cellularity, the hematopoietic cells of the kidney. T, tubules; G, glomeruli. May-Grunwald–Giemsa stain. 10× objective.

part of the body wall, particularly in areas where there may be lesions, and sections of fins, especially those involved with lesions. Remember that some fish have a urinary bladder, and try to include this sample with your necropsy tissues.

The brain can be difficult to access; however, by using large shears or sturdy necropsy scissors, the brain cavity can be opened by placing the lower blade into the oral cavity of the fish, directing it ventrally with the upper blade along the midline on the dorsum of the head of the fish. By cutting down and adding a slight twist, this, in many fish, will break open the braincase, allowing access to the central nervous system. The eyes can also have significant pathology, and if an eye lesion had been noted on antemortem examination, the eye should be collected and placed in formalin. It is advised to carefully remove the globe intact, as rupturing the globe can complicate processing by the pathology lab.

If the tissues need to be cleaned for proper evaluation or for photographs, use physiological saline as a rinse. Tissue specimens are sensitive to hydrostatic and osmotic pressures. Rinsing specimens with tap water may cause histomorphological artifacts.

Fixed tissues and cytology preparations should be submitted for evaluation to a pathologist who either has experience in fish tissues or has a dedicated interest in learning. Properly label all containers. It is also helpful to identify organs and place them in labeled cassettes. Cassettes should be marked with a lead pencil or special histology markers, as tissue processing steps will remove ink.

Important features of internal organs

Swim bladder

This is the glistening white sac in the retroperitoneal dorsal body cavity, just ventral to the kidney, and can have one or two chambers depending on the species. The swim bladder is used as an equilibrium-ballast device (buoyancy control). The cichlid family, physoclists, regulate amount of gas in the swim bladder by using one or more countercurrent capillary beds (rete mirabile) located in the wall of the swim bladder. Physostomous fish (such as koi) have a pneumatic duct and will swallow air. Some bottom-dwelling fish do not have swim bladders. Metazoan and protozoan parasites may be found encapsulated or free-living in the swim bladder.

Gonads

The gonads will vary in size with the breeding condition of the fish. The reproductive organs are ribbonlike strips that lie just ventral to the swim bladder. The testes are generally white and smooth, close to the distal portion of the large intestine. In the gravid female, the eggs will fill a major portion of the coelomic cavity. Primary diseases of the gonads are rare. Some systemic diseases caused by mycobacteria or nocardia, or systemic fungal (*Ichthyophonus*) infections may involve the gonads.

Gastrointestinal tract

The digestive tract is similar to mammals, with the length depending on diet type (herbivores, carnivores, or omnivores). Herbivorous fish tend to have longer intestines than carnivores. In some species there are extensions of the pyloric portion of the stomach called pyloric cecae. These are blind sacs used for digestion and absorption. Cyprinids, such as koi and goldfish, do not have a true stomach; they have a swelling of the proximal intestine. There is usually abundant fat deposited around the intestinal tract. Many parasites can be found in the intestinal tract as well as embedded within the fat surrounding the intestines.

Liver and gallbladder

The liver is yellow-brown to dark red in coloration and is lobed. It will be involved in most systemic infections. Granulomas of mycobacterium, encysted nematodes, and metacercariae of digenetic trematodes may be found in the liver. MMCs can be prominent. The gallbladder is a saclike structure embedded in the liver tissue. It may be small or large depending on the species and whether the fish has eaten or not. Aspiration and cytology should be considered, as protozoa can sometimes be found in the gall bladder.

Spleen

The spleen is usually bright red in color, species-dependent in shape, and located near the fundic portion of the stomach. In fish subject to chronic stress, increased numbers of MMCs can be seen on cytology. The spleen is also the site for granulomas.

Heart

The heart is a two-chambered organ, although there are four divisions; the sinus venosus, atrium, ventricle, and bulbous arteriosus. It is located cranial to the liver and adjacent to the gills (in the "throat" of the animal). Cysts of tapeworms, intermediates, and nematodes and granulomas can be seen in the heart.

Kidneys

The kidney is divided into two unique portions: the head or anterior kidney and the posterior kidney. The head kidney, located dorsally and caudal to the gill arches, is the major lymphoid and hematopoietic organ of the fish. The posterior kidney is located dorsal to the swim bladder and is the site of renal excretion and adrenal hormone secretion (interrenal tissue). The kidney is the organ of choice for isolating bacteria from systemic infections.

Glands

The majority of the glandular tissues of fish may only be detectable histologically except for the thymus. Thymic tissue is located in the dorsal commissure of the operculum. The analogs for the adrenal gland, of interrenal cells and chromaffin cells, are found in the kidney. Exocrine and endocrine pancreas can be found throughout the mesentery or may be part of the liver and/or spleen. Thyroid tissue is usually identified around the ventral aorta but can also be identified in the kidney, spleen, and occasionally, the mesenteries.

Zoonotic diseases

As with all postmortem examinations, care should be taken to prevent exposure to potential zoonotic pathogens. With fish, these are primarily bacterial infections. Aeromonads, *Vibrio* sp., and *Edwardsiella tarda* can infect the skin as well as result in gastroenteritis. Mycobacterium, which is not an uncommon bacterial infection of many fish, is the cause of "fish-tank granulomas," a chronic infection usually limited to the fingers and hands (Passantino et al., 2008).

References

Agius, C. and Roberts, R.J. (2003) Melano-macrophage centres and their role in fish pathology. *Journal of Fish Diseases* **26** (9): 499–509.

Anderson, K.A. (1996) A micro-digestion and analysis method for determining macro and micro elements in plant tissues by inductively coupled plasma atomic emission spectrometry. *Atomic Spectrous* **1**: 30–33.

Callahan, H.A. and Noga, E.J. (2002) Tricaine dramatically reduces the ability to diagnose protozoan ectoparasite (*Ichthyobodo necator*) infections. *Journal of Fish Diseases* **25** (7): 433–437.

Fedewa, L.A. and Lindell, A. (2005) Inhibition of growth for select gram-negative bacteria by tricaine methane sulfonate (MS-222). *Journal of Herpetological Medicine and Surgery* **15** (1): 13–17.

Miller, O., Fuller, F.J., Gebreyes, W.A., et al. (2007) Phylogenetic analysis of spring viremia of carp virus reveals distinct subgroups with common origins for recent isolates in North America and the UK. *Diseases of Aquatic Organisms* **76** (3): 193–204.

Noga, E.J. (1996) *Fish Disease: Diagnosis and Treatment*. St. Louis. MO: Mosby.

Passantino, A., Macrì, D., Coluccio, P., et al. (2008) Importation of mycobacteriosis with ornamental fish: medico-legal implications. *Travel Medicine and Infectious Diseases* **6** (4): 240–244.

Roberts, H. and Palmeiro, B.S. (2008) Toxicology of aquarium fish. *Veterinary Clinics of North America: Exotic Animal Practice* **11** (2): 359–374.

Wacharapluesadee, S., Ruangvejvorachai, P., and Hemachudha, T. (2006) A simple method for detection of rabies viral sequences in 16-year old archival brain specimens with one-week fixation in formalin. *Journal of Virological Methods* **134** (1–2): 267–271.

Westenend, P.J. (2004) Incidental freezing artifacts in sentinel lymph node biopsies masquerading as lymphangiography artifacts. *Journal of Clinical Pathology* **57**: 670–672.

Chapter 20
Neoplasia in Fish

Drury Reavill

Introduction

Neoplastic diseases occur with some frequency in fish, both in wild populations and captive animals. However, published information regarding prognosis and therapy of specific neoplasms in the pet fish population is limited. With the increasing use of veterinarians by the fish-owning public to provide disease diagnosis and therapy options, the pool of information should improve. This review will cover some basic tumor information and will reference the few reports of neoplastic diseases in privately owned fish (Table 20.1). A brief mention of the tumors recognized in wild and commercially important populations, as well as those fish used as models for tumor development, will be provided. Many excellent reviews cover tumor formation in commercially important fish as well as in those developed for tumor models (Schlumberger and Lucke, 1948; Mearns and Sherwood, 1978; Harshbarger, 1984, 2001; Hawkins et al., 1985; Harshbarger and Clark, 1990; Stoletov and Klemke, 2008).

General diagnostics

There are several diagnostic methods to consider when faced with a fish for examination. Detailed discussions are to be found in other chapters in this book. When presented with a mass lesion, either on the surface or identified by radiographs or ultrasound, an exfoliative cytology can be a rapid and reasonably safe diagnostic test.

For most external masses, aspiration cytology can be done during an office visit. This usually provides an in-house evaluation to differentiate inflammatory lesions from neoplasia. However, fish tumors may have a prominent inflammatory response, and neoplastic cell determination may prove problematic. Benign neoplasia can be virtually indistinguishable from that of tissue hyperplasia. The cells in both benign or hyperplastic lesions are immature, exhibit cytoplasmic basophilia, and have pale vesicular nuclei. With malignant neoplasms, the sample may be highly cellular, with loss of normal cell-to-cell interactions in malignancy. Neoplastic cells tend to be highly polymorphic, and there will be marked variations in nuclear size and nucleus-to-cytoplasm ratios. Some malignancies will have a high mitotic index and the cell nuclei may have irregular chromatin (coarse, hypochromatic, irregularly clumped).

If an apparent inflammatory lesion fails to respond with adequate therapy, the lesion should be reassessed and a biopsy for histological examination considered. In fish, granulomatous diseases can closely mimic tumors. This difficulty in correctly classifying lesions as inflammatory versus neoplasms is a more common occurrence in fish than in mammals (Harshbarger, 1984; Groff, 2004).

Radiographic studies with or without contrast are useful in evaluating the degree of organ involvement, searching for metastases, and providing important information about the integrity of adjacent tissues. Computerized tomography and ultrasonography also are useful tools. All of these modalities can provide information about prognosis and can be used for guidance in obtaining an excisional or aspiration biopsy.

The definitive diagnosis usually relies on an appropriate biopsy. Performing an excisional

Table 20.1 Tumors of pet fish.

Tumor	Location	Fish	Reference
Erythrophoroma	Cornea	Goldfish	Groff (2004)
Fibroma	Cornea	Goldfish	Lewbart (1998)
Fibroma	Cornea	Goldfish	Lewbart (1998)
Branchioblastoma	Gill	Koi	Wildgoose and Bucke (1995)
Adenocarcinoma	Intestines	Koi	Lewbart (1998)
Adenoma	Kidney	Oscar	Gumpenberger et al. (2004)
Mesonephric duct adenoma	Kidney	Oscar	Lewbart (1998)
Hepatoma	Liver	Koi	Garland et al. (2002)
Lip fibroma	Oral cavity	Freshwater angelfish	Francis-Floyd et al. (1993)
Papilloma	Oral cavity	Koi	Lewbart (1998)
Ovarian granulosa-theca cell tumor	Ovary	Koi	Lewbart (1998)
Ovarian tumor	Ovary	Koi	Raidal et al. (2006); Ishikawa et al. (1976); Ishikawa and Takayama (1978)
Adenocarcinoma	Pancreas	Goldfish	Lewbart (1998)
Adenocarcinoma	Renal collecting ducts	Oscar	Petervary et al. (1996)
Hemangioma	Retrobulbar	Goldfish	O'Hagan and Raidal (2006)
Chromatophoroma	Skin	Butterfly fish	Okihiro (1988)
Chromatophoroma	Skin	*Corydoras* catfish	Noga (1996)
Erythrophoroma	Skin	Koi	Murchelano and Edwards (1981)
Erythrophoroma	Skin	Goldfish	Harshbarger (2001)
Erythrophoroma	Skin	Platyfish (*Platypoecilus maculates* var. rubra)	Ghadially and Whiteley (1951)
Fibroma	Skin	Common carp (*Cyprinus carpio*)	Manier et al. (1984)
Fibroma	Skin	Goldfish	Finkelstein (2002)
Fibrosarcoma	Skin	Goldfish	Ahmed and Egusa (1980)
Papilloma	Skin	Goldfish	Lewbart (1998)
Squamous cell carcinoma	Skin and liver	Hybrid sunfish	Fitzgerald et al. (1991)
Malignant lymphoma	Skin, frontal dome	*Pseudotropheus* cichlid	Lewbart (1998)
PNST	Skin/subcutaneous	Goldfish	Harshbarger (2001)
PNST	Skin/subcutaneous	Buffalo sculpin.	Miller (2000)
Disgerminomas, seminomas, leiomyomas, and Sertoli cell tumors	Testes	Carp hybrids	Granado-Lorencio et al. (1987)
Seminoma	Testes	Black sea bass	Weisse et al. (2002)
Thymic lymphoma	Thymus	Black fin pearl fish	Harshbarger (2001)
Carcinoma	Urinary bladder	Oscar	Harshbarger (2001)
Papillary cystadenoma	Urinary bladder	Oscar	Harshbarger (2001)

PNST = peripheral nerve sheath tumors.

biopsy can also be an important part of the treatment, as the tumor may be completely removed by the procedure or will at least be debulked prior to exploring other forms of therapy. For fish, surgical removal of tumor masses, even if only partially resected, can provide a significant improvement in the quality of life.

Tumors of skin and soft tissues

Papillomas

Papillomas are one of the most common cutaneous neoplasms reported in both wild and captive fish (Schlumberger and Lucke, 1948; Roberts,

1989; Noga, 1996). These are similar to papillomas described in other species. In fish, they are generally benign with a discrete growth. Papillary formations are raised soft to firm growths that may have a narrow to broad base or pedicle, as well as presenting a slightly raised flat cutaneous plaques. These may appear anywhere on the fish body. Lesions around the mouth and growths on the head can interfere with feeding and breathing. Some papillomas, such as smelt papillomatosis, have been associated with Cowdry-type herpesvirus intranuclear inclusions (Anders and Möller, 1985). It is felt that while papillomas may have a primary viral etiology, there is usually chronic trauma or irritation to the integument that leads to development of the lesion.

In koi, there is a virally induced cutaneous papilloma (Fig. 20.1). This is commonly called carp pox and may appear as milky white epidermal proliferative lesions that have a candle-waxlike appearance. This particular lesion is caused by a temperature-sensitive herpesvirus. As the water temperature rises, the papilloma cells containing the virus particles will lyse, and an inflammatory response is produced, and these tumors will slough. During the cold season, these infected epidermal cells will start to proliferate again. This is considered a hyperplastic lesion, although some feel this is a neoplastic change. These lesions have progressed to form large squamous cell carcinomas in some conditions (Wildgoose, 1992; Harschbarger, 2001).

Occasionally, the term epithelioma is found in the literature (Schlumberger and Lucke, 1948; Rosskopf et al., 1985; Lewbart, 1998). This is described as a benign tumor arising from epithelial cells. When reviewed, it appears that these lesions may represent squamous papillomas or, in the more invasive lesions, squamous cell carcinomas (Schlumberger and Lucke, 1948).

Squamous cell carcinoma

Squamous cell carcinomas, which are neoplastic proliferations of the squamous epithelial cells, have been reported in individual pet fish as well as in wild populations. There is no site predilection. These tumors can present grossly similar to papillomas and may originate from papillomatous lesions. Some tumors are infiltrative and will have associated erosion and ulceration of the skin, with frequent involvement of the underlying subcutaneous tissues. In a hybrid sunfish, there was a metastatic tumor within the liver (Fitzgerald et al., 1991).

Chromatophoromas (pigment cell tumors)

These tumors, which are common on some species, arise from the specialized pigment-producing cell and generally exhibit the color of the cell of origin (Fig. 20.2). For example, melanomas are black, whereas iridophoromas are silver, erythrophoromas are red, and xanthophoromas are typically orange. These can be multicolored because the neoplastic pigment cells may differentiate into several pigment phenotypes. Generally, pigment tumors are all classified as chromatoblastomas, as without electron microscopy or further studies, it may not be possible to definitively identify all the populations of pigment-producing neoplastic cells.

Melanomas are best studied in the platy cross swordtail hybrids. These crosses will selectively eliminate the suppressor genes that regulate

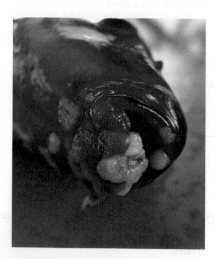

Fig. 20.1 The white, proliferative mass on the head of this koi is a papilloma, consistent with the papillomas induced by a herpesvirus (photo courtesy of Walt Oldenburg).

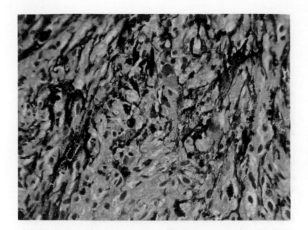

Fig. 20.2 A malignant chromatophoroma from a koi. Note the brown pigmentation in the neoplastic cell. H&E stain. 40× objective.

the activated pigment oncogene carried by the platy. Melanomas arise spontaneously in the offspring (Roberts, 1989). These tumors can also be induced by exposure to ultraviolet (UV) light or carcinogenic chemicals (Masahito et al., 1989; Roberts, 1989). The primary differential for these pigmented tumors is the inflammatory response to metacercariae of trematode parasites. The parasites will induce proliferation of melanophores, resulting in a black color to the lesion.

Erythrophoromas are reported as the most common type of pigmented tumor of goldfish and koi (Murchelano and Edwards, 1981; Masahito et al., 1989; Harshbarger, 2001). They are focal to multifocal cutaneous proliferative skin masses. In general, these neoplasms are benign but can be locally invasive and may recur without complete surgical excision (Groff, 2004). A more invasive erythrophoroma is briefly described in a red platyfish (*Platypoecilus maculatus* var. *rubra*) (Ghadially and Whiteley, 1951). Chromatophoromas have also been identified on two species of Hawaiian butterfly fish (Okihiro, 1988). The tumors from the brown-barred butterfly fish (*Chaetodon multicinctus*) were predominantly iridophoromas, and those of the lemon butterfly fish (*Chaetodon miliaris*) were melanophoromas. Both species also had mixed chromatophoromas. *Corydoras* catfish have also been listed as developing chromatophoromas (Noga, 1996).

Mesenchymal tumors

Spindle cell tumors

Fibromas generally have a discrete, expansile growth and are composed of dense collagen and neoplastic fibrocytes. Some may mineralize, giving these a hard, gritty texture (Manier et al., 1984; Harshbarger, 2001). These tumors can become large, and if they become ulcerated, removal is recommended. Complete surgical removal is expected to be curative (Lewbart, 1998; Finkelstein, 2002).

Spindle cell sarcomas are a broad category of variably differentiated tumors characterized by elongated to spindle-shaped cells arranged in streaming to interlacing bundles. Fibrosarcomas, peripheral nerve sheath tumors (PNSTs), pigment cell tumors (chromatophoromas), and leiomyosarcomas (rare in fish) can all have a similar histological appearance. In other species, immunohistochemistry and electron microscopy can help determine specific classification. Fortunately, the behavior for all the spindle cell sarcomas is similar. They are locally aggressive but have a variable growth rate.

The tumors morphologically consistent with fibrosarcomas are invasive, firm masses that may disfigure the fish. Fibrosarcomas and other mesenchymal sarcomas are associated with viral infections and chemical agents in wild and laboratory fish (Schwab et al., 1978; Roberts, 1989; Kazianis et al., 2001). These are also commonly described tumors of pet fish, particularly goldfish and koi (Schlumberger and Lucke, 1948; Ahmed and Egusa, 1980; Clyde et al., 1995; Lewbart, 1998; Groff, 2004). There have been no reports on a possible viral or chemical agent responsible for their development in this population of fish. At this time, surgical debulking or removal, if possible, is the treatment of choice (Clyde et al., 1995).

Myxosarcoma is a variation of a fibrosarcoma that has abundant glycosaminoglycans widely separating the individual neoplastic cells. These tumors are locally aggressive and have the potential to metastasize, although they are rarely reported in fish (Schlumberger and Lucke, 1948).

Peripheral Nerve Sheath Tumors (PNSTs)

Some authors have reported that neoplasms arising from the peripheral nerves are common in fish (Schlumberger, 1952, 1957). However, as previously discussed about spindle cell sarcomas, it is difficult to differentiate the different tumor types (fibrosarcomas, PNSTs, nonpigmented chromatophoromas, and some of the muscle tumors) without further testing and examination (Clyde et al., 1995). Further controversy exists concerning benign and malignant PNSTs. Classically, schwannoma (and the malignant version) is used when the tumor is solely derived from Schwann cells (these cells form the myelin sheath of nerve fibers). Neurofibroma/sarcoma is used to describe a tumor composed of Schwann cells and perineural cells. Unfortunately, even with immunohistochemistry, it has been difficult to determine the cell of origin. These tumor types will be lumped together and will be referred to as PNSTs.

PNSTs can be induced by chemical and viral agents in fish, and several species are used as tumor models (Schmale et al., 1994; Harshbarger and Slatick, 2001). They are commonly reported in goldfish and they appear to arise spontaneously (Schlumberger, 1952; Duncan and Harkin, 1969; Harshbarger 2001). There are rare reports of these tumors in other noncommercial fish. One case in a buffalo sculpin was successfully surgically removed (Miller, 2000). The tumor masses are generally present within the subcutaneous tissues and are firm.

Lipoma/liposarcoma

Lipomas are benign neoplasms arising of mature adipocytes. They can appear as single or multiple well-circumscribed masses generally within the dermal or hypodermal tissues. Rarely, they have been recognized within the liver and coelomic membranes (Harshbarger, 2001; Groff, 2004). Tumors within the dermis may present with a dermal ulceration due to the enlarging mass. Some lipomas may have areas of vascular (angiolipoma) or fibrous (fibrolipoma) tissue embedded with them (Harshbarger and Bane, 1969). The majority of reports in the literature have been in cultured fish, including a channel catfish, largemouth

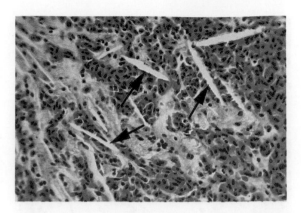

Fig. 20.3 An H&E-stained section through a cutaneous xanthoma from an eel. The arrows identify cholesterol crystals. 40× objective.

bass (Noga, 1996), Pacific halibut (Roberts, 1989), and brown bowhead (Hayes and Ferguson, 1989). Liposarcomas are not reported in the literature.

Xanthoma

Xanthomas are not neoplastic, although they are locally invasive mass lesions. The lesion has only rarely been described in fish. Internal masses in the mesentery were found in a wolf eel (*Anarrhichthys ocellatus*). Cutaneous xanthomatous lesions have been identified in two other eels, a California moray eel (*Gymnothorax mordax*) and a snowflake eel (*Echidna nebulosa*). The lesions in all three of the eels supported numerous acicular clefts (cholesterol clefts), surrounded by multinucleate giant cells, and a scattering of vacuolated macrophages (Fig. 20.3). Multiple xanthomas are suspected to be due to altered fat metabolism, and in species examined, they have had alterations in blood lipids and cholesterols (Reavill et al., 2006).

Tumors of the gills

Only rare spontaneous neoplasms have been reported involving the gills. These are primarily in commercially important fish. These rare tumors have been induced in medaka fish when exposed to N-methyl-N′-nitro-N-nitrosoguanidine (MGGN) (Brittelli et al., 1985). A spontaneous branchioblastoma was described in a koi (*Cyprinus carpio*) (Wildgoose and Bucke, 1995). The fish had been ill and had developed edema and bilateral exophthalmia. Firm masses were present in the dorsal area of the gills. Branchioblastoma is defined as a benign tumor of blast cells possibly arising from the connective tissue of the gills (Wildgoose and Bucke, 1995).

Tumors of hematopoietic origin

The hematopoietic organs of fish include the spleen, renal interstitium, and in some fish, the periportal areas of the liver, the intestinal submucosa, and the only specialized lymphoid organ, the thymus. Fish lack lymph nodes and bone marrow. The lymphoid, myeloid, and erythroid cell series are all derived from the pluripotent hematopoietic stem cells of the hematopoietic organs. The vast majority of tumors are derived from the lymphoid cell lines. Rare cases of granulocytic tumors (Anderson and Luther, 1987) and plasma cell tumors (Roberts, 1989) have been described.

Many different fish species of commercial value have been reported with these tumors, including tilapia, rainbow trout, pike, muskellunge, brook trout Atlantic salmon, grayling, coho salmon, and channel catfish (Hayes and Ferguson, 1989; Roberts, 1989). The lymphomas described in epizootic outbreaks in groups of pikes as well as muskellunge were associated with a retrovirus (Roberts, 1989). The neoplastic lesions were disseminated, and some fish were leukemic. The lymphomas of the northern pike originated on the head and mouth as well as the subcutaneous tissues before multiple foci were recognized in other organs. Another group of northern pike in the New York Aquarium developed tumors that originated in the kidney. The lymphomas from the muskellunge occurred primarily in the subcutaneous tissue, with subsequent identification in the liver, kidney, and spleen. The tumors apparently started within the skin as small nodules invading into the musculature and finally being identified in the spleen, liver, and kidney. The cellular morphology of the lymphomas were pleomorphic; primarily of highly undifferentiated blast cells, although immature lymphocytes could be identified. They commonly had the appearance of an inflammatory cellular response (Roberts, 1989).

Thymic-origin lymphoma has also been reported in salmonids, and the tumor is leukemic (Hayes and Ferguson, 1989). From a review of the lymphocytic neoplasms on file with the Registry of Tumors in Lower Animals, the salmonid group represents the largest and most diverse group of species affected with this tumor. However, salmonids are also the most extensively cultivated and examined.

It is curious that this particular tumor is uncommon in aquarium fish. A thymic lymphoma is briefly described in a black fin pearl fish. It presented as a large white mass protruding from the opercular cavity (Harshbarger, 2001). A male *Pseudotropheus* cichlid presented with an asymmetrical ulcerated swelling of the frontal dome, which on biopsy and cytology supported neoplastic lymphocytes. At postmortem examination, no other foci of malignant lymphoma were recognized (Lewbart, 1998). In cases examined by the author, lymphoma has only been identified in a blue gill and a walleye. In the walleye, it was involved with the thymus.

Tumors of the alimentary tract

Several tumors types have been described involving the oral tissues of fish. Neoplasms of tooth germ origin (odontomas, ameloblastomas) are reported in a variety of commercial fish (Schlumberger and Katz, 1956; Harshbarger et al., 1976; McAllister et al., 1978). In most cases, the masses distort the lips and dental plates. The tumors are generally a combination of variably differentiated tooth structures supported in dense fibrous connective tissue. Several authors have reported the lip fibromas of freshwater angelfish as odontomas or odontogenic hamartomas (Lewbart, 1998; Harshbarger, 2001; Groff, 2004). These particular growths are associated with retroviral-like particles within the stromal cells (Francis-Floyd et al., 1993). The proliferative masses, which affected the upper and lower lids along the mucocutaneous junction, are firm, multinodular, and elevated. Histologically, the growths are of dense fibrous connective tissue covered by a thickened stratified squamous epithelium and associated with immature teeth. The presence of these immature teeth and epithelial-lined crypts prompted the possible interpretation that these are odontogenic hamartomas. In one particular report, it was felt that the teeth were secondarily entrapped within the neoplastic lesions (Francis-Floyd et al., 1993). The therapy for affected pet fish is surgical debulking or removal. No tumor regrowth occurred with complete removal when followed for 12 months (Francis-Floyd et al., 1993). Given the association with the retrovirus, isolation from other angelfish is suggested.

Papillomas, which are lesions of hyperplastic epithelium supported on fibrovascular stromal cores, are described involving the oral cavity of many commercial fish (Schlumberger and Lucke, 1948; McAllister et al., 1978; Roberts, 1989). Many etiologies have been proposed as a cause for many of these papillomas, but it is felt that a combination of environmental factors and infectious agents of disease may best explain the lesions. One buccal cavity papilloma supported on a narrow stalk from the dorsal pharyngeal wall in a koi was successfully removed surgically (Lewbart, 1998). The fish presented as having difficulty eating.

Tumors of the liver are best described in commercial fish living in polluted environments (Roberts, 1989; Harshbarger and Clark, 1990). The hepatic tumors include those of hepatocyte origin (hepatomas and hepatocellular carcinoma) and those from the biliary epithelium (cholangioma, cholangiocarcinoma). Hepatocellular carcinomas are one of the few tumors that metastasize (Noga, 1996). Pancreatic and hepatic tumors have developed after exposure to chemical mutagens in several laboratory fish models (Hawkins et al., 1985; Fourni and Hawkins, 2002; Stoletov and Klemke, 2008). These tumors are rarely described in aquarium fish. A hepatoma was diagnosed with a computed tomographic (CT) scan and biopsy in an adult Japanese koi (C. carpio). The fish presented with an abdominal swelling and failure to thrive (Garland et al., 2002). Additional clinical signs associated with hepatic tumors include coelomic cavity fluid accumulation and edema of the scales (Lewbart, 1998).

Rare tumors of the alimentary tract are described. An asymmetrical abdominal swelling in a koi was due to an adenocarcinoma in the intestines (Lewbart, 1998). Adenocarcinomas of the pancreas will also distend the coelomic cavity of goldfish (Lewbart, 1998; Harshbarger, 2001).

Reproductive system

The tumors of the testes can arise from germ cells (seminoma, teratoma) or sex-cord stromal elements (Leydig or interstitial ell tumors and Sertoli cell tumors). Testicular tumors reported in fish are rare but include Sertoli cell neoplasms in cyprinids (Leatherland and Sonstegard, 1978) and seminomas in African lungfish and sea bass. African lungfish have been overrepresented with seminomas in the literature (Masahito et al., 1984; Hubbard and Fletcher, 1985; Roberts, 1989). The lesions were of smooth encapsulated nodules and located within the mid-testes. Sheets of large neoplastic spermatocytes and eosinophilic cells with large nuclei infiltrated into the normal tissue were identified. The most important clinical sign noted of these tumor masses were of coelomic cavity distention and adjacent compression of organs. Possibly, due to the popularity of these fish, goldfish and carp hybrids appear to have a high incidence of gonadal tumors (Hayes and Ferguson, 1989; Noga 1996; Harshbarger, 2001). A wild population of carp hybrids (Carassius carassius × C. carpio) developed a significant number of testicular tumors (Granado-Lorencio et al., 1987). The tumors identified in these fish include disgerminomas, seminomas, leiomyomas, Sertoli cell tumors, and spermatocytic seminomas. The result was many of the fish died during spawning, resulting in a significant reduction in the population in this reservoir. There is a report of a surgical removal of a seminoma from a black sea bass (Centropristis striata) (Weisse et al., 2002). This fish presented with the typical clinical signs of a gonadal tumor with coelomic cavity distention. Positive contrast radiography was used to confirm that the mass was not within the gastrointestinal tract. No tumor regrowth was noted at least 8 weeks after surgical removal.

Ovarian neoplasms have been induced in laboratory fish exposed to chemicals (Roberts, 1989). In ornamental koi, gonadal neoplasms occur with

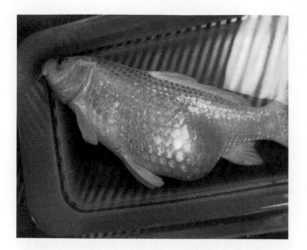

Fig. 20.4 Coelomic cavity distension in a female koi (photo courtesy of Dr. Helen Roberts).

some frequency and do not appear to be associated with toxic exposures (Ishikawa et al., 1976; Ishikawa and Takayama, 1978; Groff, 2004). These neoplasms are common in sexually mature female koi. They appear to originate from the ovary, although generally, at the time of diagnosis they are large poorly differentiated tumors, and the cellular origin is often difficult to determine (Raidal et al., 2006). These fish will present with coelomic distention, ascites, and subcutaneous edema (Lewbart, 1998; Groff, 2004) (Fig. 20.4). The tumors will be located in the dorsal caudal coelomic cavity. The difficulty in identifying these tumors early is that, during breeding season, koi fish will commonly appear distended. These tumors can become large, and some have resulted in the rupture of the body wall (Ishikawa et al., 1976; Groff, 2004). Successful surgical removal has been described (Raidal et al., 2006).

Urinary system

Tumors arising from within the urinary system are uncommon in fish. In commercial fish, nephroblastomas are described in many species, including rainbow trout, smelt, Japanese eel, and striped bass (Hayes and Ferguson, 1989; Roberts, 1989; Groff, 2004). These arise from pluripotent embryonal cells and are composed of variable amounts of epithelial and fibrous and/or cartilaginous components.

Oscars (*Astronotus* sp.) seem to commonly develop renal tumors. An adenocarcinoma developed in the collecting ducts of an oscar (Petervary et al., 1996). A renal adenoma was diagnosed in a red oscar and was evaluated by radiographic, ultrasonographic, and CT examination. This tumor resulted in abdominal swelling, and the diagnosis was made at necropsy (Gumpenberger et al., 2004). Urinary bladder tumors are also more commonly identified in oscars, which will present with a swollen abdomen, prolapsing of tissues of the anus, and lethargy. The mass is generally retroperitoneal in the caudal abdomen. It will appear cystic, with brown to yellow fluid. Histologically, most tumors are papillary cystadenomas and carcinomas of the urinary bladder epithelium (Harshbarger, 2001).

As the kidney is also one of the hematopoietic organs of fish, tumors from these cell lines also commonly involve the kidney.

Special senses

Tumors arising from the tissues of the eye have been induced in fish when exposed to methylazoxymethanol acetate (MAM-Ac) (Hawkins et al., 1986) and N-methyl-N-nitrosourea (MNU), as well as in fish living in polluted waters (Mearns and Sherwood, 1978). Medulloepitheliomas developed in Japanese medaka (*Oryzias latipes*) exposed to MAM-Ac. A retinoblastoma associated with exophthalmos is briefly mentioned in an aquarium fish. The fish species is not provided (Harshbarger, 2001). This tumor has been induced by exposure to the carcinogen MNU in a platyfish model (Kazianis et al., 2001).

Corneal sarcomas have been described on goldfish (Lewbart, 1998; Groff, 2004). These have included fibromas and chromatophoromas. Corneal chromatophoromas have been recognized in Pacific rockfish (*Sebastes* spp.) exposed to environmental pollutants (Okihiro et al., 1993).

A retrobulbar hemangioma was associated with marked exophthalmia in a goldfish. The tumor and eye were successfully removed (O'Hagan and Raidal, 2006).

Thyroid gland

The thyroid gland is generally a diffuse organ located along the floor of the gill chamber as well as in the spleen, heart, and cranial kidney. Thyroid hyperplasia, as well as thyroid adenoma/carcinoma, will present as large bilateral nodular swellings at the base of the gills extending along the lower gill arches. These masses will distend the opercula. These have been described both in fish and sharks (Hoover, 1984; Gridelli et al., 2003). It is suspected that in marine fish and sharks, there may be exposure to dietary goitrogenic substances, although many factors may influence thyroid growth (Sonstegard and Leatherland, 1976). A biopsy sample is relatively easy to collect from these masses to help differentiate between hyperplastic lesions and tumors (Groff, 2004).

References and further reading

Ahmed, A.T.A. and Egusa, S. (1980) Dermal fibrosarcoma in goldfish Carassius auratus (L.). Journal of Fish Diseases 3 (3): 249–254.

Anders, K. and Möller, H. (1985) Spawning papillomatosis of smelt, Osmerus eperlanus L., from the Elbe estuary. Journal of Fish Diseases 8 (2): 233–235.

Anderson, W.H. and Luther, P.B. (1987) Poorly differentiated granuloplastic leukaemia in a bowfish (Amia calva L.). Journal of Fish Diseases 10: 411–413.

Brittelli, M.R., Chen, H.H., and Muska, C.F. (1985) Induction of branchial (gill) neoplasms in the medaka fish (Oryzias latipes) by N-methyl-N'-nitro-N-nitrosoguanidine. Cancer Research 45 (7): 3209–3214.

Clyde, V.L., Schultze, A.E., and Donnell, R. (1995) What is your diagnosis? Body wall mass from a goldfish. Veterinary Clinical Pathology 24 (1): 173–175.

Duncan, T.E. and Harkin, J.C. (1969) Electron microscopic studies of goldfish tumors previously termed neurofibromas and schwannomas. American Journal of Pathology 55 (2): 191–202.

Finkelstein, A. (2002) Neoplasia and surgical management in a pet goldfish. Exotic DVM 4 (2): 15–16.

Fitzgerald, S.D., Carlton, W.W., and Sandusky, G. (1991) Metastatic squamous cell carcinoma in a hybrid sunfish. Journal of Fish Diseases 14 (4): 481–487.

Fourni, J.W. and Hawkins, W.E. (2002) Exocrine pancreatic carcinogenesis in the guppy Poecilia reticulata. Diseases of Aquatic Organisms 52 (3): 191–198.

Francis-Floyd, R., Bolon, B., Fraser, W., et al. (1993) Lip fibromas associated with retrovirus-like particles in angel fish. Journal of the American Veterinary Medical Association 202 (3): 427–429.

Garland, M.R., Lawler, L.P., Whitaker, B.R., et al. (2002) Modern CT applications in veterinary medicine. Radiographics 22 (1): 55–62.

Ghadially, F.N. and Whiteley, H.J. (1951) An invasive red-pigmented tumour (erythrophoroma) in a red male platy fish (Platypoecilus maculatus var. rubra). British Journal of Cancer 5 (4): 405–408.

Granado-Lorencio, C., Garcia-Novo, F., and Lopez-Campos, J. (1987) Testicular tumors in carp-funa hybrid: annual cycle and effect on a wild population. Journal of Wildlife Diseases 23 (3): 422–427.

Gridelli, S., Diana, A., Parmeggiani, A., et al. (2003) Goitre in large and small spotted dogfish, Scyliorhinus stellaris (L.) and Scyliorhinus canicula (L.). Journal of Fish Disease 26 (11–12): 687–690.

Groff, J.M. (2004) Neoplasia in fishes. Veterinary Clinics of North America: Exotic Animal Practice 7 (3): 705–756.

Gumpenberger, M., Hochwartner, O., and Loupal, G. (2004) Diagnostic imaging of a renal adenoma in a red oscar (Astronotus ocellatus Cuvier, 1829). Veterinary Radiology and Ultrasound 45 (2): 139–142.

Harshbarger, J.C. (1984) Pseudoneoplasms in ectothermic animals. National Cancer Institute Monograph 65: 251–273.

Harshbarger, J.C. (2001) Neoplasia and developmental anomalies. In BSAVA Manual of Ornamental Fish, 2nd Edition (Wildgoose, W.H., ed.), pp. 219–224. Gloucester: British Small Animal Veterinary Association.

Harshbarger, J.C. and Bane, G.W. (1969) Case report of a fibrolipoma on a rockfish, Sebastodes diploproa. National Cancer Institute Monograph 31: 219–221.

Harshbarger, J.C. and Clark, J.B. (1990) Epizootiology of neoplasms in bony fish of North America. The Science of the Total Environment 94 (1–2): 1–32.

Harshbarger, J.C. and Slatick, M.S. (2001) Lesser known aquarium fish tumor models. Marine Biotechnology 3: S115–S129.

Harshbarger, J.C., Shumway, S.E., and Bane, G.W. (1976) Variably differentiating oral neoplasms, ranging from epidermal papilloma to odontogenic ameloblastoma, in cunners ((Tautogolabrus adspersus) Osteichthyes; Perciformes: Labridae). Progress in Experimental Tumor Research 20: 113–128.

Hawkins, W.E., Overstreet, R.M., Fournie, J.W., et al. (1985) Development of aquarium fish models for environmental carcinogenesis: tumor induction in seven species. Journal of Applied Toxicology 5 (4): 261–264.

Hawkins, W.E., Fournie, J.W., Overstreet, R.M., et al. (1986) Intraocular neoplasms induced by methylazoxymethanol acetate in Japanese medaka (Oryzias latipes). Journal of the National Cancer Institute 76 (3): 453–465.

Hayes, M.A. and Ferguson, H.W. (1989) Neoplasia in fish. In Systemic Pathology of Fish (Ferguson, H., ed.), pp. 23–247. Ames: Iowa State University Press.

Hoover, K.L. (1984) Hyperplastic thyroid lesions in fish. National Cancer Institute Monograph 65: 275–289.

Hubbard, G.B. and Fletcher, K.C. (1985) A seminoma and a leiomyosarcoma in an albino African lungfish (*Protopterus dolloi*). *Journal of Wildlife Diseases* **21** (1): 72–74.

Ishikawa, T. and Takayama, S. (1978) Ovarian neoplasia in ornamental hybrid carp (Nishikigoi) in Japan. *Annals of the New York Academy of Sciences* **298**: 330–341.

Ishikawa, T., Kuwabara, N., and Takayama, S. (1976) Spontaneous ovarian tumors in domestic carp (*Cyprinus carpio*): light and electron microscopy. *Journal of the National Cancer Institute* **57** (3): 579–584.

Kazianis, S., Gimenez-Conti, I., Setlow, R.B., et al. (2001) Laboratory investigation: a journal of technical methods and pathology MNU induction of neoplasia in a platyfish model. *Laboratory Investigation* **81** (9): 1191–1198.

Leatherland, J.F. and Sonstegard, R.A. (1978) Structure of normal testis and testicular tumors in cyprinids from Lake Ontario. *Cancer Research* **38** (10): 3164–3173.

Lewbart, G.A. (1998) *Self-Assessment Colour Review of Ornamental Fish*. London: Manson Publishing.

Manier, J.F., Raibaut, A., Lopez, A., et al. (1984) A calcified fibroma in the common carp, *Cyprinus carpio* L. *Journal of Fish Diseases* **7** (4): 283–292.

Masahito, P., Ishikawa, T., and Takayama, S. (1984) Spontaneous spermatocytic seminoma in African lungfish. *Journal of Fish Diseases* **7**: 169–172.

Masahito, P., Ishikawa, T., and Sugano, H. (1989) Pigment cells and pigment cell tumors in fish. *Journal of Investigative Dermatology* **92** (Suppl. 5): 266S–270S.

McAllister, P.E., Nagabayashi, T., and Wolf, K. (1978) Viruses of eels with and without stomatopapillomas. *Annals of the New York Academy of Sciences* **29** (298): 233–244.

Mearns, A.J. and Sherwood, M.J. (1978) Distribution of neoplasms and other diseases in marine fishes relative to the discharge of waste water. *Annals of the New York Academy of Sciences* **298**: 210–224.

Miller, S.M. (2000) Surgical excision of a schwannoma in a buffalo sculpin. *Exotic DVM* **2** (2): 41–43.

Murchelano, R.A. and Edwards, R.L. (1981) An erythrophoroma in ornamental carp, *Cyprinus carpio* L. *Journal of Fish Diseases* **4** (3): 265–268.

Noga, E.J. (1996) *Fish Disease: Diagnosis and Treatment*. St. Louis, MO: Mosby.

O'Hagan, B.J. and Raidal, S.R. (2006) Surgical removal of retrobulbar hemangioma in a goldfish (*Carassius auratus*). *Veterinary Clinics of North America: Exotic Animal Practice* **9** (3): 729–733.

Okihiro, M.S. (1988) Chromatophoromas in two species of Hawaiian butterflyfish, *Chaetodon multicinctus* and *C. miliaris*. *Veterinary Pathology* **25** (6): 422–431.

Okihiro, M.S., Whipple, J.A., Groff, J.M., et al. (1993) Chromatophoromas and chromatophore hyperplasia in Pacific rockfish (*Sebastes* spp.). *Cancer Research* **53** (8): 1761–1769.

Petervary, N., Gillette, P.N., Lewbart, G.A., et al. (1996) A spontaneous neoplasm of the renal collecting ducts in an oscar, *Astronotus ocellatus* (Cuvier), with comments on similar cases in this species. *Journal of Fish Diseases* **19**: 279–281.

Probasco, D., Noga, E.J., Marcellin, D., et al. (1994) Dermal fibrosarcoma in a goldfish: a case report. *Journal of Small and Exotic Animal Medicine* **2**: 173–175.

Raidal, S.R., Shearer, P.L., Stephens, F., et al. (2006) Surgical removal of an ovarian tumour in a koi carp (*Cyprinus carpio*). *Australian Veterinary Journal* **84** (5): 178–181.

Reavill, D.R., Adams, L., Hoech, J., et al. (2006) Xanthomatous lesions in three eels. Proceedings of the International Association for Aquatic Animal Medicine, Nassau, Bahamas, May, p. 85.

Roberts, R.J. (1989) Neoplasia of teleosts. In *Fish Pathology* (Roberts, R.J., ed.), pp. 153–171. London: Bailliere Tindall.

Rosskopf, W.J., Woerpel, R.W., and Huffman, E. (1985) Tumor removal in a goldfish. *Avian and Exotic Practice* **2** (2): 34–36.

Schlumberger, H.G. (1952) Nerve sheath tumors in an isolated goldfish population. *Cancer Research* **12**: 890–899.

Schlumberger, H.G. (1957) Tumors characteristic for certain animal species. *Cancer Research* **17**: 823–832.

Schlumberger, H.G and Katz, M. (1956) Odontogenic tumors of salmon. *Cancer Research* **16** (4): 367–370.

Schlumberger, H.G. and Lucke, B. (1948) Tumors of fishes, amphibians, and reptiles. *Cancer Research* **8**: 657–754.

Schmale, M.C., Gill, K.A., Cacal, S.M., et al. (1994) Characterization of Schwann cells from normal nerves and from neurofibromas in the bicolour damselfish. *Journal of Neurocytology* **23** (11): 668–681.

Schwab, M., Abdo, S., Ahuja, M.R., et al. (1978) Genetics of susceptibility in the platyfish/swordtail tumor system to develop fibrosarcoma and rhabdomyosarcoma following treatment with N-methyl-N-nitrosourea (MNU). *Zeitschrift für Krebsforschung und klinische Onkologie. Cancer Research and Clinical Oncology* **91** (3): 301–315.

Sonstegard, R. and Leatherland, J.F. (1976) The epizootiology and pathogenesis of thyroid hyperplasia in coho salmon (*Oncorhynchus kisutch*) in Lake Ontario. *Cancer Research* **36** (12): 4467–4475.

Stoletov, K. and Klemke, R. (2008) Catch of the day: zebrafish as a human cancer model. *Oncogene* **27** (33): 4509–4520.

Weisse, C., Weber, E.S., Matzkin, Z., et al. (2002) Surgical removal of a seminoma from a black sea bass. *Journal of the American Veterinary Medical Association* **221** (2): 280–283.

Wildgoose, W.H. (1992) Papilloma and squamous cell carcinoma in koi carp (*Cyprinus carpio*). *Veterinary Record* **130** (8): 153–157.

Wildgoose, W.H. and Bucke, D. (1995) Spontaneous branchioblastoma in a koi carp (*Cyprinus carpio*). *Veterinary Record* **136**: 418–419.

Chapter 21

Specific Syndromes and Diseases

William H. Wildgoose and Brian Palmeiro

Buoyancy and swim bladder disorders

Buoyancy disorders are common in ornamental fish and in goldfish (*Carassius auratus*), in particular. Affected fish often present following a sudden onset and are found lying on the bottom of the tank or pond or floating at the surface. Most are single cases and they often deteriorate due to skin damage through desiccation from exposure to air if at the surface or trauma from contact with the substrate. Few cases ever improve, but despite the poor prognosis, owners often want some investigation and treatment, particularly if they are emotionally attached to their pets.

There are very few references in the scientific literature, but there is much comment and speculation in the hobby literature and on several Internet Web sites, most of which use the term "swim bladder disease." Poor genetics, poor water quality, poor nutrition, a rapid drop in water temperature, or constipation are often cited as the underlying cause. One of the few scientific papers on swim bladder disorders in goldfish describes buoyancy problems affecting young short-bodied goldfish (Tanaka et al., 1998). This was given the name "tenpuku" by Japanese farmers, which means "capsized." Affected fish develop the problem after a marked drop in temperature or in winter. Many fish were affected at the same time; there was a wide range in the size of the posterior chamber of the swim bladder in both affected and unaffected fish. Many anatomical aspects of the swim bladder were studied, but the authors were unable to explain the pathogenesis of the abnormal swimming and buoyancy of affected fish. Elsewhere, a significant number of cases seen in general practice have been reviewed, and it

was noted that chronic conditions such as granulomatous disease, kidney enlargement, and fluid accumulation in the swim bladder are common causes of buoyancy disorders (Wildgoose, 2007).

Swim bladder anatomy

The bones and muscle tissues of fish are denser than water, and fish control their depth in the water column by storing gas or oils and lipids. In many species, buoyancy is controlled by the amount and distribution of gas within the body. This is primarily enclosed within a gas-filled buoyancy organ, the swim bladder or gas bladder. In some fish, physostomes, there is a patent pneumatic duct that connects the swim bladder to the anterior esophagus, which permits air to be swallowed and forced into the swim bladder or expelled. In other fish, physoclists, there is no patent connection and the swim bladder is inflated by the release of gas from arterial blood by a vascular rete in the wall of the swim bladder; this also occurs in some physostomes. In addition, various parts of the brain are thought to be involved in balance and buoyancy control.

In goldfish, the swim bladder is a two chambered organ located dorsally within the body cavity, adjacent to the ventral margin of the spine. The anterior chamber is lined with epithelial cells, supported by several tissue layers and has an outer layer of dense connective tissue (tunica externa). The anterior chamber is cuboid in shape and has limited capacity to change in volume. At the anterior pole, the tunica externa is firmly attached to the Weberian ossicles and a flattened bony process at the base of the fourth vertebra to assist in sound reception (hearing). The posterior chamber is thin-walled and is thus capable

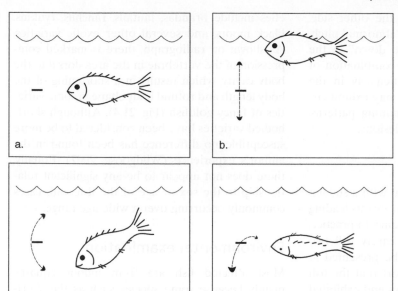

a.   b.   c.   d.

Fig. 21.1 Diagram of position and posture: (a) neutral buoyancy and normal posture, (b) excessive positive buoyancy, (c) abnormal pitch with "head down," (d) abnormal listing with rotation of the body along the longitudinal axis.

of significant volume change because it does not have a tunica externa. There is a diffuse vascular rete mirabile system that is involved in gas secretion and absorption into the posterior chamber, which assists in buoyancy control. The posterior chamber connects to the left side of the proximal esophagus by a long patent pneumatic duct and to the anterior chamber by the ductus communicans. The total volume of the swim bladder is about 5%–10% of the total body volume. The posterior or body kidney is a compact organ situated dorsally between the two chambers and is responsible for the excretion of fluid and some nitrogenous wastes.

Clinical presentation

A significant proportion of phone calls from fish keepers involve buoyancy disorders, and many clients will seek professional investigation. This may be influenced by their emotional attachment to their pets, the absence of any obvious visible lesions, or the lack of response to proprietary medicines available in pet stores. Clinically, fish with buoyancy disorders present with abnormal position in the water column and abnormal body posture (Fig. 21.1). Fish may be floating at the

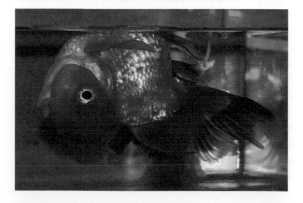

Fig. 21.2 A fancy variety of goldfish (oranda) presenting with excessive positive buoyancy and floating upside down at the surface. Radiographically, this fish had an overinflated swim bladder (reprinted with permission from Wildgoose, 2007).

surface (positive buoyancy; Fig. 21.2) or lying at the bottom on the substrate (negative buoyancy). In the latter, fish may still attempt to swim upward at times but will then sink to the bottom when not actively swimming. Many cases will exhibit varying degrees of listing or rolling to one side, and some may be completely upside down. Some fish rotate back to their original abnormal position when rolled over onto the other side. Small numbers may present with abnormal pitch, most of which are usually "head down" in the water. In many cases, there is a combination of abnormal pitch and listing, particularly in the short-bodied varieties. Some fish may exhibit circling behavior or abnormal swimming patterns, and this is often related to brain lesions.

Clinical history

Typically, affected fish will present with a sudden onset; there are seldom any specific events leading up to the start of buoyancy problems. In practice, most are single cases, and only rarely will two or more from the same facility be presented at the same time. Owners may report that the fish had been not eating for a few days and exhibited behavior typical of a sick fish such as becoming less active or preferring to isolate itself away from the others in a group. The duration of clinical signs prior to examination may range from hours to months, depending on the owner's ability or determination to seek professional advice.

The distribution of species affected may be influenced more by the popularity of those kept by hobbyists rather than genuine species differences. However, goldfish, which have a more diverse range of body shapes than any other species, appear to be particularly susceptible to buoyancy disorders. The long-bodied varieties consist mainly of common goldfish and comet-tailed goldfish (Fig. 21.3). The short-bodied vari-

eties include orandas, fantails, ranchus, ryukins, black moors, and several other exotic varieties. As shown on radiograph, there is marked compression of the vertebrae in the area dorsal to the body cavity, which results in a shortening of the body length and rotund body shape in some varieties of fancy goldfish (Fig. 21.4). Although short-bodied varieties have been considered to be more susceptible, no difference has been found in the author's experience (Wildgoose, 2007). Equally, there does not appear to be any significant relationship to the sex or age of the fish, with cases commonly occurring over a wide age range.

Environmental examination

Most affected fish are from indoor aquaria, mainly because some species such as the short-bodied fancy varieties of goldfish are not suitable for keeping in outdoor ponds. Fish kept indoors often receive more attention due to a more frequent and greater level of observation. In many cases, water quality parameters are acceptable and other fish in the tank are unaffected. Where solitary fish are affected and there are no other fish in contact, water quality should be tested for routine parameters and a detailed clinical history taken to eliminate the possibility of contamination with neurotoxins such as environmental insecticides.

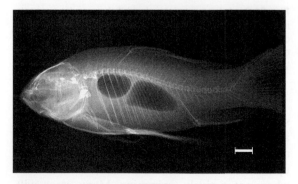

Fig. 21.3 Radiograph of a long-bodied goldfish (comet-tailed) showing the normal shape and position of the two-chambered swim bladder. Bar = 1 cm (reprinted with permission from Wildgoose, 2007).

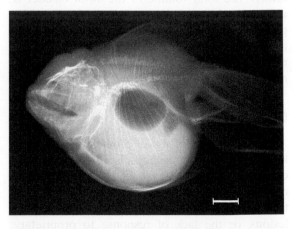

Fig. 21.4 Radiograph of short-bodied goldfish (oranda) showing marked compression of the vertebrae dorsal to the body cavity. This fish had an enlarged ovary full of eggs. Bar = 1 cm (reprinted with permission from Wildgoose, 2007).

Clinical examination

The clinical examination of affected fish is often unrewarding, with few exhibiting any clinical signs other than abnormal position and posture. Fish should be anaesthetized and removed from the water for a detailed examination and palpation of the abdomen. In some, there may be abdominal swelling and this is often asymmetrical: Affected goldfish are prone to polycystic kidneys or "kidney enlargement disease," and oscars (*Astronotus ocellatus*) commonly develop a renal tumor. Some fish exhibit exophthalmos, particularly if they have fluid following systemic disease or granulomas behind the globe of the eye. Hyphema and generalized hyperemia with engorged blood vessels in the fins or skin is sometimes observed. In general, clinical signs are usually of limited value in determining the underlying pathology.

Diagnostic imaging

Radiography has proved to be the most useful nonlethal method of investigating cases and clearly demonstrates the distribution of gas and space-occupying lesions within the body cavity. The procedure requires only brief anesthesia to remove the fish from water and utilizes standard radiographic equipment and techniques. The radiographic appearance of the swim bladder varies significantly among some species, and it is essential to have images of normal fish in order to compare and accurately identify what are often subtle abnormalities. In goldfish, there are slight differences between the long- and short-bodied varieties, and the posterior chamber is often much smaller or nonexistent in the latter. A horizontal beam view is useful where there is partial filling of the swim bladder with fluid. Contrast radiography using barium or other radiopaque media given by gavage can be used to delineate the intestinal tract and help localize space-occupying lesions. Although ultrasonography is of limited benefit when examining the swim bladder and kidney due to the echoes generated by the swim bladder, it is very useful for identifying diseases of the other abdominal organs and fluid accumulation in polycystic kidneys.

Several radiographic abnormalities can be identified in fish with buoyancy disorders and these include abnormalities of the swim bladder such as overinflation, displacement, fluid accumulation and rupture, and intestinal tympany. In some cases, there may be a combination of radiographic abnormalities, complicating the interpretation and diagnosis.

Overinflation of the swim bladder

In goldfish, the most common abnormality is overinflation of the swim bladder (Fig. 21.5), although in some cases this may be difficult to assess because of the variable appearance of the posterior chamber in the different varieties of goldfish. In oscars, renal papillary cystadenomas are common and cause abdominal swelling in the posterior part of the body cavity, often resulting in excessive positive buoyancy due to overinflation of the thin membranous swim bladder.

Displacement of the swim bladder

In goldfish, the posterior chamber may become displaced and requires both lateral and dorsoventral radiographic views in order to correctly assess its location. The anterior chamber of the swim

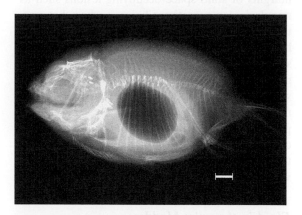

Fig. 21.5 Lateral view radiograph of a fancy goldfish (ranchu) with overinflation of the anterior chamber of the swim bladder. Despite aspiration and antibiotic treatment, this fish deteriorated over 4 months and was found to have systemic granulomatous disease on postmortem examination. Bar = 1 cm (reprinted with permission from Wildgoose, 2007).

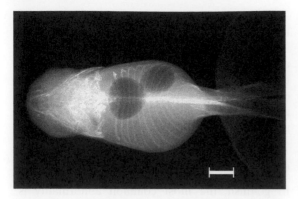

Fig. 21.6 Dorsoventral view radiograph of a fancy goldfish (oranda) showing displacement of the posterior chamber of the swim bladder to the right side due to a polycystic kidney disease. This fish was originally presented after floating at the surface with its right side uppermost for 2 weeks. Bar = 1 cm (reprinted with permission from Wildgoose, 2007).

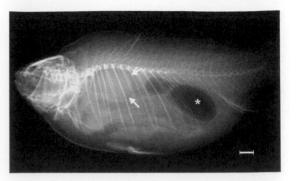

Fig. 21.7 Radiograph of a common goldfish with rupture of the posterior chamber of the swim bladder and free gas in the retroperitoneal space (asterisk). The anterior chamber (indicated by arrows) is full of fluid and has a homogeneous radiodensity. This fish had presented 4 days after it developed a "head down" posture, with its tail above the water surface. Bar = 1 cm (reprinted with permission from Wildgoose, 2007).

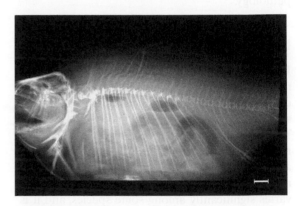

Fig. 21.8 Horizontal beam radiograph of a common goldfish with fluid partially filling both chambers of the swim bladder. Excess gas is also present within the bowel. This fish had exhibited negative buoyancy and a "head down" posture for 10 days. Bar = 1 cm (reprinted with permission from Wildgoose, 2007).

bladder has a thick tunica externa and is firmly attached to a bony vertebral process at its anterior pole: this is a useful landmark when interpreting radiographs of goldfish and koi (*Cyprinus carpio*). The posterior chamber is only attached to the anterior chamber by the narrow ductus communicans and is easily displaced laterally from its normal midline position or ventrally into the body cavity by space-occupying lesions (Fig. 21.6). The margins of solid space-occupying lesions such as neoplasia can sometimes be seen when they partially overlie the gas-filled chambers of the swim bladder. The gap between the two chambers is small, usually about 1–2 mm, but this is widened in goldfish with enlargement of the posterior kidney with polycystic kidney disease, extensive granulomas, or neoplasia. Equally common, a mass in the posterior body cavity may displace the posterior chamber forward, reducing the gap and causing it to overlap the anterior chamber on radiographic views.

Fluid in the swim bladder

There is rarely any fluid seen in the normal swim bladder, although the epithelial cells produce a surfactant that is thought to have an antiadhesive and protective function. The radiographic appearance of fluid in the swim bladder varies

depending on the amount present. When full of fluid, the swim bladder is barely visible and has a homogeneous radiodensity similar to the surrounding tissues (Fig. 21.7). When partially filled, a faint area of radiolucency is seen in the center of the affected swim bladder chambers when radiographed in lateral recumbency: the gas lies above the fluid and a fluid line can be detected more readily on a horizontal beam image (Fig. 21.8). Abnormal fluid may vary from a clear straw color to a white purulent material, occasionally containing granulomas and acid-fast bacteria.

Rupture of the swim bladder

The absence of a thick tunica externa in the posterior chamber allows significant volume change, and in extreme cases, predisposes it to rupture. Although an uncommon cause of buoyancy disorder, this has been seen in orfe (*Leuciscus idus*) and goldfish (Fig. 21.7) in winter, suggesting that low water temperatures may be a contributing factor.

Intestinal tympany

The similar radiodensity of bowel, liver, and body fat make it difficult to differentiate the abdominal tissues. Normally, little detail is seen within the bowel, but occasionally, there may be small amounts of radiopaque foreign matter such as sand or grit in pond fish or radiolucent gas. Some affected fish have excessive amounts of gas in the bowel (Fig. 21.8), which will result in excessive positive buoyancy.

Laboratory procedures

Microscopic examination of skin and gill scrapes should be performed on all cases to identify ectoparasitic infestations that may cause severe debility. Similarly, fresh fecal samples should be examined for heavy burdens of endoparasites such as flagellates and nematodes. If a significant amount of fluid is present in the swim bladder, a sample can be obtained by pneumocystocentesis using a syringe and needle directed carefully through the lateral body wall. Cytological examination, Ziehl–Neelsen staining, and bacterial culture and sensitivity can provide useful information about the nature of the fluid.

Laparotomy and laparoscopy

Invasive investigations such as laparotomy and laparoscopy should be undertaken with care since many fish have chronic and extensive disease (see later under the section on postmortem examination). A complete workup, including radiographic examination, is essential to determine the

best approach and likely benefit of any surgical intervention.

Treatment

The response of abnormal buoyancy cases to treatment is often poor due to the severity of the underlying disease. Euthanasia is indicated in most instances, but in the absence of obvious pathology, some owners may request treatment. Depending on the clinical signs and radiographic findings, some of the following treatments may be of benefit in some cases. Those that are not treated often deteriorate over a period of days or weeks, depending on the severity of the underlying pathology.

Environmental management

- Ensure that the water quality is acceptable, and if necessary, perform partial water changes every 2–3 days to reduce any buildup of metabolic wastes or contaminants.
- Sodium chloride salt added to the water at 2–5 g/l as a permanent bath is often physiologically beneficial to affected freshwater fish.
- Increasing or decreasing the water temperature by a few degrees, provided it is within the fish's tolerance range, may alter the fish's metabolic rate and assist in recovery in some cases.
- Starving for 3–4 days allows the bowel to empty and eliminate any gas-producing contents.
- Feeding a lightly crushed green pea (canned or cooked) once daily is thought to have a mild purgative effect that may dislodge gas in the bowel (Lewbart, 2000).

Medical therapy

- A few proprietary pet shop medicines claim to treat swim bladder disorders, although some manufacturers have not disclosed the ingredients, making it difficult to assess which cases may benefit from these products.
- Antibiotics given by immersion, by injection, or in the food for 14–21 days may be effective in some cases where bacterial infections are involved.
- Metronidazole given in the food has been used to treat enteric flagellate infestations.

- Carbonic anhydrase inhibitors such as acetazolamide have been used by injection at 6–10 mg/kg to treat gas bubble disease in seahorses and may be beneficial in fish with overinflated swim bladders by reducing the production of new gas from the vascular rete.

Surgery

A few surgical procedures have been performed in an attempt to improve buoyancy control, but some require an advanced approach, and success often depends on the underlying cause of the disorder.

- Fish with negative buoyancy due to an under-inflated swim bladder have had various flotation devices fitted, including the use of slings with cork or polystyrene floats, and Floy® tags (Floy Tag, Seattle, WA) with limited success (Lewbart et al., 2005).
- Fish with an overinflated swim bladder can have some gas removed by aspiration using a needle and syringe (pneumocystocentesis) to adjust their buoyancy. These often improve temporarily, but in many cases, the swim bladder becomes overinflated again within a few days. In some cases, repeated aspiration may eventually resolve the problem.
- A partial pneumocystectomy can be performed to remove part of the swim bladder and reduce its size, and hence, the buoyancy of the fish (Lewbart et al., 1995; Britt et al., 2002).
- Coelomic implants placed inside the body cavity have been described on the Internet as a method of adding extra ballast to fish that are excessively buoyant.

Postmortem examination

Detailed postmortem examination of affected fish often reveals various pathological changes. It is essential that samples are taken from the brain and all major organs in order to appreciate the extent and nature of the disease. In the author's experience (Wildgoose, 2007), the most common causes of buoyancy disorders found at postmortem examination are listed as follows:

- Granulomatous disease, probably due to mycobacteria, is found primarily in fish kept in aquaria.

Many will have lesions within the cranial cavity, but only some may reveal acid-fast bacteria.
- Fluid in the swim bladder often contains bacteria such as *Aeromonas*, *Pseudomonas* spp., and mycobacteria. It is not known how bacteria enter the swim bladder, but this may be via the patent pneumatic duct or bloodborne and enter through the vascular rete.
- Polycystic kidney disease is common in goldfish cases, which may produce massive enlargement of the posterior kidney, causing it to occupy up to 80% of the body cavity.
- Major diseases of other organs in advanced stages can affect the general health of the fish and result in apparent buoyancy disorders due to debility. These may include ovarian disorders, renal disease, and neoplasia.
- In some cases, no visible pathology may be identified, and therefore, small but significant lesions may have been overlooked elsewhere such as in the brain.

Conclusion

Despite the relatively common occurrence, there is still a poor understanding of buoyancy disorders in fish, and detailed investigations should be performed at every opportunity. Many cases show no consistent clinical features that relate to the pathology found, and the abnormal buoyancy may simply be a terminal clinical sign. Despite the sudden onset, many cases seen in general veterinary practice have chronic diseases with which they have coped for months. These may differ from young fish with similar buoyancy disorders that are culled by farmers and retailers prior to sale and that may have other underlying causes such as genetic or congenital defects as suggested in the hobby literature. It is clear that more detailed research is required to improve our understanding of this common disorder.

Head and lateral line erosion (HLLE)

HLLE is an important, idiopathic clinical syndrome seen in both marine and freshwater fish. HLLE occurs in private collections and public

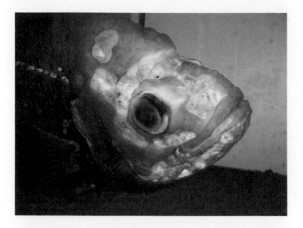

Fig. 21.9 Severe head and lateral line erosion lesions in an oscar. Note the deep coalescing depigmented ulcers.

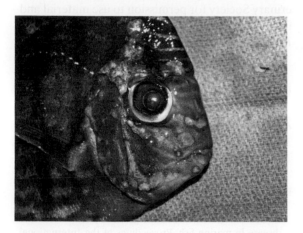

Fig. 21.10 Head and lateral line erosion in a discus.

aquaria but not in wild fish. This syndrome is also referred to as "hole-in-the-head" in the ornamental fish industry. The disorder causes progressive, often symmetrical, depigmented erosions and ulcerations that coalesce to produce large crateriform lesions and pits on the head, and in some cases, extending down the lateral line (Figs. 21.9 and 21.10). Freshwater cichlids (discus, oscars, other South American cichlids) are commonly affected. Marine fish that are commonly affected include surgeonfishes and tangs (family Acanthuridae) and marine angelfish (family Pomacanthidae). Secondary bacterial, fungal, and parasitic infections may occur. Affected fish may eventually become anorexic, lethargic, and thin.

Contributing factors

Stressors such as overcrowding, poor water quality, or poor nutrition may predispose fish to HLLE. The exact etiology of this syndrome is unknown. Proposed causative agents include hexamitid parasites (such as *Spironucleus vortens*), activated carbon/carbon dust, heavy metals such as copper, stray electrical voltage, ozone, ultraviolet (UV) radiation products, nutrient deficiencies of vitamins A and/or C and minerals, and various other stressors (Palmeiro, 2009). There may not be one particular inciting cause, and the syndrome may represent a clinical response to various stressors. *S. vortens* has been isolated from lesional skin and internal organs of discus affected with HLLE (Paull and Matthews, 2001). In one study, a reovirus was isolated from a moribund marine angelfish with initial HLLE lesions (Varner and Lewis, 1991). One report that evaluated the effects of in-line UV radiation and carbon in ocean surgeons (*Acanthurus bahianus*) found that only carbon use produced skin lesions in consistent areas (Stamper et al., 2005). No significant difference in development of HLLE was found between ocean surgeonfish fed diets containing varying concentrations of vitamin C (Croft et al., 2005). The author has evaluated numerous freshwater cichlids with this syndrome and found underlying disease such as mycobacteriosis and cryptobiosis in many affected fish.

Diagnosis

Diagnosis of HLLE is typically based on history and clinical signs. The environment/husbandry should always be evaluated for possible nutritional and environmental stresses. Wet mount exam of the skin should be performed to evaluate for secondary bacterial, fungal, and parasitic infections. Fecal examination is recommended to evaluate for the presence of intestinal parasitism. Histopathology of affected areas can vary significantly. Typically, an erosive to ulcerative dermatitis is seen with epidermal spongiosis (intercellular edema), vesicle formation, or inflammatory cell exocytosis (infiltration into the epidermis); chronic lesions may contain dermal fibrosis (scarring) (Stamper et al., 2005; Morrison et al., 2007; Palmeiro,

2009). One study reported keratinocyte ballooning degeneration (Stamper et al., 2005). In Nile tilapia, *Oreochromis niloticus*, the most severe lesions were posterior to the eye. In histological sections of this region in fish without lesions, previously unreported small canals arising from the lateral line canals were found running parallel to the epidermis and opening at the surface through pores; it was proposed that these canals may serve as an entry route for pathogens and toxins that could infiltrate into surrounding tissues through the simple epithelium lining the canals (Morrison et al., 2007).

Treatment

The husbandry should be improved by maintaining excellent water quality, performing frequent water changes, reducing overcrowding, and providing a balanced/varied diet. There are anecdotal reports of treating HLLE with various vitamin supplements. A grounding device can be installed to remove stray voltage from the system. If present, activated carbon should be removed from the system. Concurrent hexamitid (*Spironucleus/Hexamita*) infestations should be treated with metronidazole. HLLE has been successfully treated in marine tropical fish with 0.01% becaplermin (Regranex®, Ortho-McNeil Pharmaceutical Inc., Raritan, NJ). The fish is sedated and the lesions are debrided with a sterile scalpel blade and gently flushed. Regranex is applied with sterile cotton applicators. Various recommendations have been proposed for contact time; the author typically allows a contact time of 2–3 minutes prior to placing the fish back into the water.

Various protocols with Regranex have been shown to be effective in marine fish:

- Once weekly applications for 8 weeks was successful in sailfin tangs (Boerner et al., 2003).
- Successful treatment has been reported in juvenile ocean surgeons with a single application of Regranex, or with one treatment every 3 weeks. However, fish placed in water that was known to induce lesions consistent with HLLE did not improve with Regranex treatment (Fleming et al., 2005).

- Regranex has also been diluted with 0.9% sodium chloride to a concentration of 50% or 25%, with similar healing rates to fish treated with the full concentration (Adams and Michalkiewicz, 2005).

In a controlled study, the author has applied Regranex biweekly to HLLE-affected freshwater cichlids with only minimal improvement. However, most fish in that study had underlying disease caused by *Mycobacterium* or *Cryptobia* (Palmeiro and Weber, in press).

Acknowledgment

William H. Wildgoose is grateful to the Fish Veterinary Society for permission to use material and images from his paper previously published in the *Fish Veterinary Journal* (2007; 9: 22–37).

References and further reading

Adams, L. and Michalkiewicz, J. (2005) Effect of Regranex® gel concentration or post application time on the healing rate of head and lateral line erosions in marine tropical fish. Proceedings of the International Association of Aquatic Animal Medicine, Seward, Alaska, May 14.

Boerner, L., Dube, K., Peterson, K., et al. (2003) Angiogenic growth factor therapy using recombinant platelet-derived growth factor (Regranex®) for lateral line disease in marine fish. Proceedings of the International Association of Aquatic Animal Medicine, Waikoloa, Hawaii, May 10.

Britt, T., Weisse, C., Weber, E.S., et al. (2002) Use of pneumocystoplasty for overinflation of the swim bladder in a goldfish. *Journal of the American Veterinary Medical Association* 221: 690–693.

Croft, L., Francis-Floyd, R., Petty, B.D., et al. (2005) The effect of dietary vitamin c levels on the development of head and lateral line erosion syndrome in ocean surgeonfish (*Acanthurus bahianus*). Proceedings of the International Association of Aquatic Animal Medicine, Seward, Alaska, May 14.

Fleming, G., McCoy, J., Corwin, A., et al. (2005) Treatment factors influencing the use of recombinant platelet-derived growth factor (Regranex) for head and lateral line erosion syndrome in ocean surgeons (*Acanthurus bahianus*). Proceedings of the International Association of Aquatic Animal Medicine, Seward, Alaska, May 14.

Francis-Floyd, R., Tilghman, G.C., et al. (2005) Captive nutritional management of Atlantic surgeon fish: effect of dietary vitamin A on development of head and lateral line erosion lesions. Proceedings of the International Association of Aquatic Animal Medicine. Seward, Alaska, May 14.

Lewbart, G.A. (2000) Green peas for buoyancy disorders. *Exotic DVM* **2** (2): 7.

Lewbart, G.A., Stone, E.A., and Love, N.E. (1995) Pneumocystectomy in a Midas cichlid. *Journal of the American Veterinary Medical Association* **207**: 319–321.

Lewbart, G.A., Christian, L.S., and Dombrowski, D. (2005) Development of a minimally invasive technique to stabilize buoyancy-challenged goldfish Carassius auratus. Proceedings of the International Association for Aquatic Animal Medicine, May 14.

Morrison, C.M., O'Neil, D., and Wright, J.R. (2007) Histopathology of "hole-in-the-head" disease in the Nile tilapia, *Oreochromis niloticus. Aquaculture* **273**: 427–433.

Palmeiro, B. (2009) Head and lateral line erosion. In *Clinical Veterinary Advisor: Exotic Medicine* (Mayer, J., ed.), In press.

Palmeiro, B. and Weber, S. Treatment of HLLE in freshwater cichlids with 0.01% becaplermin (Regranex®). Unpublished manuscript.

Paull, G. and Matthews, R.A. (2001) Spironucleus vortens, a possible cause of hole-in-the-head disease in cichlids. *Diseases of Aquatic Organisms* **45**: 197–202.

Stamper, M.A., McCoy, A.J., and Corwin, A. (2005) Head and lateral line erosion syndrome in ocean surgeons (*Acanthurus bahianus*): current efforts to determine etiologies. Proceedings of the International Association of Aquatic Animal Medicine, Seward, Alaska, May 14.

Tanaka, D., Wada, S., and Hatai, K. (1998) Gross, radiological and anatomical findings of goldfish with tenpuku disease. *Suisanzoshoku* **46**: 293–299.

Varner, P.W. and Lewis, D.H. (1991) Characterization of a virus associated with head and lateral line erosion syndrome in marine angelfish. *Journal of Aquatic Animal Health* **3**: 198–205.

Wildgoose, W.H. (2007) Buoyancy disorders of ornamental fish: a review of cases seen in veterinary practice. *Fish Veterinary Journal* **9**: 22–37.

Index

Note: Page numbers in *italics* refer to Figures or Tables.

Printed and bound by CPI Group (UK) Ltd, Croydon, CR0 4YY

27/10/2024

14580243-0004